APhA NAPLEX®
QUICK REVIEW GUIDE

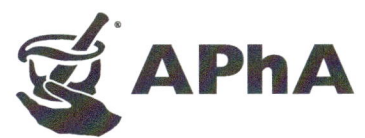

APhA NAPLEX®
QUICK REVIEW GUIDE

BRITTANY HOFFMANN-EUBANKS,
PharmD, MBA

Founder and CEO
Banner Medical, LLC
Frankfort, Illinois

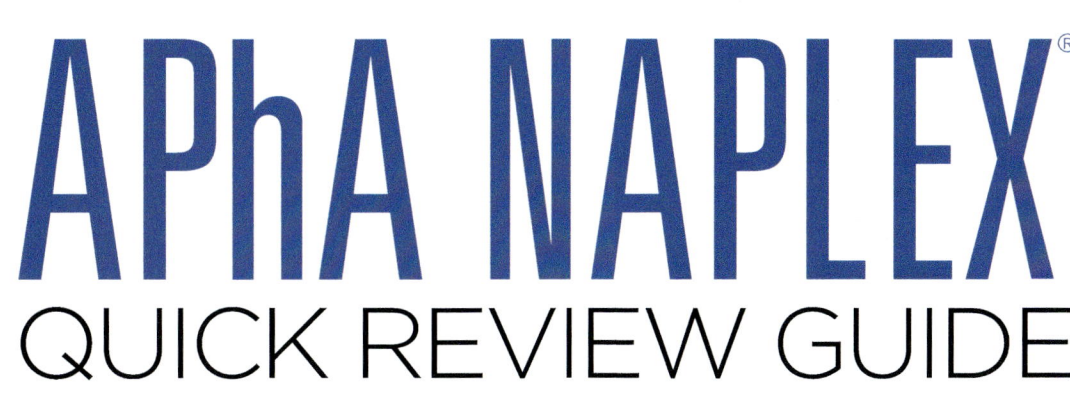

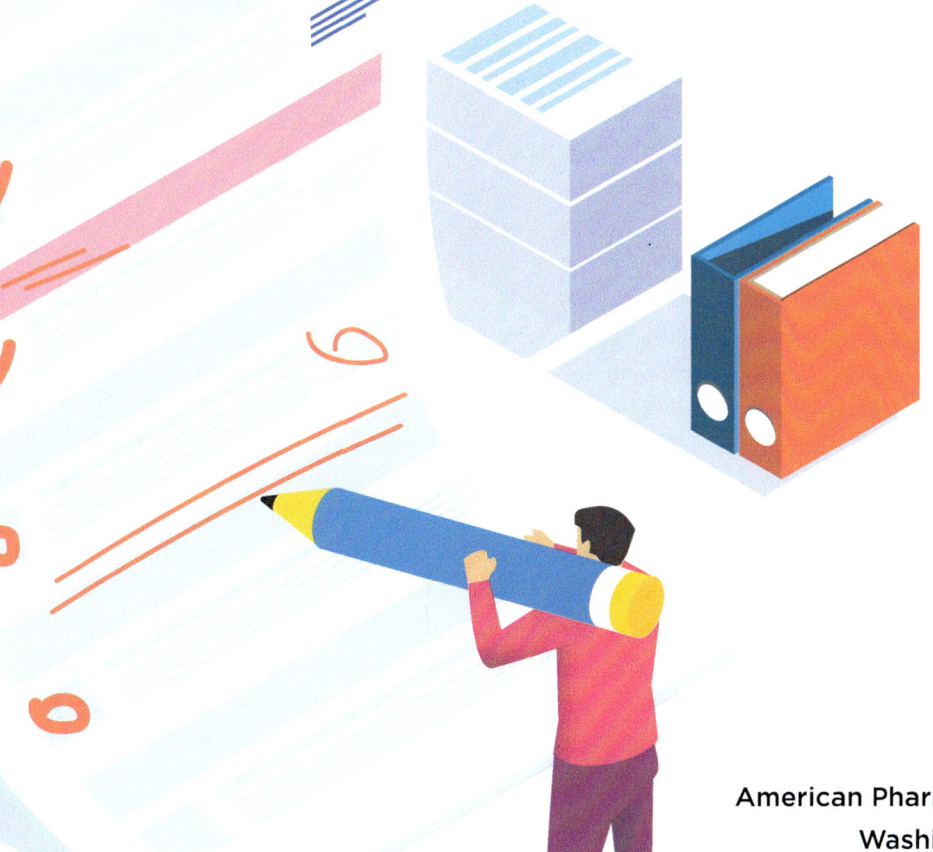

American Pharmacists Association
Washington, DC

Senior Director, Books and Digital Publishing: Janan Sarwar, PharmD
Editorial Director: Jesse Vineyard
Production Editor: Brittany Williams
Editorial Services: Circle Graphics, Inc.
Cover Design: Scott Neitzke, APhA Integrated Design and Production
Concept Development: Drew Register, PharmD, APhA Member Relations

Medical writing support provided by Banner Medical LLC Writers:
Jennifer Miller, PharmD, BCOP
Miriam Opara, PharmD
Milena Murray, PharmD, MSc, BCIDP, AAHIVP
Tomasz Jurga, PharmD, BCPS, BCACP, CDCES

Published by the American Pharmacists Association
2215 Constitution Avenue, NW
Washington, D.C. 20037-2985
www.pharmacist.com
www.pharmacylibrary.com

To comment on this book by e-mail, send your message to the publisher at aphabooks@aphanet.org.

Library of Congress Control Number: 2020951667

ISBN-13: 978-1-58212-367-7

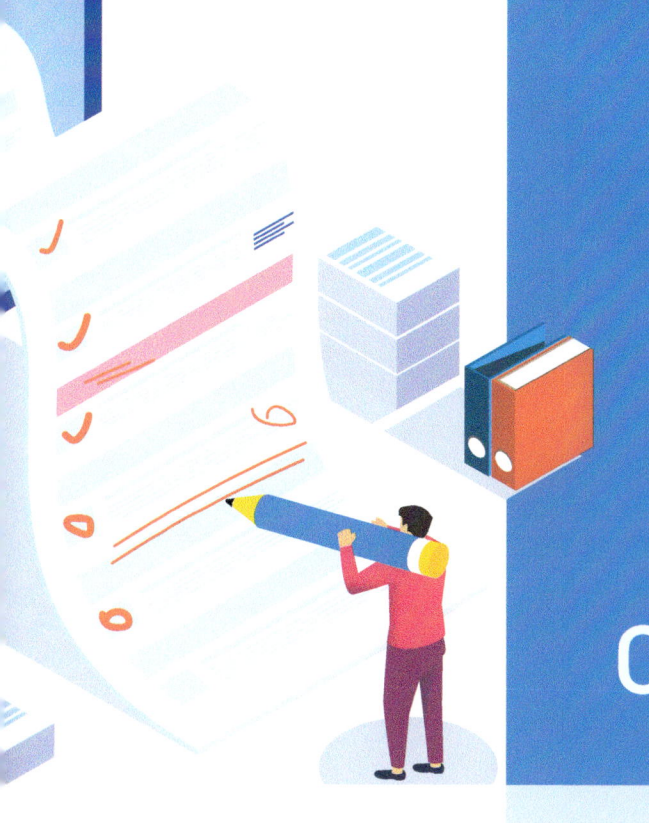

Contents

CHAPTER 1

Pharmacy Foundations

With medical writing support provided by
Banner Medical LLC Writer: Miriam Opara

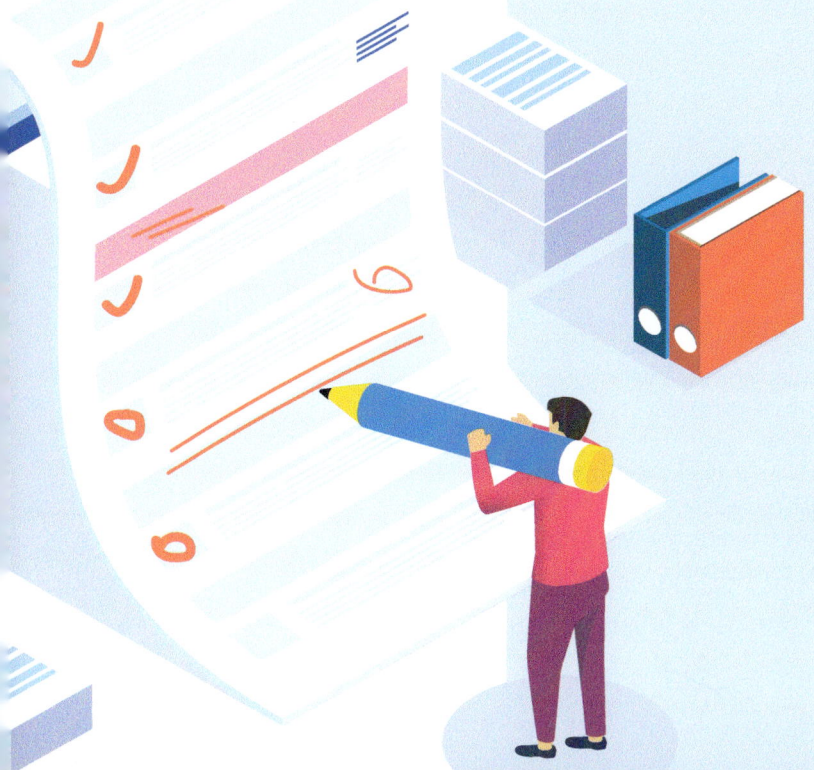

Medication safety and quality

The goal of medication therapy is to optimize the patient's quality of life and minimize harm. Mishaps associated with medication therapy include[1]

- **Medication errors:** inappropriate medication use or patient harm (preventable)
- **Adverse drug events:** harm or injury resulting from medication intervention (generally unpreventable)

Medication errors typically occur as a result of flaws in the medical system, not from an individual error. Table 1-1 lists common types of medication errors.[1]

Strategies for preventing medication errors are important to establish. Systems for ordering, dispensing, and administering medications should be established to minimize errors. The "5 Rights" (patient, drug, dose, time, and route) should be verified before giving medications. Recommended strategies to reduce medication errors include[1]

- Computerized provider–order entry
- Automated dispensing cabinets
- Barcode medication administration
- Smart IV infusion pumps
- Robotic dispensing systems
- Patient-controlled analgesia devices

Pharmacokinetics

Pharmacokinetics is what the body does to a drug, including its absorption, distribution, metabolism, and excretion.

Absorption

Absorption is the process by which a drug moves from its site of administration to the bloodstream. Absorption with oral drugs occurs mostly through

- Passive diffusion: high concentration to low concentration
- Active transport: drug moves into circulation via transporter proteins

The **rate of dissolution** is how quickly an oral medication dissolves and the active ingredient is released. The amount (or fraction) of the drug that reaches systemic circulation is called bioavailability (F). Intravenous route skips absorption and is directly administered into systemic circulation; therefore, the bioavailability is 100%. The following equation is used to determine the bioavailability of other routes of administration:

$$F(\%) = 100 \times \frac{AUC_{extravascular}}{AUC_{intravenous}} \times \frac{Dose_{intravenous}}{Dose_{extravascular}}$$

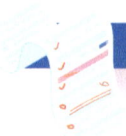

Table 1-1	Types of Medication Errors[1]

ERROR	EXAMPLES
Prescribing error	Incorrect drug selection or illegible prescriptions
Omission error	Drug not administered or therapy missing for a disease state
Wrong time error	Drug administered too soon or too late
Dosage error	Dose is too high or too low
Route error	Drug administered in different route than prescribed
Administration error	Improper administration technique
Monitoring error	Missing laboratory data or failure to review patient's regimen
Adherence error	Patient not taking drug appropriately

Distribution

The **volume of distribution (Vd)** is the volume that accounts for the concentration in the blood, depending on the amount of drug administered; it indicates whether a drug is more likely to stay in the blood or distribute into tissues and organs.[2] The Vd is a hypothetical value as it can exceed body size. Various factors affect the distribution of a drug:

- **Lipophilicity**—high lipophilicity increases passage into the tissues
- **Molecular weight**—low molecular weight allows drugs to pass membranes easier
- **Ionization**—un-ionized drugs have increased distribution
- **Protein binding**—low protein binding in blood is important for increased distribution
- **Membranes**—increased membrane permeability increases distribution into the tissues

The Vd can be calculated using the following equation:

$$Vd = \frac{amount\ of\ drug\ in\ body}{concentration\ of\ drug\ in\ plasma}$$

Metabolism

Metabolism is the process by which a drug is broken down by the body for elimination or activation (e.g., prodrugs). The majority of drugs on the market are metabolized by the liver. First-pass metabolism refers to hepatic metabolism before an oral drug reaching systemic circulation. First-pass metabolism can reduce the bioavailability of a drug. Enzyme metabolism includes the following:

- Phase I reactions: oxidation, reduction, hydrolysis
- Phase II reactions: conjugation, glucuronidation

Cytochrome (CY)P450 enzymes catalyze reactions and drugs break them down to facilitate excretion.[3] Multiple CYP450 enzymes metabolize drugs, and genetic variation of some CYP450s can affect the rate of metabolism (poor metabolizer, intermediate metabolizer, rapid metabolizer, or ultra-metabolizer).[3]

Drugs that are **enzyme inducers** increase enzyme production and increase metabolism rate.

- In**D**ucers—**D**ecrease drug levels
  - Prodrugs—inducers increase levels of the active form
  - Ultra-metabolizers have the same effect on drug levels

Drugs that are **enzyme inhibitors** decrease functional enzymes and decrease metabolism rate.

- **IN**hibitors—**IN**crease drug levels (adverse drug reactions, toxicities)
  - Prodrugs—inhibitors decrease levels of the active form
  - Poor metabolizers have the same effect on drug levels

Drug inducers or inhibitors (Table 1-2) are categorized as strong, moderate, or weak based on the effect on metabolism of the enzyme's substrate drug.

Excretion

Excretion is the removal of drugs from the body. Excretion occurs through the kidneys, liver, gut (P-glycoprotein efflux pumps), lungs, and sweat. The **clearance** (Cl) of a drug is the volume of blood cleared of the drug over time. It is a function of the rate of drug removal from the body. Clearance determines the steady-state concentration for a particular dosage rate. Steady state occurs when the rate of elimination equals the rate of administration. Calculating Cl and elimination rate (ke) is done using the following equations:

$$Cl = \frac{F \times dose}{AUC} \quad | \quad Cl = ke \times Vd \quad | \quad ke = \frac{Cl}{Vd}$$

The **half-life** of a drug is calculated to determine the time required for 50% of the drug to be eliminated.

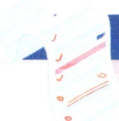

Table 1-2   Common Drug Inducers and Inhibitors[3]

COMMON INDUCERS: "SUPERCOPS"	COMMON INHIBITORS: "CAMPAIGN"
Smoking	**C**imetidine, cobicistat, cyclosporine
U	**A**zoles
Phenytoin	**M**acrolides (except azithromycin)
E	**P**rotease inhibitors
Rifampin	**A**miodarone
Carbamazepine (autoinducer)	I
Oxcarbazepine	**G**rapefruit
Phenobarbital	**N**on-DHP CCB
St. John's Wort	

Note: Azoles—fluconazole, itraconazole, ketoconazole, voriconazole; macrolides—clarithromycin, erythromycin; non-DHP CCB (Non-dihydropyridine calcium channel blockers)—diltiazem, verapamil; protease inhibitors—darunavir, atazanavir, lopinavir, ritonavir.

Half-life is proportional to the Vd (larger volumes = larger half-life) and is inversely proportional to Cl (larger Cl = lower half-life). It takes 5 half-lives to reach steady state. The half-life ($t_{1/2}$) can be calculated using ke:

$$t_{1/2} = \frac{0.693}{ke}$$

A **loading dose (LD)** may be necessary to rapidly achieve steady state or therapeutic concentrations. When the half-life of a drug is long, a LD is usually given; an IV bolus LD can be calculated using the following equation:

$$LD = \frac{desired\ concentration \times Vd}{F}$$

Loading doses for other routes can be estimated by using the maintenance dose and the accumulation factor (Ra).

$$LD = Maintenance\ dose \times Ra$$

Pharmacokinetics and pharmacogenetics contribute to patient-specific drug allergies, drug metabolism, and drug removal from the body. **Pharmacodynamics** is the relationship between the concentration of the drug and the response in the patient (i.e., what the drug does to the body). These aspects of medication therapy enable pharmacists to identify common drug–drug interactions and monitor patients appropriately.

Renal excretion—the majority of drugs are excreted in the urine as a metabolite or their unmetabolized form.[3] Drugs are usually metabolized into an ionized (water-soluble) form to be excreted in the urine.

Gut excretion—P-glycoprotein (P-gp) efflux pumps[3]

- P-gp efflux pumps are in various tissues and transport the drug out of the cell
- In the gut, P-gp efflux pumps keep the drug in the gut lumen where it can be excreted in the feces
- Many drugs that act as metabolism inducers and inhibitors are also P-gp inducers or inhibitors

Pharmacogenomics

Pharmacogenetics (PG) determines the genetic variations in a patient that affect drug efficacy and safety.[4] The goal of PG is to individualize therapy based on genotype.

Nucleotide bases: adenine (A), guanine (G), cytosine (C), thymidine (T), uracil (U)

- DNA Pairs—A-T and G-C AND RNA Pairs—A-U and G-C

Gene: sequence of nucleotides that code for a specific protein

Genotype: sequence of genes that determines a specific trait

Allele: sequence of nucleotides within the chromosome
- Homozygous (2 identical alleles) and hetero-zygous (2 different alleles)

Phenotype: outward expression of the genotype
- Poor metabolizer—2 nonfunctional alleles

- Intermediate metabolizer—1 nonfunctional allele and one decreased functional allele
- Normal metabolizer—2 normal functioning alleles
- Rapid metabolizer—1 normal functional allele and 1 increased functional allele
- Ultra-metabolizer—2 increased functional alleles

Table 1-3 summarizes the common pharmacogenetic testing and applies the results to individualized patient therapy.

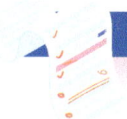

| **Table 1-3** | Common Pharmacogenetic Testing[4] |

TEST	DRUG AGENT	RESULT
DISEASE-ASSOCIATED GENES		
HLA-B	Abacavir	Positive HLA-B*5701; ↑ risk for hypersensitivity, do not use
	Carbamazepine	Positive HLA-B*1502; ↑ risk for SJS and TEN, do not use
	Phenytoin	
Factor V Leiden Mutation	Estrogen-containing oral contraceptives	Variation in Factor V Leiden; ↑ risk of thromboembolic disorders
CYP450 POLYMORPHISMS		
CYP2C19	Clopidogrel (prodrug)	CYP2C19*2 and *3 alleles are poor metabolizers; consider alternative therapy
	Proton pump inhibitors	CYP2C19*17 are rapid metabolizers; require a higher dose
CYP2D6	Codeine (prodrug)	Ultra-rapid metabolizers; ↑ toxicity
		Poor metabolizers; ↓ efficacy
	Tramadol	Ultra-rapid metabolizers; ↓ efficacy
		Poor metabolizers; ↑ toxicity
CYP2C9	Warfarin	CYP2C9*2 and *3 are intermediate or poor metabolizers; ↑ risk of bleeding
CYP2A6	Nicotine	Poor metabolizers; easier time quitting; ↓ dependency
OTHER		
UGT1A1	Irinotecan	UGT1A1 promoter; ↑ the risk of neutropenia
HER2	Trastuzumab	Overexpression of HER2 is required for these drugs; if HER2 is negative, do not use
	Pertuzumab	
	Lapatinib	
KRAS	Cetuximab	If KRAS is positive, do not use
	Panitumumab	

Abbreviations used: SJS, Steven Johnson's syndrome; TEN, toxic epidermal necrolysis.

Common drug interactions

Drug interactions may cause unexpected side effects, increase toxicity, or decrease drug efficacy. Table 1-4 reviews common drug interactions (not all-inclusive).

Drug formulations

Different drug formulations are available to accommodate individual patient needs. Multiple factors should be taken into account when selecting a dosage form: adherence, abuse potential, palatability, route

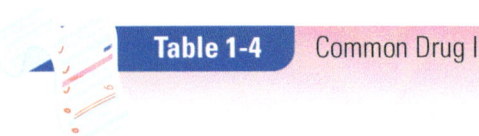

| **Table 1-4** | Common Drug Interactions[5] |

DRUG AGENT	RECOMMENDATIONS	INTERACTION EFFECTS
ANTICHOLINERGICS		
First-generation antihistamines First-generation antipsychotics TCAs Benztropine Muscle relaxants Bladder antimuscarinics	Use an alternative or use a low dose to decrease toxicity	Sedation, dry mouth, blurry vision, constipation, urinary retention
CNS DEPRESSION		
Antiepileptic drugs Benzodiazepines Hypnotics Muscle relaxants Opioids Trazodone	Do not use together, do not use with alcohol, use caution when operating heavy machinery or driving	Somnolence, dizziness, confusion, delirium, gait instability
HYPERKALEMIA RISK		
Amiloride or triamterene RAAS inhibitors Spironolactone or eplerenone Sulfamethoxazole/Trimethoprim	Do not use ACE inhibitors and ARBs, monitor potassium	Weakness, heart palpitations, arrhythmias
INCREASED BLEEDING RISK		
Anticoagulants Antiplatelets NSAIDs SSRIs/SNRIs Statins 5Gs: garlic, ginger, ginkgo, ginseng, glucosamine	Avoid combining drugs if possible, monitor bleeding risk and INR	↑ risk of bleeding
OTOTOXICITY		
Aminoglycosides Loop diuretics Vancomycin	Avoid combining drugs if possible, monitor with hearing assessments	Hearing loss, tinnitus, vertigo
QT-INTERVAL PROLONGATION		
Antiarrhythmics Antibiotics Antidepressants Antipsychotics Anti-emetics	Avoid concurrent use if possible, use lower doses	↑ risk of torsades de pointes

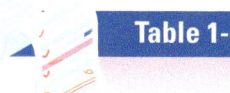

Table 1-4 Common Drug Interactions[5] (*Continued*)

DRUG AGENT	RECOMMENDATIONS	INTERACTION EFFECTS
SEROTONIN SYNDROME		
Antidepressants MAO inhibitors Dextromethorphan Lithium Metoclopramide Opioids Triptans	Avoid concurrent use if possible, separate initiating drugs	Confusion, delirium, tremor, tachycardia, agitation, diarrhea, mydriasis
OTHERS		
Calcium channel blockers + statins	↓ maximum dose of statins	↑ risk of muscle toxicity
PDE-5 inhibitors + nitrates	Do NOT use together	Vasodilation: hypotension, orthostasis, dizziness, falls
PDE-5 inhibitors + alpha blockers	Start with low doses	↑ risk of hypotension, orthostasis, dizziness, falls
Quinolones, tetracyclines + antacids, multivitamins, sucralfate	Separate by 2–6 h	Drugs chelate together and ↓ absorption and efficacy
Warfarin + antibiotics, amiodarone	Monitor INR, may ↓ warfarin dose	↑ INR, ↑ risk of bleeding

Abbreviations used: ACE, angiotensin converting enzyme; ARB, angiotensin receptor blocker; INR, international normalized ratio; MAO, monoamine oxidase; NSAID, nonsteroidal anti-inflammatory drugs; PDE-5, phosphodiesterase-5; RAAS, renin-angiotensin-aldosterone system; SNRI, serotonin-norepinephrine reuptake inhibitors; SSRI, selective serotonin reuptake inhibitors; TCA, tricyclic antidepressant.

of administration, local vs. systemic absorption, and so forth. The different dosage forms available include the following:[6]

- **Tablets**—come in multiple forms (e.g., chewable, buccal, effervescent, ODT); some may be crushed or dissolved in liquid
- **Capsules**—come in hard and soft shell; some may be broken and sprinkled on food
- **Liquid**—delivered as suspensions, syrups, or solutions
- **Suppositories/enemas**—administered in the rectum
- **Eye/ear/nasal drops**—localized administration to the affected area
- **Inhalers/nebulizers**—delivered directly to the lungs
- **Injections**—delivered intravenously, intramuscularly, or subcutaneously

- **Creams/lotions/gels/ointments**—localized administration to the affected area
- **Patches**—applied to the upper chest, back, upper arm, or abdomen for various lengths of time

Emergency preparedness, toxicology, and antidotes

Emergency preparedness is essential for pharmacy staff to respond to disasters (e.g., natural disasters, chemical agents, radioactive or nuclear devices, pandemics). A well-developed distribution and response plan should be in place and discourage unnecessary stockpiling.

Toxicology is the study of poisonous chemicals. Drug poisoning is an adverse effect of taking an excessive amount of the drug. Poisoning can be intentional or unintentional.

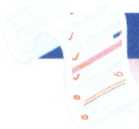

Table 1-5 Child-Resistant Closures[7]

Acetaminophen
Aspirin
Diphenhydramine
Ethylene glycol
Glue removers containing acetonitrile
Ibuprofen
Iron
Kerosene
Methyl Salicylate
Mouthwash
Naproxen
Sodium hydroxide

Prevention strategies[7]

The **Poison Prevention Packaging Act of 1970** mandated the development of packaging that is difficult for children under age 5 to open. **Child-resistant containers** are not "childproof." Table 1-5 lists products that require child-resistant closures.

Treatment strategies[7]

- Ensure ABCs—airway, breathing, circulation
- Ipecac syrup—no longer recommended
- Activated charcoal—most effective if given within 1 hour of ingestion (dose: 1 g/kg)

Commonly used antidotes are reviewed in Table 1-6.

ADDITIONAL RESOURCES

Southwood R, Fleming V, Huckaby G. *Concepts in Clinical Pharmacokinetics.* 7th ed. Bethesda, MD: American Society of Health-System Pharmacists; 2018.

Centers for Disease Control and Prevention. Genomics & precision health. Available at: https://www.cdc.gov/genomics/default.htm. Accessed June 30, 2020.

Byrd LB, Asuka E, Martin N. Antidotes. In: StatPearls. National Center for Biotechnology Information Web site. Available at: https://www.ncbi.nlm.nih.gov/books/NBK539884/. Updated May 17, 2020. Accessed June 10, 2020.

REFERENCES

1. Weber RJ. Medication safety principles and practices. In: DiPiro JT, Yee GC, Posey LM, Haines ST, Nolin TD, Ellingrod V, eds. *Pharmacotherapy: A Pathophysiologic Approach.* 11th ed. New York, NY: McGraw-Hill; 2020:13–14.

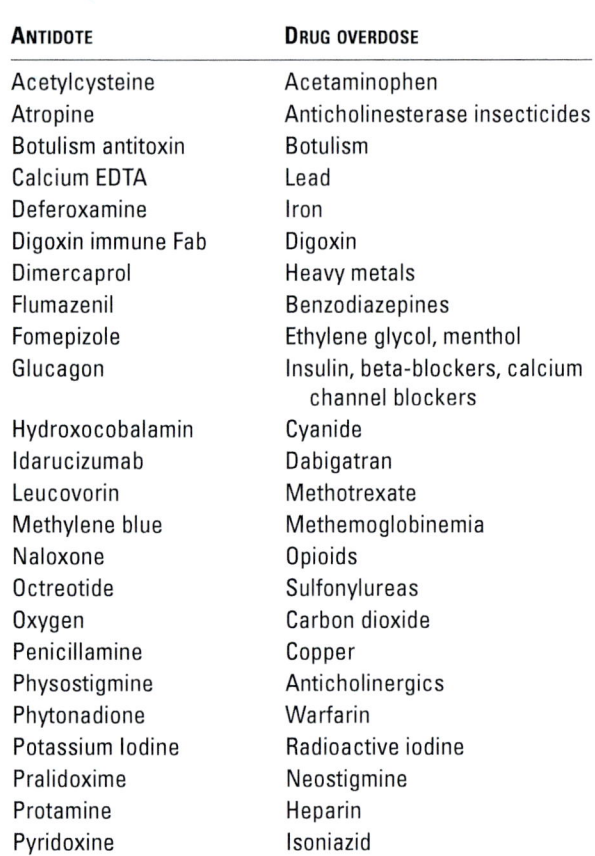

Table 1-6 Common Antidotes[7]

ANTIDOTE	DRUG OVERDOSE
Acetylcysteine	Acetaminophen
Atropine	Anticholinesterase insecticides
Botulism antitoxin	Botulism
Calcium EDTA	Lead
Deferoxamine	Iron
Digoxin immune Fab	Digoxin
Dimercaprol	Heavy metals
Flumazenil	Benzodiazepines
Fomepizole	Ethylene glycol, menthol
Glucagon	Insulin, beta-blockers, calcium channel blockers
Hydroxocobalamin	Cyanide
Idarucizumab	Dabigatran
Leucovorin	Methotrexate
Methylene blue	Methemoglobinemia
Naloxone	Opioids
Octreotide	Sulfonylureas
Oxygen	Carbon dioxide
Penicillamine	Copper
Physostigmine	Anticholinergics
Phytonadione	Warfarin
Potassium Iodine	Radioactive iodine
Pralidoxime	Neostigmine
Protamine	Heparin
Pyridoxine	Isoniazid
Succimer	Lead

2. Bauer LA. Clinical pharmacokinetics and pharmacodynamics. In: DiPiro JT, Yee GC, Posey LM, Haines ST, Nolin TD, Ellingrod V, eds. *Pharmacotherapy: A Pathophysiologic Approach.* 11th ed. New York, NY: McGraw-Hill; 2020:15–16.

3. U.S. Food & Drug Administration. Drug development and drug interactions: table of substrates, inhibitors and inducers. Available at: https://www.fda.gov/drugs/drug-interactions-labeling/drug-development-and-drug-interactions-table-substrates-inhibitors-and-inducers. Accessed June 18, 2020.

4. Cavallari LH, Lam YWF. Pharmacogenetics. In: DiPiro JT, Yee GC, Posey LM, Haines ST, Nolin TD, Ellingrod V, eds. *Pharmacotherapy: A Pathophysiologic Approach.* 11th ed. New York, NY: McGraw-Hill; 2020:17–18.

5. Carpenter M, Berry H, Pelletier AL. Clinically relevant drug-drug interaction in primary care. *Am Fam Physician.* 2019;99(9):558–564.

6. Pharmacy Xpress. Different formulations of medicines. Available at: https://www.pharmacy-xpress.co.uk/manuals/training-handbook/2-different-formulations-medicines. Accessed June 19, 2020.

7. Hayes BD, Chyka PA. Clinical toxicology. In: DiPiro JT, Yee GC, Posey LM, Haines ST, Nolin TD, Ellingrod V, eds. *Pharmacotherapy: A Pathophysiologic Approach.* 11th ed. New York, NY: McGraw-Hill; 2020:19–20.

CHAPTER 2

Calculations

With medical writing support provided by
Banner Medical LLC Writer: Miriam Opara

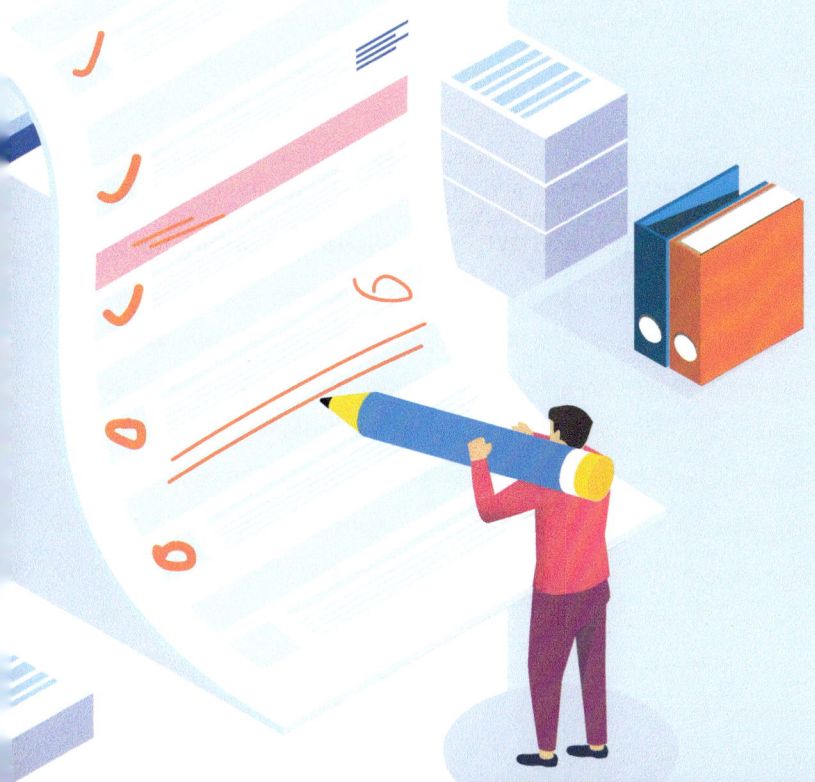

Basic math calculations
Common conversions[1]

LIQUID CONVERSIONS

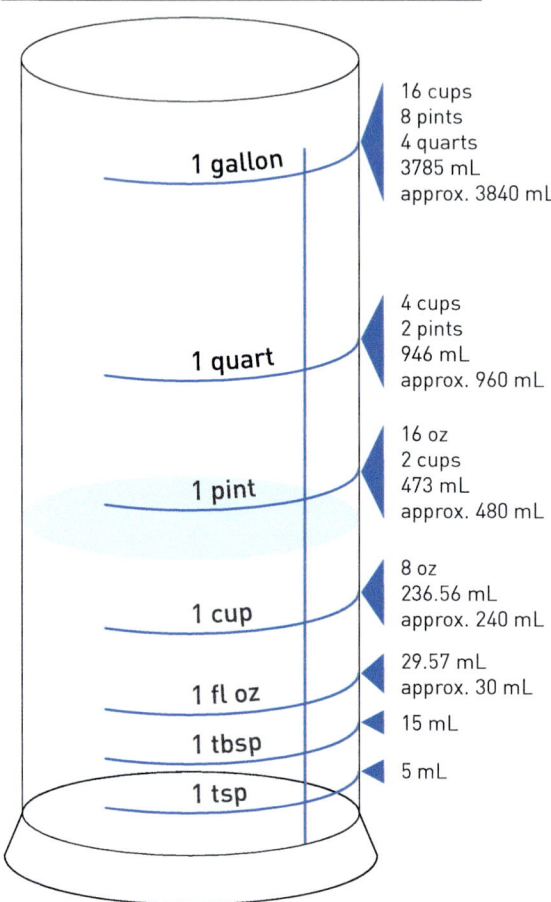

1 gallon
- 16 cups
- 8 pints
- 4 quarts
- 3785 mL
- approx. 3840 mL

1 quart
- 4 cups
- 2 pints
- 946 mL
- approx. 960 mL

1 pint
- 16 oz
- 2 cups
- 473 mL
- approx. 480 mL

1 cup
- 8 oz
- 236.56 mL
- approx. 240 mL

1 fl oz
- 29.57 mL
- approx. 30 mL

1 tbsp
- 15 mL

1 tsp
- 5 mL

SOLID CONVERSIONS

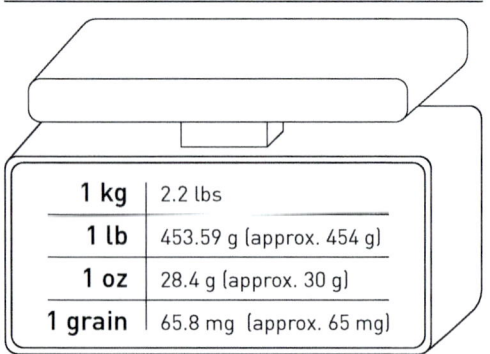

1 kg	2.2 lbs
1 lb	453.59 g (approx. 454 g)
1 oz	28.4 g (approx. 30 g)
1 grain	65.8 mg (approx. 65 mg)

HEIGHT CONVERSIONS

1 inch	2.54 cm
1 foot	12 inches
1 meter	100 cm

TEMPERATURE CONVERSIONS

$$°C = \frac{°F - 32}{1.8} \qquad °F = (°C \times 1.8) + 32$$

Proportions and dimensional analysis[1]

Proportions are two fractions that are set equal: matching the units in the denominators or matching the units in the numerator and denominator. Dimensional analysis is set up to cancel out the same units diagonally.

Method 1:

$$\frac{200\ lbs}{X\ kg} = \frac{2.2\ lbs}{1\ kg} = 90.9\ kg$$

$$\frac{2\ L}{X\ mL} = \frac{1\ L}{1000\ mL} = 2000\ mL$$

Method 2:

$$\frac{200\ lbs}{2.2\ lbs} = \frac{X\ kg}{1\ kg} = 90.9\ kg$$

$$\frac{2\ L}{1\ L} = \frac{X\ mL}{1000\ mL} = 2000\ mL$$

Method 3: dimensional analysis

$$200\ lbs \times \frac{1\ kg}{2.2\ lbs} = 90.9\ kg$$

$$2\ L \times \frac{1000\ mL}{1\ L} = 2000\ mL$$

Compounding calculations

Percentage strength is used to describe the amount of ingredient to the total amount of the product.[1]

$$\%\frac{w}{v} = \frac{X\ g}{100\ mL} \qquad \%\frac{w}{w} = \frac{X\ g}{100\ g}$$

$$\%\frac{v}{v} = \frac{X\ mL}{100\ mL}$$

Ratio strength is a comparison between two numbers (i.e., 3:1); a ratio looks at the relationship of a part to the whole. Converting between ratio and percentage strength is common in compounding.[1]

$$Percentage\ strength = \frac{100}{ratio\ strength}$$

$$Ratio\ strength = \frac{100}{percentage\ strength}$$

Parts per million (PPM) is used to express the concentration of extremely dilute solutions. Converting between PPM and percentage strength is common in compounding.[1]

- PPM → percentage strength: move the decimal **left** 4 places (30 PPM = 0.003%)
- Percentage strength → PPM: move the decimal **right** 4 places (3% = 30,000 PPM)

Specific gravity is a ratio of the density of a substance to the density of water.[1]

$$Specific\ gravity = \frac{g}{mL}$$

Dilution and concentration

Increasing or decreasing the strength of a product is done by changing the quantity when combining two concentrations.[1] (Important: make sure the units on each side match.)

$$Q1 \times C1 = Q2 \times C2$$

Q1 = original quantity
C1 = original concentration
Q2 = final quantity
C2 = final concentration

Alligation is used with three concentrations, compounding two concentration strengths to find a new concentration strength.[1]

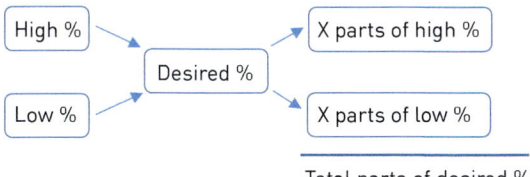

Setup alligation:
- High goes high; low goes low
- Desired concentration in the middle
- Subtract diagonally to obtain number of parts (absolute value)
- Add the no. of parts to get total parts of desired concentration

Osmolarity is the measure of the total number of particles per liter of solution.[1] Table 2-1 summarizes the number of particles in common compounds.

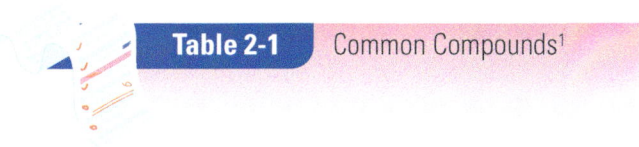

Table 2-1 Common Compounds[1]

COMPOUND	NUMBER OF PARTICLES
Dextrose	1
Mannitol	1
Potassium chloride (KCl)	2
Sodium chloride (NaCl)	2
Calcium chloride (CaCl$_2$)	3

$$mOsmol/L = \frac{Wt\ of\ substance\ (g/L)}{MW\ (g)} \times (\#\ of\ particles)$$
$$\times 1000$$

Isotonicity

Solutions can be isotonic, hypotonic, or hypertonic. Isotonic is when the osmotic pressure (osmolality) of the solution is the same as the blood (300 mOsmol/kg).[1] Normal saline (0.9% NaCl) is the most common isotonic solution used. When making a medication to infuse into the body, the drug provides solutes to the solvent, which can create a hypertonic solution. To avoid hypertonicity, the relationship between the amount of drug that produces a specific osmolarity and the amount of NaCl that produces the same osmolarity is determined by the **E-value** formula.[1]

(i = dissociation factor based on the percentage that ions dissociate in solution [see Table 2-2])

$$E = \frac{(58.5)(i)}{(MW\ of\ drug)(1.8)}$$

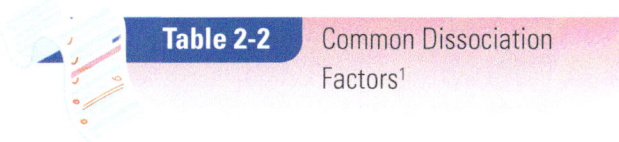

Table 2-2 Common Dissociation Factors[1]

NUMBER OF DISSOCIATED IONS	DISSOCIATION FACTOR
1	1
2	1.8
3	2.6

Mole and millimole represent the molecular weight of the substance in grams or milligrams, respectively.[1]

$$mols = \frac{g}{MW} \quad | \quad mmols = \frac{mg}{MW}$$

Milliequivalents (mEq) represent the relationship between the amount (mg) of a solute to the molecular weight of the compound, taking into account the valence charge of each ion.[1] Table 2-3 summarizes the valence of common compounds.[1]

$$mEq = \frac{mg \times valence}{MW} \quad | \quad mEq = mmols \times valence$$

Nutrition calculations

Parenteral nutrition is when calories are given through a peripheral (max 900 mosm/L) or central (>900 mosm/L) line when the patient's GI tract is not functioning.[1] Calories (interchangeable with kilocalories [kcal]) are provided by three components:

carbohydrates (i.e., dextrose), **protein** (i.e., amino acids), and **fats** (i.e., lipids). The following equations are used to determine the amount of each component needed for a patient's calorie intake.[1]

$$Dextrose = \frac{3.4\ kcal}{g} \quad | \quad Fat\ 10\% = \frac{1.1\ kcal}{mL}$$

$$Protein = \frac{4\ kcal}{g} \quad | \quad Fat\ 20\% = \frac{2\ kcal}{mL}$$

Daily fluid needs are used to ensure the patient is receiving adequate fluids to maintain hydration.[1] (Use patient's actual weight in kilograms.)

$$If\ weight > 20\ kg: 1500\ mL + (20\ mL)(weight - 20)$$

Dehydration is determined by evaluating the patient's blood urea nitrogen (BUN) with the serum creatinine (SCr).

$$BUN:SCr > 20:1$$

Calcium replacement. Half of serum calcium (Ca) is bound to albumin. Therefore, if albumin levels are low (<3.5 g/dL), calcium levels may be falsely low and must be corrected before providing calcium replacement.

$$Ca_{corrected} = serum\ Ca + [(4.0 - albumin) \times 0.8]$$

Calcium and phosphate replacement. Calcium (Ca^{++}) and phosphate (PO_4) can bind together and precipitate. Remember the following:[1]

- Add PO_4 first, then Ca^{++}
- Use calcium gluconate versus calcium chloride
- Ca^{++} and PO_4 added together should **not** exceed 45 mEq/L

Clinical calculations

Body mass index (BMI) is used to determine if a patient is classified as normal weight, low weight, or overweight.[1] Table 2-4 shows the classification of weight based on a patient's BMI.

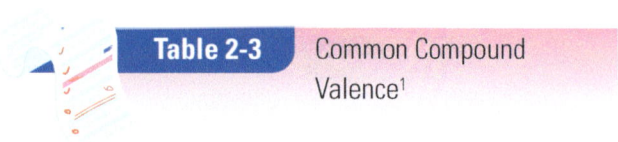

Table 2-3	Common Compound Valence[1]

COMPOUND	VALENCE
Ammonium chloride (NH_4Cl)	1
Potassium chloride (KCl)	1
Sodium chloride (NaCl)	1
Calcium chloride ($CaCl_2$)	2
Ferrous sulfate ($FeSO_4^{2-}$)	2
Magnesium sulfate ($MgSO_4^{2-}$)	2

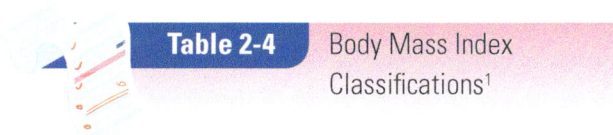

Table 2-4 | Body Mass Index Classifications[1]

BMI (KG/M²)	CLASSIFICATION
<18.5	Underweight
18.5–24.9	Normal weight
25–29.9	Overweight
≥30	Obese

Abbreviation used: BMI, body mass index.

$$BMI(kg/m^2) = \frac{weight(kg)}{[height(m)]^2}$$

OR

$$BMI(kg/m^2) = \frac{weight(lb)}{[height(inches)]^2} \times 703$$

Ideal body weight (IBW) is the healthy weight for a person.[1]

$$IBW(males) = 50\,kg + (2.3\,kg)(inches\ over\ 5\ feet)$$

$$IBW(females) = 45.5\,kg + (2.3\,kg)(inches\ over\ 5\ feet)$$

Adjusted body weight (AdjBW) is used when patients are >20% of the IBW.[1]

$$AdjBW = IBW + 0.4(Actual\ BW - IBW)$$

Creatinine clearance (CrCl) is used to determine kidney function. As kidney function declines, CrCl will decrease.

$$CrCl(mL/min) = \frac{(140 - age) \times weight(kg)}{72 \times SCr}$$
$$\times 0.85(if\ female)$$

Flow rates (drops/min) are used to specify the amount of drug a patient will receive over a given period.[1]

$$\frac{\#\ drops}{mL} \times \frac{mL}{hr} \times \frac{hr}{60\ mins} = \frac{\#\ drops}{min}$$

Anion gap is the difference between the cations and anions in the blood. An anion gap is used to help determine the cause of acidosis. A high anion gap is >12 mEq/L = acidosis.

$$Anion\ Gap = Na - Cl - HCO_3$$

Absolute neutrophil count (ANC). Neutrophils are the body's main defense against infection. Therefore, calculating the ANC will allow us to determine if the patient is more susceptible to infection.

Normal ANC = 2,200 – 8,000 cells/mm³

$$ANC = WBC \times \frac{(\%segs + \%bands)}{100}$$

Certain disease states require drug calculations to convert between oral and IV or vice versa. Loop diuretics are commonly used in treating chronic heart failure. The loop diuretic dose conversion is listed in Table 2-5.

Patients with diabetes who are prescribed insulin must be able to correct for carbohydrate intake or correct the insulin dose based on blood glucose readings (see Table 2-6).[3] The correction factor determines how much insulin is needed to cover the increase in blood sugar.[3]

Phenytoin is highly bound to albumin; when phenytoin levels are reported, they account for bound and unbound levels.[4] Disease states that decrease albumin concentration (e.g., burns, hepatic

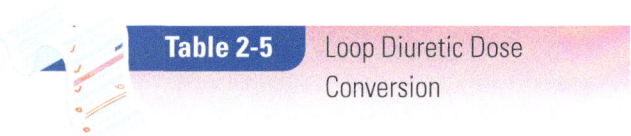

Table 2-5 | Loop Diuretic Dose Conversion

DIURETIC	DOSE
Ethacrynic acid	50 mg
Furosemide	40 mg
Torsemide	20 mg
Bumetanide	1 mg

Note: Furosemide IV:PO = 1:2; Ethacrynic acid, Torsemide, Bumetanide IV:PO = 1:1

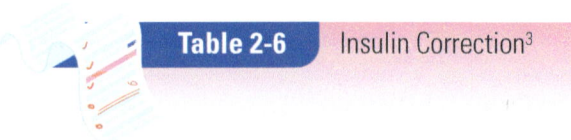

Table 2-6   Insulin Correction[3]

RULE of 500: Insulin-to-carb ratio with rapid-acting insulin

$$\frac{500}{TDD} = grams\ of\ carbs\ covered\ by\ 1\ unit\ of\ insulin$$

RULE of 1800: Correction factor with rapid-acting insulin

$$\frac{1800}{TDD} = correction\ factor\ for\ 1\ unit\ of\ insulin$$

RULE of 1500: Correction factor with regular insulin

$$\frac{1500}{TDD} = correction\ factor\ for\ 1\ unit\ of\ insulin$$

Correction dose

$$Correction\ dose = \frac{(actual\ blood\ glucose) - (target\ blood\ glucose)}{correction\ factor}$$

Abbreviation used: TDD, total daily dose of insulin.

cirrhosis, cystic fibrosis) eventually lead to increased unbound phenytoin levels. Since the reported levels are a total phenytoin level, we must use the phenytoin correction calculation to predict the level of unbound phenytoin when albumin levels are ≤3.5 g/dL.[4]

$$Phenytoin\ correction = \frac{Total\ phenytoin}{(albumin \times 0.2) + 0.1}$$

Body surface area (BSA) is used in medication dosing of chemotherapy drugs.[1]

$$BSA(m^2) = \sqrt{\frac{Ht(cm) \times wt(kg)}{3600}}$$

Pharmacokinetics describes the absorption, distribution, metabolism, and elimination of drugs.[5] Table 2-7 lists the main calculations needed to determine the pharmacokinetics and individualize drug treatment.[5]

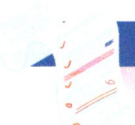

Table 2-7   Pharmacokinetics Calculations[5]

BIOAVAILABILITY

$$F(\%) = 100 \times \frac{AUC_{extravascular}}{AUC_{intravenous}} \times \frac{Dose_{intravenous}}{Dose_{extravascular}}$$

VOLUME OF DISTRIBUTION[6]

$$Vd = \frac{amount\ of\ drug\ in\ body}{concentration\ of\ drug\ in\ plasma}$$

CLEARANCE (CL)

$$Cl = \frac{F \times dose}{AUC} \qquad | \qquad Cl = ke \times Vd$$

ELIMINATION RATE (KE)

$$ke = \frac{Cl}{Vd}$$

HALF-LIFE (T_{1/2})

$$t_{1/2} - \frac{0.693}{ke}$$

LOADING DOSE

$$LD = \frac{desired\ concentration \times Vd}{F}$$

Abbreviations used: AUC, area under the curve; F, fraction of drug absorbed into systemic circulation (also called bioavailability).

ADDITIONAL RESOURCES

Zatz JL, Teixeira MG. *Pharmaceutical Calculations.* 5th ed. Hoboken, NJ: Wiley; 2017.

Southwood R, Fleming V, Huckaby G. *Concepts in Clinical Pharmacokinetics.* 7th ed. Bethesda, MD: American Society of Health-System Pharmacists; 2018.

REFERENCES

1. Zatz JL, Teixeira MG. *Pharmaceutical Calculations.* 5th ed. Hoboken, NJ: Wiley; 2017.
2. Ternacle J, Krapf L, Mohty D, et al. Aortic stenosis and cardiac amyloidosis: *JACC* review topic of the week. *J Am Coll Cardiol.* 2019;74(21):2638–2651.
3. Howard-Thompson A, Khan M, Jones M, George C. Type 2 diabetes mellitus: outpatient insulin management. *Am Fam Physician.* 2018;97(1).
4. Millares-Sipin CA, Alafris A, Cohen H. Phenytoin and fosphenytoin. In: Cohen H, ed. *Casebook in Clinical Pharmacokinetics and Drug Dosing.* New York, NY: McGraw-Hill; 2015.
5. Southwood R, Fleming V, Huckaby G. *Concepts in Clinical Pharmacokinetics.* 7th ed. Bethesda, MD: American Society of Health-System Pharmacists; 2018.
6. Klukowska A, Laguna P, Svirin P, Shiller E, Vdovin V. Efficacy and safety of OCTANINE F in children with haemophilia B. *Haemophilia.* 2008;14(3):531–538.

CHAPTER 3

Lab Values and Drug Monitoring

With medical writing support provided by
Banner Medical LLC Writer: Miriam Opara

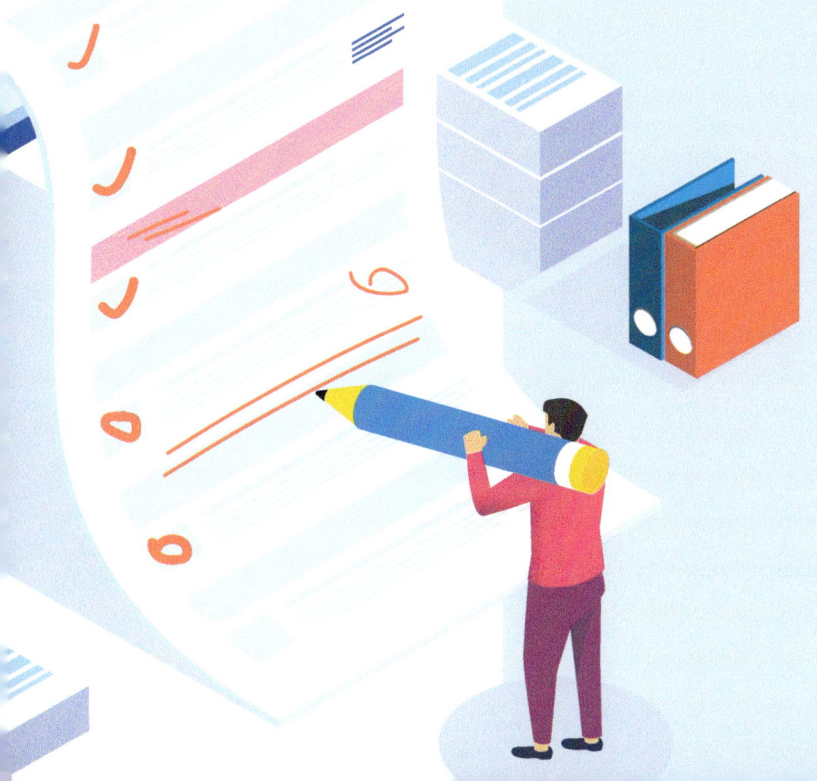

Common lab values

Laboratory values are used to diagnose disease, guide therapy, and monitor disease and drug treatment. Laboratory values may vary slightly depending on the lab used.

A comprehensive metabolic panel evaluates the body's metabolism, blood sugar, electrolytes, and health of the kidney and liver (see Table 3-1)[1].

Complete blood count (CBC) evaluates red blood cells, white blood cells, and platelets to detect infections and conditions such as anemia, infection, inflammation, and leukemia (see Table 3-2).[4]

Evaluating specific lab values will help in the diagnosis and treatment of specific diseases. The following is a list of common laboratory values used for further disease state evaluation:

Acid-base disorders[5]

Respiratory acidosis

- Compensation: kidney $\uparrow HCO_3$ retention and excretion of acid
- $\downarrow pH$, $\uparrow HCO_3$, $\uparrow PCO_2$

Respiratory alkalosis

- Compensation: kidney $\downarrow HCO_3$ retention and excretion of acid
- $\uparrow pH$, $\downarrow HCO_3$, $\downarrow PCO_2$

Metabolic acidosis

- Compensation: hyperventilation to $\uparrow CO_2$ elimination
- $\downarrow pH$, $\downarrow HCO_3$, $\downarrow PCO_2$

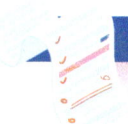

Table 3-1 Comprehensive Metabolic Panel[1–3]

LABORATORY VALUE	REFERENCE RANGE	NOTES
Glucose*	70–99 mg/dL	Primary energy source for cells
PROTEINS		
Albumin	3.5–5 g/dL	Small protein made by the liver
Total protein	60–83 g/L	Measures all proteins in the body
ELECTROLYTES		
Bicarbonate	22–29 mEq/L	Maintenance of acid-base balance
Calcium	8.5–10.5 mg/dL	Essential for functioning of muscles, nerves, and heart; required for blood clotting and bone formation
Chloride	95–106 mEq/L	Maintenance of acid-base balance
Potassium	3.5–5 mEq/L	Essential for cell metabolism and muscle function
Sodium	135–145 mEq/L	Essential for nerve and muscle function
KIDNEY TESTS		
BUN	7–20 mg/dL	Waste product filtered by the kidney
SCr	0.6–1.3 mg/dL	Waste product produced by the muscles and filtered by the kidney
LIVER TESTS		
ALP	33–131 IU/L	Enzyme in bone, liver, and tissue
ALT	10–40 units/L	Enzyme in liver and kidney
AST	10–40 units/L	Enzyme in the heart and liver
Bilirubin	0.1–1.2 mg/dL	Waste product produced by heme breakdown

Abbreviations used: ALP, alkaline phosphatase; ALT, alanine aminotransferase; AST, aspartate aminotransferase; BUN, blood urea nitrogen; SCr, serum creatinine.
*Fasting glucose (consult Ch. 13 for more information on elevated glucose levels).

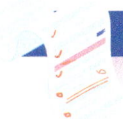

Table 3-2	Complete Blood Count[2-4]

LABORATORY VALUE	REFERENCE RANGE	NOTES
RBC TESTS		
RBC count	$4.1–5.9 \times 10^6$ cell/mcL	Total number of RBC in blood sample
Hemoglobin	12–17.5 g/dL	Amount of oxygen-carrying protein in the blood
Hematocrit	36–50%	Percentage of total blood volume consisting of RBCs
Mean corpuscular volume	80–96 fL	Average size of your RBCs
Mean corpuscular hemoglobin	27–31 pg/cell	Average amount of hemoglobin inside your RBCs
Mean corpuscular hemoglobin concentration	33–36 g/dL	Average concentration of hemoglobin inside your RBCs
WBC TESTS		
WBC count	4500–11000 cells/mcL	Total number of WBC in blood sample
Neutrophils	45–73%	First-line defense for immune response
Eosinophils	0–5%	Attack parasites, respond to allergies
Basophils	0–1%	Small cells that respond to blood infection
Bands	3–5%	Immature segments of neutrophils
Segs	40–60%	Segmented neutrophils
Lymphocytes	20–40%	Create antibodies
PLATELET TESTS		
Platelet count	150000–450000/mcL	Total number of platelets in blood sample

Abbreviations used: RBC, red blood cell; WBC, white blood cell.

Metabolic alkalosis

- Compensation: hypoventilation to $\downarrow CO_2$ elimination
- $\uparrow$ pH, $\uparrow HCO_3$, $\uparrow PCO_2$

Anemia (see Ch. 11 for more information)[6]

B12 deficiency → Macrocytic anemia
- Hgb $\downarrow$, MCV $\uparrow$, reticulocyte count $\downarrow$

Folic acid deficiency → Macrocytic anemia
- Hgb $\downarrow$, MCV $\uparrow$, reticulocyte count $\downarrow$

Iron deficiency → Microcytic anemia
- Hgb $\downarrow$, MCV $\downarrow$, reticulocyte count $\downarrow$

Anemia of chronic disease → Normocytic anemia
- Hgb $\downarrow$, MCV $\downarrow$ (or no change), reticulocyte count $\downarrow$

- C-reactive protein for inflammation
- Erythropoietin for chronic kidney anemia

Bleeding disorders (see Ch. 11 for more information)[7]

- CBC
- D-dimer—evaluate blood clot formation during bleeding, monitor for deep vein thrombosis
- Prothrombin time and International Normalized Ratio—monitor warfarin
- Activated partial thromboplastin time—monitor heparin
- Antifactor Xa activity—monitor low molecular weight heparin 4 hours after dosing
- Platelet function—monitor for heparin induced thrombocytopenia and risk of bleeding

Congestive heart failure (see Ch. 10 for more information)[8]

- B-type natriuretic peptide (BNP) or N-terminal pro-BNP (NT-proBNP)—hormone produced by the left ventricle
- BMP and CBC
- Thyroid levels

Hypercholesterolemia and atherosclerosis (see Ch. 10 for more information)[9,10]

Lipid panel measures the level of lipids in the blood and is used to evaluate atherosclerosis risk and various additional health conditions.

- Total cholesterol (TC; <200 mg/dL) measures all the cholesterol in all the lipoproteins
- High-density lipoprotein (HDL; women: 50–59 mg/dL, men: 40–50 mg/dL) takes up excess cholesterol for removal
- Low-density lipoprotein (LDL; <100 mg/dL) → deposits excess cholesterol in walls of blood vessels
- Triglycerides (<150 mg/dL) measures all triglycerides in all the lipoproteins
- Non-HDL (<130 mg/dL), non-LDL (<100 mg/dL) → total cholesterol minus HDL or LDL
- TC/HDL ratio (<4.5:1) → ↑ ratio = ↑ risk of heart disease

Myocardial infarction and acute coronary syndrome (see Ch. 10 for more information)[11]

- Troponin is elevated during myocardial infarction

- Creatinine Kinase-MB is found mostly in the heart and is elevated in heart damage
- BNP or NT-proBNP is found in the heart and elevated with heart failure

Kidney disease (see Ch. 8 for more information)[12]

- Urine albumin and albumin/creatinine ratio detect albumin in the urine
- Urinalysis detects protein, red blood cells, and white blood cells in the urine
- Estimated glomerular filtration rate → creatinine test or a cystatin C test

Rheumatoid arthritis and osteoarthritis (see Ch. 17 for more information)[13]

- Rheumatoid factor is positive in rheumatoid arthritis (RA) and negative in osteoarthritis
- Erythrocyte sedimentation rate detects inflammation, ↑ in RA
- C-reactive protein detects inflammation, ↑ in RA
- Antinuclear antibody screens for autoimmune disorders including RA

Therapeutic drug monitoring

Therapeutic drug monitoring utilizes drug levels to optimize care by monitoring efficacy and safety (see Table 3-3). Drug monitoring is especially important for narrow therapeutic index drugs. A narrow therapeutic index is when there is a small difference in drug concentration for a therapeutic level and a toxic level.[14]

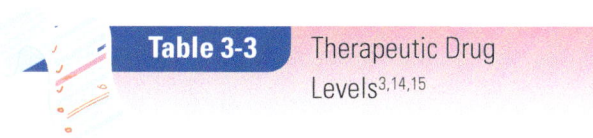

Table 3-3 Therapeutic Drug Levels[3,14,15]

DRUG AGENT	THERAPEUTIC RANGE
ANTIBIOTICS	
Amikacin	Peak: 20–35 mcg/mL
	Trough: <8 mcg/mL
Gentamycin	Peak: 6–10 mg/L
	Trough: <1–2 mg/L
Vancomycin	Trough: 10–15 and AUC/MIC >400 (infections)
	Trough:[16] 15–20 and AUC/MIC: 400–600
	(serious infections: bacteremia, endocarditis, meningitis, osteomyelitis, pneumonia)
Anticoagulants	
Warfarin	INR goal 2–3
	INR goal 2.5–3.5 with mechanical valve
ANTIEPILEPTICS	
Carbamazepine	4–12 mg/L
Phenytoin	10–20 mg/L
Free phenytoin	1–2 mg/L
Valproic acid	50–100 mg/L
BRONCHODILATORS	
Theophylline	5–15 mg/L
CARDIAC DRUGS	
Digoxin	Atrial fibrillation: 0.8–2 mcg/L
	Heart failure: 0.5–0.9 mcg/L
MOOD STABILIZERS	
Lithium	Acute management: 0.5–1.2 mEq/L
	Maintenance: 0.6–0.8 mEq/L

Abbreviations used: AUC, area under the curve; INR, international normalized ratio; MIC, minimum inhibitory concentration.

ADDITIONAL RESOURCES

Lee M. *Basic Skills in Interpreting Laboratory Data*. Bethesda, MD: ASHP publications; 2017.

Blix HS, Viktil KK, Moger TA, Reikvam A. Drugs with narrow therapeutic index as indicators in the risk management of hospitalized patients. *Pharm Pract (Granada)*. 2010;8(1):50–55.

REFERENCES

1. American Association of Clinical Chemistry. Comprehensive metabolic panel (CMP). Available at: https://labtestsonline.org/tests/comprehensive-metabolic-panel-cmp. Accessed June 21, 2020.
2. University of California San Francisco Health. Medical tests. Available at: https://www.ucsfhealth.org/medical-tests. Accessed August 15, 2020.
3. Mayo Clinic Laboratories. Test information. Available at: https://www.mayocliniclabs.com/test-catalog/index.html. Accessed August 15, 2020.
4. American Association of Clinical Chemistry. Complete blood count (CBC). Available at: https://labtestsonline.org/tests/complete-blood-count-cbc. Accessed June 21, 2020.
5. American Association of Clinical Chemistry. Acidosis and alkalosis. Available at: https://labtestsonline.org/conditions/acidosis-and-alkalosis. Accessed June 21, 2020.
6. American Association of Clinical Chemistry. Anemia. Available at: https://labtestsonline.org/conditions/anemia. Accessed June 21, 2020.
7. American Association of Clinical Chemistry. Bleeding disorders. Available at: https://labtestsonline.org/conditions/bleeding-disorders. Accessed June 21, 2020.
8. American Association of Clinical Chemistry. Congestive heart failure. Available at: https://labtestsonline.org/conditions/congestive-heart-failure. Accessed June 21, 2020.
9. Millán J, Pintó X, Muñoz A, et al. Lipoprotein ratios: physiological significance and clinical usefulness in cardiovascular prevention. *Vasc Health Risk Manag*. 2009;5:757–765.
10. DiPiro J, Talbert R, Yee G, Matzke G, Wells B, Posey L. Dyslipidemia. In: *Pharmacotherapy: A Pathophysiologic Approach*. 8th ed. McGraw-Hill; 2011:365–388.
11. American Association of Clinical Chemistry. Heart attack and acute coronary syndrome. Available at: https://labtestsonline.org/conditions/heart-attack-and-acute-coronary-syndrome. Accessed June 21, 2020.
12. American Association of Clinical Chemistry. Kidney disease. Available at: https://labtestsonline.org/conditions/kidney-disease. Accessed June 21, 2020.
13. American Association of Clinical Chemistry. Rheumatoid arthritis. Available at: https://labtestsonline.org/conditions/rheumatoid-arthritis. Accessed June 21, 2020.
14. Blix HS, Viktil KK, Moger TA, Reikvam A. Drugs with narrow therapeutic index as indicators in the risk management of hospitalised patients. *Pharm Pract (Granada)*. 2010;8(1):50–55.
15. Lee M. *Basic skills in interpreting laboratory data*. Bethesda, MD: ASHP; 2017.
16. Rybak MJ, Le J, Lodise TP, et al. Therapeutic monitoring of vancomycin for serious methicillin-resistant Staphylococcus aureus infections: a revised consensus guideline and review by the American Society of Health-System Pharmacists, the Infectious Diseases Society of America, the Pediatric Infectious Diseases Society, and the Society of Infectious Diseases Pharmacists. *Am J Health Syst Pharm*. 2020;77(11):835–864.

Biostatistics

With medical writing support provided by Banner Medical LLC writers: Miriam Opara and Milena Murray

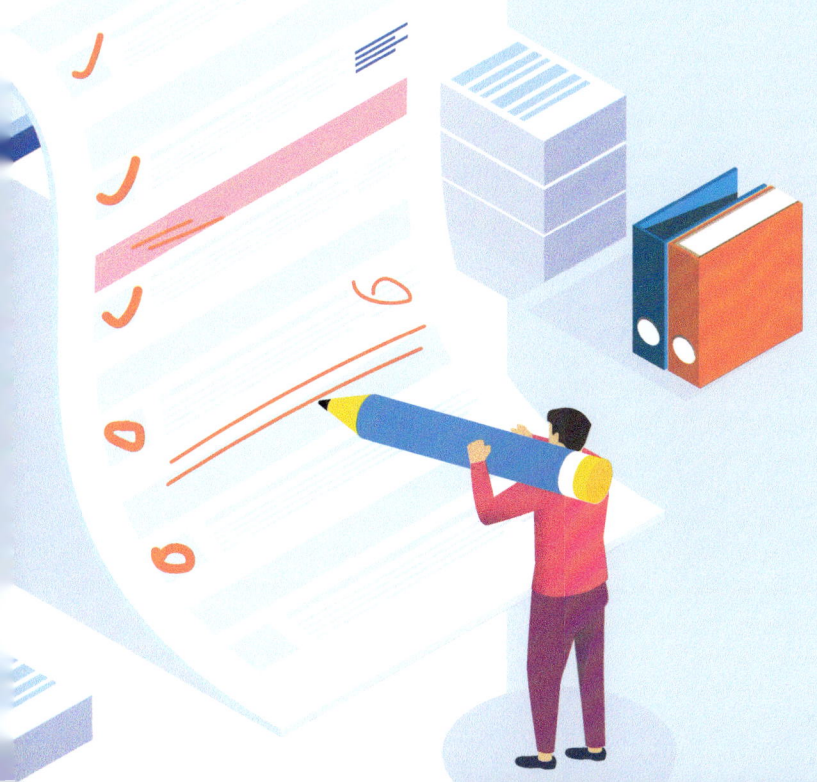

Biostatistics utilizes statistical analysis and methods to provide the interpretation of data related to medicine and human biology.

Variables[1]

- Dependent variable: the outcome resulting from changes in the independent variable
- Independent variable: responsible for the change in the observed situation
  - Control variables (confounding): additional variables that may affect changes in the dependent variable
  - Active variables: under the control of the researcher (e.g., amount of drug administered)

- Attribute variables: cannot be manipulated by the researcher (e.g., gender, age, blood pressure)

Hypothesis testing[2]

- Null hypothesis (H_0): no difference between groups
- Alternative hypothesis: difference between groups

Types of data and common statistical tests

Data are collected throughout a study to analyze the differences and relationships between variables. The type of data and question being asked determines the appropriate statistical test to evaluate if differences or relationships between the treatment and control groups are statistically significant (Figure 4-1).[3, 4]

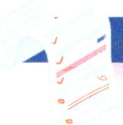

| **Figure 4-1** | Types of Study Data and Common Statistical Tests for Data[3, 4] |

CONTINUOUS DATA

Interval Data	**Ratio Data**
No true zero	True zero
0 ≠ none	0 = none
Ex: height, blood pressure	Ex: age, weight

STATISTICAL TESTS:

One group:
One-sample t-test

Two groups (treatment and control):
Independent/unpaired student t-test

Three or more groups:
ANOVA

Paired groups:
Dependent/paired t-test (used if one group has before and after data)

CATEGORICAL DATA

Nominal Data	**Ordinal Data**
No order (yes/no)	Ranked order
Ex: gender, mortality	Ex: 0-10 pain scale

STATISTICAL TESTS:

One group:
Chi-Square test

Two groups (treatment and control):
Chi-Square or Fisher's exact test
Mann-Whitney-U (also called Wilcoxon Rank-Sum)

Three or more groups:
Kruskal-Wallis test

Paired groups:
Wilcoxon Signed-Rank test (used if one group has before and after data)

Random sampling[4]

- Simple random sampling: each member of the population has an equal chance to be part of the sample, a list of all members of a population is prepared, and N items are chosen among the population size
- Systematic random sampling: every k^{th} participant is selected; k is determined by the total number of participants divided by the desired sample size
- Stratified random sampling: participants are divided into subgroups, and a random sample is selected from each subgroup
- Cluster random sampling: clusters of participants, based on natural groupings, are selected to randomly sample

Study blinding[4]

- Open-label: both participants and investigators are aware of treatment group allocations
- Single-blinded: either participants or investigators are not aware of treatment group allocations
- Double-blinded: both participants and investigators are not aware of treatment group allocations

Data analysis

- Intention to treat: includes all participants originally starting in the active or control groups, regardless if they completed the trial
- Per protocol: includes only participants who completed the trial

Types of studies

The type of study chosen by the investigator determines the quality of the study. Each design has strengths and weaknesses (Table 4-1).[5] Evidence-based medicine looks at the validity and reliability of the study design. Figure 4-2 shows the hierarchy of evidence, with the most reliable evidence at the top to the least reliable evidence at the bottom.[5]

Table 4-2 outlines common statistical measures used to analyze and interpret biological data obtained in experimental and observational studies.

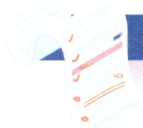

| **Table 4-1** | Strengths and Weaknesses of Study Designs[6, 7] |

TYPE OF STUDY	STRENGTHS	WEAKNESSES
EXPERIMENTAL DESIGN		
RCT Compares an experimental treatment to a control	▪ Less potential for bias ▪ Determines cause and effect, noninferiority, or superiority	▪ Time-consuming ▪ Expensive
OBSERVATIONAL DESIGN		
Case-control ▪ Compares patients with a disease to those without the disease ▪ Retrospective	▪ Inexpensive ▪ Useful when an active trial is unethical ▪ Less time required	▪ Potential for interfering confounding factors ▪ Potential for selection bias
Case report ▪ Investigates a single case when a patient exhibits reaction or condition ▪ Retrospective	▪ Inexpensive ▪ Useful for rare diseases ▪ Less time required	▪ Conclusions cannot be drawn from a single case

(*continued on next page*)

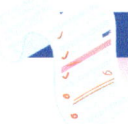 **Table 4-1** Strengths and Weaknesses of Study Designs[6, 7] (*Continued*)

TYPE OF STUDY	STRENGTHS	WEAKNESSES
Case series ■ Investigates multiple similar cases ■ Retrospective	■ Inexpensive ■ Useful for rare diseases ■ Smaller sample size ■ Less time required	■ Incomplete historical data ■ Potential for selection bias
Cohort ■ Patients placed into groups based on exposure/risk factor and followed over time to observe outcomes ■ Prospective or retrospective	■ Simple ■ Large sample size ■ Follow patients over a long period of time	■ Expensive ■ Time-consuming ■ Potential loss to follow up ■ Potential for selection bias
Cross-sectional ■ Collection of data at a single point in time from a sample population ■ Prevalence studies	■ Quick and inexpensive ■ Useful for quality improvement	■ No distinction of cause and effect
ANALYSIS		
Meta-analysis Combines results of multiple studies	■ Greater statistical power ■ Less time required	■ Potential for selection bias ■ Heterogeneity of studies

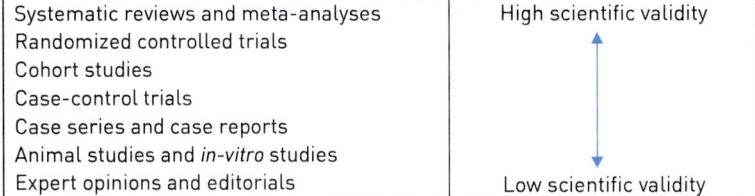 **Figure 4-2** Hierarchy of Evidence[5]

Systematic reviews and meta-analyses Randomized controlled trials Cohort studies Case-control trials Case series and case reports Animal studies and *in-vitro* studies Expert opinions and editorials	High scientific validity ↑ ↓ Low scientific validity

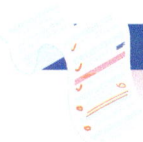

Table 4-2   Common Statistical Measures Used in Biostatistics[1, 8]

STATISTICAL MEASURE	DESCRIPTION	EQUATION
Absolute risk	Size of the risk	# exposed group − # unexposed group
Absolute risk reduction	Includes risk reduction and incidence rate of the outcome	% risk control group − % risk treatment group
Alpha (α)	Probability of a type I error	—
Attributable fraction	Fraction of all cases of a disease or adverse event in a population attributable to a specific exposure	$\dfrac{RR - 1}{RR} \times 100$
Beta (β)	Probability of a type II error	—
Confidence interval	For a 95% CI, it is interpreted that there is a 95% confidence that the population value lies within the interval	$CI = 1 - \alpha$
Correlation	Number between −1 and 1+ that describes the linear association between two variables	—
Hazard ratio	Rate an unfavorable event occurs within a short period of time	$\dfrac{HR\ treatment\ group}{HR\ control\ group}$
Incidence rate	Frequency of some event over a specified time period	$\dfrac{\#\ of\ cases}{\#\ of\ at\text{-}risk\ experience}$
Interquartile range or middle 50% of data	Interval between the 25th and 75th percentile	—
Mean	The average value	$\dfrac{Sum\ of\ all\ scores}{Number\ of\ scores}$
Median	Data midpoint	50% of values above and 50% of values below
Mode	Most commonly occurring value	—
Normal distributions	The curve is symmetrical, 68% of the values are within 1 SD, 95% of values are within 2 SDs	—
Number needed to treat	Number of patients needed to be treated over a period of time for 1 patient to benefit	$\dfrac{1}{\%\ risk\ CG - \%\ risk\ TG} \qquad \dfrac{1}{ARR\,^*}$ Round up
Number needed to harm	Number of patients needed to be treated over a period of time for 1 patient to be harmed	$\dfrac{1}{\%\ risk\ CG - \%\ risk\ TG} \qquad \dfrac{1}{ARR\,^*}$ Round down
Odds ratio	Odds of exposure in those with disease vs. odds of exposure in those without disease	$\dfrac{ad}{bc}$

EXPOSURE	DISEASE	NO DISEASE
Exposed	a	b
Unexposed	c	d

STATISTICAL MEASURE	DESCRIPTION	EQUATION
p-value	Probability of obtaining the observed result if the null hypothesis were true Determining statistical significance of *p*-values: $p < \alpha$	—

(*continued on next page*)

STATISTICAL MEASURE	DESCRIPTION	EQUATION
Power	Ability of the test to detect a difference if there is one	$1 - \beta$
Prevalence	Proportion of cases in a population over a specified period of time	$\dfrac{\textit{Number prevalent cases}}{\textit{Size of population}}$
Range	Interval between minimal and maximal value	—
Regression	The change in dependent variable when the independent variable changes Linear: continuous dependent variables Logistic: categorical dependent variables	—
Relative risk or risk ratio	Incidence for exposed group/incidence for unexposed group	$\dfrac{\textit{Risk treatment group}}{\textit{Risk control group}}$
Relative risk reduction	Ratio of treatment vs. control group	$\dfrac{\% \textit{ risk CG} - \% \textit{ risk TG}}{\% \textit{ risk CG}}$ $\quad 1 - RR*$
Risk	Probability of a disease or event	$\dfrac{\# \textit{ with unfavorable event}}{\textit{Total \# in group}}$
Risk difference	Attributable risk or excess risk	# exposed group − # unexposed group
Sensitivity	How effectively a test identifies patients with the condition, or true positives	$\dfrac{A}{A+C} \times 100$

TEST RESULT	DISEASE	NO DISEASE
Positive	A: true positives	B: false positives
Negative	C: false negatives	D: true negatives

STATISTICAL MEASURE	DESCRIPTION	EQUATION
Specificity	How effectively a test identifies patients without the condition, or true negatives	$\dfrac{D}{B+D} \times 100$

TEST RESULT	DISEASE	NO DISEASE
Positive	A: true positives	B: false positives
Negative	C: false negatives	D: true negatives

STATISTICAL MEASURE	DESCRIPTION	EQUATION
Standard deviation	How spread out the data is, and how far the data is from the mean	—
Standard error of the mean	Variation of hypothetical studies if repeated multiple times	$\dfrac{\sigma}{\sqrt{n}}$
Type 1 error	H_0 rejected when it is true	—
Type 2 error	H_0 is accepted when it should have been rejected	—

Abreviations used: #, number; σ, population standard deviation; *, expressed in decimal form; ARR, absolute risk reduction; CG, control group; CI, confidence interval; HR, hazard ratio; H_0, null hypothesis; RR, relative risk; SD, standard deviation; TG, treatment group.
Adapted from DiCenzo R. *Clinical Pharmacist's Guide to Biostatistics and Literature Evaluation*. Lenexa, KS: American College of Clinical Pharmacy; 2011; Mansournia MA, Altman DG. Population attributable fraction. *BMJ*. 2018;360:k757. doi:10.1136/bmj.k757.

ADDITIONAL RESOURCES

DiCenzo R. *Clinical Pharmacist's Guide to Biostatistics and Literature Evaluation.* Lenexa, KS: American College of Clinical Pharmacy; 2011.

REFERENCES

1. DiCenzo R. *Clinical Pharmacist's Guide to Biostatistics and Literature Evaluation.* Lenexa, KS: American College of Clinical Pharmacy; 2011.
2. White SE. Research questions about one group. *Basic & Clinical Biostatistics.* 5th ed. McGraw-Hill Education; 2020.
3. Parab S, Bhalerao S. Choosing statistical test. *Int J Ayurveda Res.* 2010;1(3):187–191.
4. White SE. Probability & related topics for making inferences about data. *Basic & Clinical Biostatistics.* 5th ed. McGraw-Hill Education; 2020.
5. Sherer JT. Principles of evidence-based medicine. In: Aparasu RR, Bentley JP, eds. *Principles of Research Design and Drug Literature Evaluation.* 2nd ed. McGraw-Hill Education; 2020:163–172.
6. Khanna R, Aparasu RR. Research design and methods. In: Aparasu RR, Bentley JP, eds. *Principles of Research Design and Drug Literature Evaluation.* 2nd ed. McGraw-Hill Education; 2020.
7. White SE. Study designs in medical research. *Basic & Clinical Biostatistics.* 5th ed. McGraw-Hill Education; 2020.
8. Mansournia MA, Altman DG. Population attributable fraction. *BMJ.* 2018;360:k757. doi:10.1136/bmj.k757

CHAPTER 5

Compounding and Hazardous Waste

With medical writing support provided by
Banner Medical LLC Writers: Jennifer Miller
and Miriam Opara

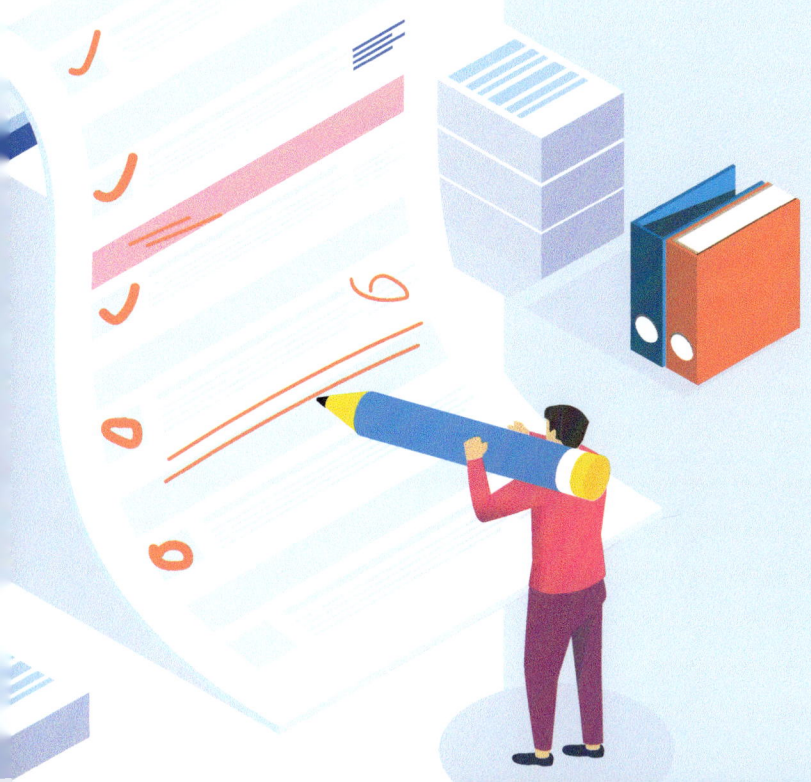

Nonsterile compounding

Compounding is when drugs are combined, mixed, or altered to create a drug specific to an individual patient need. Compounding differs from manufacturing as outlined in Table 5-1.[1]

Equipment for nonsterile compounding is essential for proper mixing and packaging.[2]

- Graduated cylinder—read the bottom of the meniscus
- Weighing balance—torsion balances have a sensitivity requirement (SR) of 6 mg
  - *Minimum weighable quantity*
    $$= \frac{SR}{acceptable\ error\,(0.05)}$$
- Mortar and pestles—grinding and blending powders

The goal of compounding with dry powders is to ensure the powder mixture is evenly distributed. Comminution is different methods of grinding, crushing, and milling to reduce powder particle size. Comminution methods include[2]

- **Trituration:** reducing particle size of a substance into a fine powder
- **Levigation:** trituration in a mortar with a pestle or with a spatula on an ointment slab with a small amount of liquid in which the substance is insoluble to make a paste
- **Spatulation:** blending powders or substances on an ointment slab with a spatula
- **Pulverization by intervention:** crystals are dissolved in a solvent and then spread out on a surface where the solvent evaporates, and

the substance then recrystallizes into smaller particles

Medications include active and inactive ingredients. Excipients (see Table 5-2) are inactive ingredients used to thicken by increasing viscosity, increase stability, prevent degradation, add flavoring, add color, and aid with absorption.

The following are excipients with multiple purposes:

- Cellulose—diluent, disintegrate
- Gelatin—coating, diluent, gelling agent
- Glycerin—diluent, sweetening agent, humectant, levigating agent, lubricant
- Lactose—diluent, sweetening agent
- Mg Stearate—glidant, lubricant
- Mineral oil—levigating agent, lubricant
- PEG—hydrophilic solvent, levigating agent, lubricant, suppository base
- Propylene glycol—humectant, levigating agent
- Starches—dry diluent, disintegrate, gelling agent
- Shellac—coating, enteric coating

Sterile compounding

Sterile compounding is a major part of a hospital pharmacy. Equipment placement is important to achieve and maintain sterility of compounded medications.[5]

- **Primary engineering controls**—hood or isolator
- **Biological safety cabinets**—used for chemotherapy and hazardous drugs

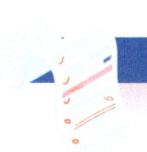

Table 5-1	Compounding vs. Manufacturing[2]

	COMPOUNDING	MANUFACTURING
Quantity	Prescription for a specific patient	Bulk quantities
Regulated by	State board of pharmacy	FDA - must follow current Good Manufacturing Practices
Expiration	Beyond use date assigned by the pharmacist	Expiration date determined by the manufacturer

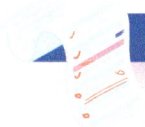 **Table 5-2** Excipients Used In Compounding[3,4]

INGREDIENT	PURPOSE	EXAMPLES
Adsorbents	Keeps powders dry	Mg oxide/carbonate Kaolin
Antifoaming agent	Breaks up and inhibits the formation of foams	Simethicone Dimethicone
Antioxidants	Prevents oxidation	Ascorbic acid Ascorbyl palmitate Sodium ascorbate/bisulfate/thiosulfate
Binders	Adhesive materials used to hold powders together	Acacia Starch paste Sucrose syrup
Buffers	Maintains pH range	Potassium phosphate Sodium acetate/citrate
Coatings	Prevents degradation from oxygen, light, and moisture and mask the unpalatable taste	Gelatin, Gluten, Shellac
Coloring agent	Provides color to the compounded product	RD&C Red No. 3 Yellow No. 6 Caramel Ferric Oxide (red)
Diluents (fillers)	Adds volume to small dosages	Liquids: water, glycerin, alcohol Dry: starches, calcium salts, lactose (mannitol, sorbitol), cellulose, gelatin Topicals: mineral oil, petrolatum, lanolin
Disintegrates	Absorbs water to cause the tablet to swell or burst	Alginic acid Polacrilin potassium (Amberlite) Cellulose products Starches, compressible sugar (Nu-Tab)

Emollient	Acts as a barrier and a vehicle for drug delivery
	  ▪ oleaginous (oil-containing)
	  ▪ aqueous (water-containing)
	  ▪ water-in-oil or oil-in-water emulsions
		Aquaphor, Aquabase
		Vaseline, Petroleum jelly (petrolatum)
		Polybase, Eucerin, Cetaphil

Enteric coating	Acid-resistant protective layer that prevents dissolution in the stomach	Cellulose acetate phthalate Shellac
Flavoring agent, sweetener	Gives sweetness to a preparation	Syrups, oils Sugarcoating for tabs: sucrose, glucose Sugar free: aspartame, saccharin Glycerin Dextrose, Mannitol, Sorbitol Phenylalanine, Stevia, Xylitol

(continued on next page)

Table 5-2 Excipients Used In Compounding[3,4] (*Continued*)

INGREDIENT	PURPOSE	EXAMPLES
Gelling (thickening) agent	Increases the viscosity of a substance and can stabilize the mixture	Agar, alginates Gums (guar, xantham, acacia) Gelatins, tragacanth Bentonite, carbomer Cellulose, starches Mg aluminum silicate (Veegum) Poloxamer (Pluronic) gels Polyvinyl alcohol (eye lubricant)
Glidant	Improves flow of properties of the powder mixture by reducing interparticle friction	Colloidal silica Mg stearate
Humectant	Prevents preparations from becoming dry and brittle	Glycerin Sorbitol Propylene glycol
Hydrophilic solvent	Liquid with high miscibility (mixes easily) with water; used to dissolve solutes	PEG Alcohols Terpenes
Hydrophobic solvent	Liquid with low miscibility (does not mix) with water; used to dissolve solutes	Oils: borage, canola, coconut, castor Fats: Omega-3, Omega-6
Levigating (wetting) agent	Liquid used in the process of reducing particle size (used to make a paste)	Mineral oil, glycerin Glycols, PEG
Lubricant	Prevents ingredients from sticking to each other and equipment	Mg stearate, calcium, PEG Glycerin, mineral oil, stearic acid, talc
Preservatives	Prevents growth of bacteria or other pathogens	Oral: parabens, sodium benzoate, benzoic acid Topical/nasal: alcohols, acids, chlorhexidine Ophthalmics: EDTA, sodium benzoate, benzoic acid, benzalkonium chloride, thimerosal
Suppository base	Stays intact for insertion but melts once inserted	Cocoa butter (theobroma oil) Hydrogenated vegetable oils PEG polymers Glycerinated gelatin
Water	Purified water Sterile water Bacteriostatic water	Purified water: nonsterile compounding unless higher purity is required Sterile water: for sterile compounding Bacteriostatic water: sterile with a preservative

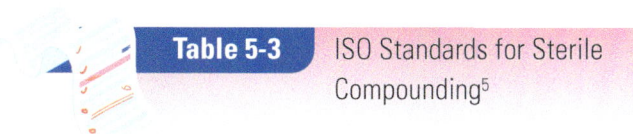

Table 5-3   ISO Standards for Sterile Compounding[5]

COMPOUNDING ROOM	ISO RATING
Hood or isolator	5
Buffer room	7
Ante area	8

Abbreviation used: ISO, International Standards Organization.

- **Segregated compounding area**—separate area for compounding when there is insufficient physical space for an IV room

Clean air is essential for reducing the risk of contamination. The International Standards Organization sets the standard for the number of particles per volume of air to determine air quality (see Table 5-3).[5]

Sterile compounding personnel must pass a gloved-fingertip test and media-fill test annually to evaluate the sterility of their garbing and aseptic technique, respectively. Garbing is donned in the ante area:[5]

1. Don shoe covers, head and facial hair covers, and face masks first.
2. Complete proper hand hygiene.

3. Don gown then enter the buffer room.
4. Use alcohol-based hand sanitizer.
5. Lastly, don gloves.

USP <797> defines three categories of contamination for compounding sterile products (see Table 5-4). The risk factors are used to determine beyond use dates.

Handling hazardous drugs

Hazardous drugs (HD) can be carcinogenic, teratogenic, cause reproductive toxicity, or cause organ toxicity and must be handled carefully. Tables 5-5 and 5-6 summarize standards for nonsterile and sterile compounding of HDs, respectively.

Personal protective equipment and handling hazardous drugs[6]

Personal protective equipment (PPE) required for compounding sterile and nonsterile HDs includes the following:

- Gowns
- Head and hair covers
- Shoe and sleeve covers
- 2 pairs of chemotherapy gloves

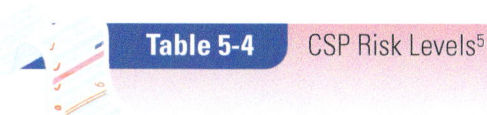

Table 5-4   CSP Risk Levels[5]

CSP RISK	AIR QUALITY	CONDITIONS	BEYOND USE DATE		
			ROOM	REFRIGERATOR	FREEZER
Low	ISO 5	Primary engineering controls	48 h	14 d	45 d
		Transfer, measuring and mixing no more than 3 ingredients			
Low with <12 h BUD	ISO 5	Segregated compounding area	12 h	12 h	—
Medium	ISO 5	Long compounding process	30 h	9 d	45 d
High	ISO 5	Nonsterile ingredients are used	24 h	3 d	45 d
		Improper garbing			

Abbreviations used: BUD, beyond use date; CSP, compounding sterile products; ISO, International Standards Organization.

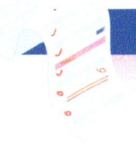

Table 5-5 — Nonsterile HD Compounding Engineering Control Standards[6]

CONTAINMENT PRIMARY ENGINEERING CONTROL	CONTAINMENT SECONDARY ENGINEERING CONTROL
Externally vented or redundant-HEPA filtered in series ■ CVE ■ Class I or II BSC ■ CACI	Externally vented ■ 12 ACPH ■ Negative pressure between 0.01-0.03 in of water column relative to neighboring areas

Abbreviations used: ACPH, air changes per hour; BSC, biologic safety cabinet; CACI, compounding aseptic containment isolator; CVE, containment ventilated enclosure; HEPA, high-efficiency particulate air.

Table 5-6 — Sterile HD Compounding Engineering Control Standards[6]

CONFIGURATION	CONTAINMENT PRIMARY ENGINEERING CONTROL	CONTAINMENT SECONDARY ENGINEERING CONTROL
ISO Class 7 buffer room and anteroom	Externally vented ■ Class II BSC ■ CACI	■ Externally vented ■ 30 ACPH ■ Negative pressure between 0.01–0.03 in of water column relative to neighboring areas
Unclassified C-SCA	Externally vented ■ Class II BSC ■ CACI	■ Externally vented ■ 12 ACPH ■ Negative pressure between 0.01–0.03 in of water column relative to neighboring areas

Abbreviations used: ACPH, air changes per hour; BSC, biologic safety cabinet; CACI, compounding aseptic containment isolator; C-SCA, containment-segregated compounding area; ISO, International Standards Organization.

PPE must be worn when handling HDs during the following

■ Receipt, storage, transport, compounding (both sterile and nonsterile), administration, deactivation/decontamination, cleaning, disinfecting, spill control, waste disposal

ADDITIONAL RESOURCES

United States Pharmacopeia and National Formulary. *USP 795 Pharmaceutical Compounding – Nonsterile Preparations.* USP42-NF37 ed. Rockville, MD: United States Pharmacopeial Convention; 2014.

United States Pharmacopeia and National Formulary. *USP 797 Pharmaceutical Compounding–Sterile Preparations.* USP42-NF37 ed. Rockville, MD: United States Pharmacopeial Convention; 2008.

United States Pharmacopeia. *USP 800 Hazardous Drugs – Handling in Healthcare Settings.* Available at: https://www.usp.org/sites/default/files/usp/document/our-work/healthcare-quality-safety/general-chapter-800.pdf.

REFERENCES

1. United States Pharmacopeia and National Formulary. *USP 795 Pharmaceutical Compounding—Nonsterile Preparations.* USP42NF37 ed. Rockville, MD: United States Pharmacopeial Convention; 2014.

2. American Society of Health-Systems Pharmacy. ASHP technical assistance bulletin on compounding nonsterile products in pharmacies. *Am J Hosp Pharm.* 1994;51(11):1441–1448.

3. Shargel L, Yu A. Impact of biopharmaceutics on drug product quality and clinical efficacy. In: Shargel L, Yu ABC, eds. *Applied Biopharmaceutics and Pharmacokinetics.* 7th ed. New York, NY: McGraw-Hill Education; 2016.

4. Suarez S, Marroum PJ, Hughes M. Biopharmaceutic considerations in drug product design and in vitro drug product performance. In: Shargel L, Yu ABC, eds. *Applied Biopharmaceutics and Pharmacokinetics.* 7th ed. New Yo 2016.

5. United States Pharmacopeia and Natio *Pharmaceutical Compounding – Sterile Pre* ed. Rockville, MD: United States Pha 2008.

6. United States Pharmacopeia. *USP Handling in Healthcare Settings.* Available sites/default/files/usp/document/our-work/healthcare safety/general-chapter-800.pdf. Accessed May 4, 2020.

CHAPTER 6

Immunizations

With medical writing support provided by Banner Medical LLC Writer: Miriam Opara

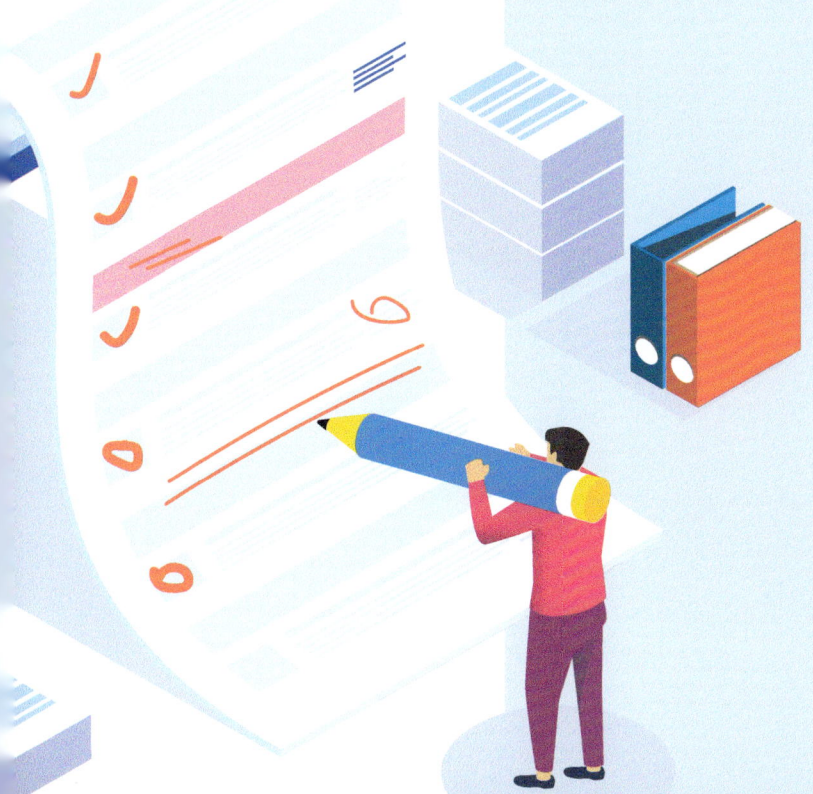

Routine vaccines

Vaccines prevent serious or potentially fatal diseases and create herd immunity (vaccinated people protect those who are unable to get vaccinated). There are two types of vaccines:[1]

1. **Live attenuated vaccines:** modified virus or bacteria to produce a strong immune response
   - Contraindicated in immunocompromised patients
   Live vaccines: **"CRAZY MOTIVE"**
     - **C**holera
     - **R**otavirus
     - **A**
     - **Z**oster (ZVL)
     - **Y**ellow fever
     - **M**MR
     - **O**
     - **T**yphoid (oral)
     - **I**ntranasal Influenza
     - **V**aricella
     - **E**
2. **Inactivated vaccines:** killed virus or bacteria that cannot replicate; a booster may be required

Vaccines should be stored properly in the original box and kept in the refrigerator or freezer per manufacturer guidelines.[1]

Simultaneous vaccine administration (≥1 vaccine at same visit or day) may occur for most vaccines with some exceptions; always consult current Advisory Committee on Immunization Practices guidelines and manufacturer guidelines prior to coadministration. For example, if two live vaccines are not administered on the same day, they must be separated by a minimum of 4 weeks.

The most common adverse effects of vaccines are injection site pain and allergic reaction. Prior to vaccine administration, screening and patient consent are required.[1] Vaccines may be administered through the following routes (depending on manufacturer guidelines):[1]

- **Intramuscular**—90° in the deltoid (see Figure 6-1)
- **Subcutaneous**—45° in fatty tissue over the triceps (see Figure 6-1)
- Gluteal
- Intranasal
- Oral

Table 6-1 includes routine vaccination recommendations including special populations (assuming there are no contraindications for administration).

Travel health

The Centers for Disease Control and Prevention provides important travel medicine updates in the *Yellow Book*. Contaminated food and water are a concern in many developing countries. Travelers may receive preventative medicine or vaccines for diseases that may be transmitted during international travel.

Traveler's diarrhea is the most common illness and can be caused by *E. coli*, *Campylobacter jejuni*, *Shigella* spp, and *Salmonella* spp.[2]

- **Prevention:** eat foods that are cooked or peeled, boil water, drink bottled water, wash hands with soap and water
- **Treatment:** hydration with salt and water, loperamide as needed, antibiotics for severe cases (≥14 days and/or dysentery)

Disease transmitted by insects

The most efficient prevention strategies against disease transmitted by insects include the following:[3]

- Sleep in screened or airconditioned rooms
- Cover skin as much as possible
- Use EPA-registered insect repellent (e.g., DEET, picaridin, IR3535, oil of lemon eucalyptus, para-menthane-diol, 2-undecanone)
- Use permethrin-treated clothing

Malaria is a parasite (*Plasmodium* spp) transmitted by Anopheles mosquitos.[3] Prevention strategies include[3]

- **Daily regimens**
  - Atovaquone/Proguanil—start 1–2 days before travel, continue 1 week after travel
  - Doxycycline—start 1–2 days before travel, continue 4 weeks after travel
  - Primaquine—start 1–2 days before travel, continue 7 days after travel
  - Tafenoquine—start 3 days before travel, continue 7 days after travel

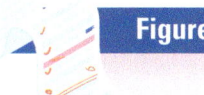
(A)

(B)

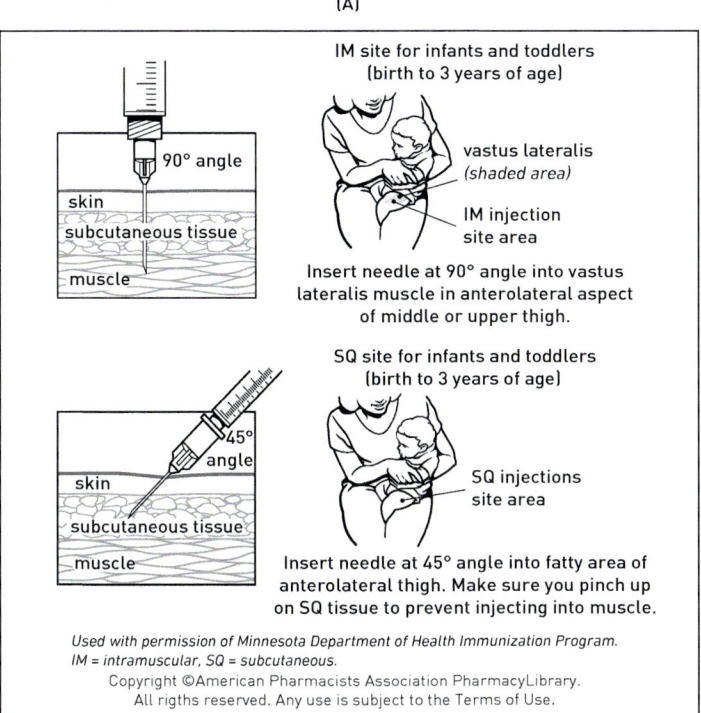

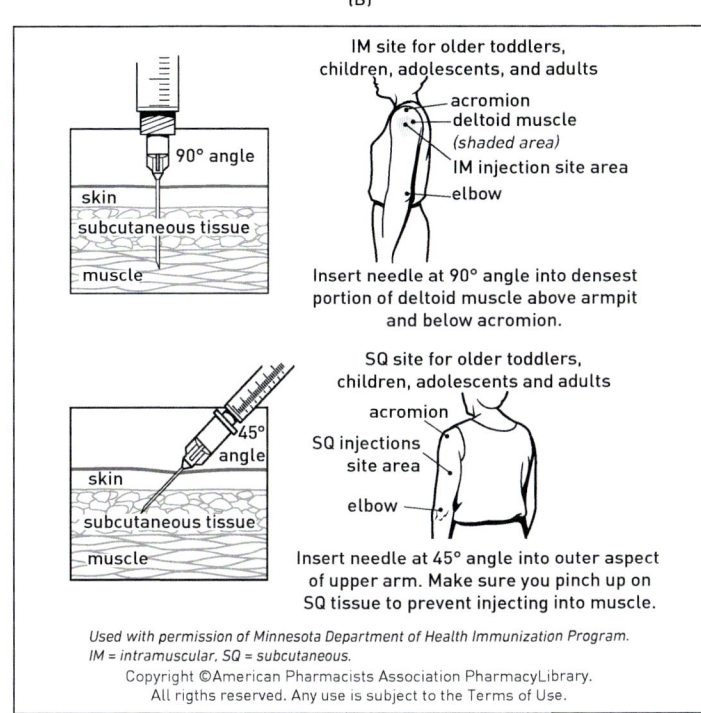

Abbreviations used: IM, intramuscular; SQ, subcutaneous. Source: Adapted with permission from the Minnesota Department of Health Immunization Program. How to Administer IM (Intramuscular) Injections; How to Administer SQ (Subcutaneous) Injections. 2018. Available at: https://www.health.state.mn.us/people/immunize/hcp/admim.pdf. Copyright © American Pharmacists Association PharmacyLibrary. All rights reserved. Any use is subject to the Terms of Use.

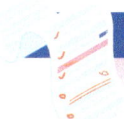 **Table 6-1** Routine Vaccination Recommendations Including Special Populations

VACCINATION	AGE ADMINISTERED	SPECIAL POPULATIONS
Hepatitis A	▪ 12–18 mo: 2-dose series	▪ Chronic liver disease ▪ HIV ▪ MSM
Hepatitis B	▪ Birth ▪ 1–2 mo ▪ 6–18 mo	▪ Chronic liver disease ▪ DM ▪ ESRD ▪ HIV ▪ MSM
Hib	▪ 2 mo ▪ 4 mo ▪ 12–15 mo	Asplenia: 1 dose HSCT: 3 doses

(*continued on next page*)

Vaccination	Age administered	Special populations
HPV	9–45 y: 2–3 doses	▪ Asplenia ▪ ESRD ▪ Chronic liver disease ▪ Heart or lung disease ▪ Healthcare personnel ▪ Immunocompromised ▪ MSM
Influenza	Annually starting at 6 mo	Not specified
Meningococcal (Serogroups A,C,W,Y)	▪ 11–12 y ▪ 16 y	▪ Asplenia ▪ HIV Special situations: traveling overseas; first year of college and military if haven't previously received
Meningococcal (Serogroups B)	▪ 16-23 y if not at increased risk	Asplenia
MMR	▪ 12–15 mo ▪ 4–6 y	Not specified
Pneumococcal (PCV13)	▪ 2 mo ▪ 4 mo ▪ 6 mo ▪ 12–18 mo ▪ ≥ 65 y: 1 dose	▪ >19 y: 1 dose ▪ Asplenia ▪ ESRD ▪ HIV ▪ Immunocompromised
Pneumococcal (PPSV23)	≥ 65 y	▪ Asplenia ▪ Chronic liver disease ▪ DM ▪ ESRD ▪ Heart or lung disease ▪ HIV
Poliovirus	▪ 2 mo ▪ 4 mo ▪ 6–18 mo ▪ 4–6 y	Not specified
Rotavirus	▪ 2 mo ▪ 4 mo	Not specified
Tdap**	▪ 2 mo ▪ 4 mo ▪ 6 mo ▪ 15–18 mo ▪ 4–5 y ▪ Booster every 10 y	1 dose every pregnancy
Varicella	▪ 12–15 mo ▪ 4–6 y	Not specified
Recombinant zoster	50 y: 2-dose series Note: ACIP prefers recombinant zoster vaccine vs. live vaccine	

Abbreviations used: ACIP, Advisory Committee on Immunization Practices; DM, diabetes mellitus; ESRD, end-stage renal disease; Hib, haemophilus influenzae type B; HPV, human papillomavirus; HSCT, hematopoietic stem cell transplant; MMR, measles, mumps, rubella; MSM, men who have sex with men; Tdap, tetanus, diphtheria, pertussis.

**Tetanus also available as DTaP, DT, and Td; consult individual prescribing information.

- **Weekly regimens**
  - Chloroquine—start 1–2 weeks before travel, continue 4 weeks after travel
  - Mefloquine—start 1–2 weeks before travel, continue 4 weeks after travel

Travelers' vaccines include the following:

- **Rabies**[4]—prevention: 3 doses, given for those traveling to high-risk areas
  - Transmitted by a virus from saliva of infected animals
  - Treatment: 2 doses (vaccinated); 4 doses (unvaccinated)
- **Typhoid**[5]—oral or intramuscular, prevention for those traveling to Asia, Africa, Caribbean, Central and South America, or the Middle East
  - Transmitted by bacteria *Salmonella typhi*
  - Live typhoid vaccine is effective for 5 years; intramuscular vaccine is effective for 2 years
- **Cholera**[6]—prevention for those traveling to Africa, Haiti, or Southeast Asia
  - Transmitted by bacteria *Vibrio cholerae*
- **Japanese encephalitis**[7]—prevention: 2 doses if traveling for >1 month to Asia
  - Transmitted by mosquito
- **Yellow fever**[8]—prevention for those traveling in tropical areas of South America and Africa
  - Transmitted by mosquito
  - No FDA-approved vaccine currently available in the U.S.
    - (There is a non–FDA-approved vaccine available to limited sites only.)
  - Yellow Fever Stamp is required to show proof of vaccination

ADDITIONAL RESOURCES

Centers for Disease Control and Prevention. Birth-18 years immunization schedule. Available at: https://www.cdc.gov/vaccines/schedules/hcp/imz/child-adolescent.html. Accessed June 15, 2020.

Centers for Disease Control and Prevention. Adult immunization schedule by vaccine and age group. Available at: https://www.cdc.gov/vaccines/schedules/hcp/imz/adult.html. Accessed June 15, 2020.

Hamborsky J, Kroger A, Wolfe S, eds. *Epidemiology and Prevention of Vaccine-Preventable Diseases*. 13th ed. Washington, DC: National Center for Immunization and Respiratory Diseases, Centers for Disease Control and Prevention; 2015.

REFERENCES

1. Hayney MS. Vaccines and immunoglobulins. In: DiPiro JT, Yee GC, Posey LM, Haines ST, Nolin TD, Ellingrod V, eds. *Pharmacotherapy: A Pathophysiologic Approach*. 11th ed. New York, NY: McGraw-Hill; 2020.

2. Roecker AM, Bates BN. Gastrointestinal infections and enterotoxigenic poisonings. In: DiPiro JT, Yee GC, Posey LM, Haines ST, Nolin TD, Ellingrod V, eds. *Pharmacotherapy: A Pathophysiologic Approach*. 11th ed. New York, NY: McGraw-Hill; 2020.

3. Centers for Disease Control and Prevention. Choosing a drug to prevent malaria. Available at: https://www.cdc.gov/malaria/travelers/drugs.html. Updated January 28, 2019. Accessed June 22, 2020.

4. Centers for Disease Control and Prevention. Rabies. Available at: https://wwwnc.cdc.gov/travel/diseases/rabies. Accessed June 21, 2020.

5. Centers for Disease Control and Prevention. Typhoid fever. Available at: https://wwwnc.cdc.gov/travel/diseases/typhoid. Accessed June 21, 2020.

6. Centers for Disease Control and Prevention. Cholera. Available at: https://wwwnc.cdc.gov/travel/diseases/cholera. Accessed June 21, 2020.

7. Centers for Disease Control and Prevention. Japanese encephalitis. Available at: https://wwwnc.cdc.gov/travel/diseases/japanese-encephalitis. Accessed June 21, 2020.

8. Centers for Disease Control and Prevention. Yellow fever. Available at:https://wwwnc.cdc.gov/travel/diseases/yellow-fever. Accessed June 21, 2020.

9^+ x

9^+ x

9^+ x

CHAPTER 7

Infectious Disease

With medical writing support provided by
Banner Medical LLC Writer: Miriam Opara

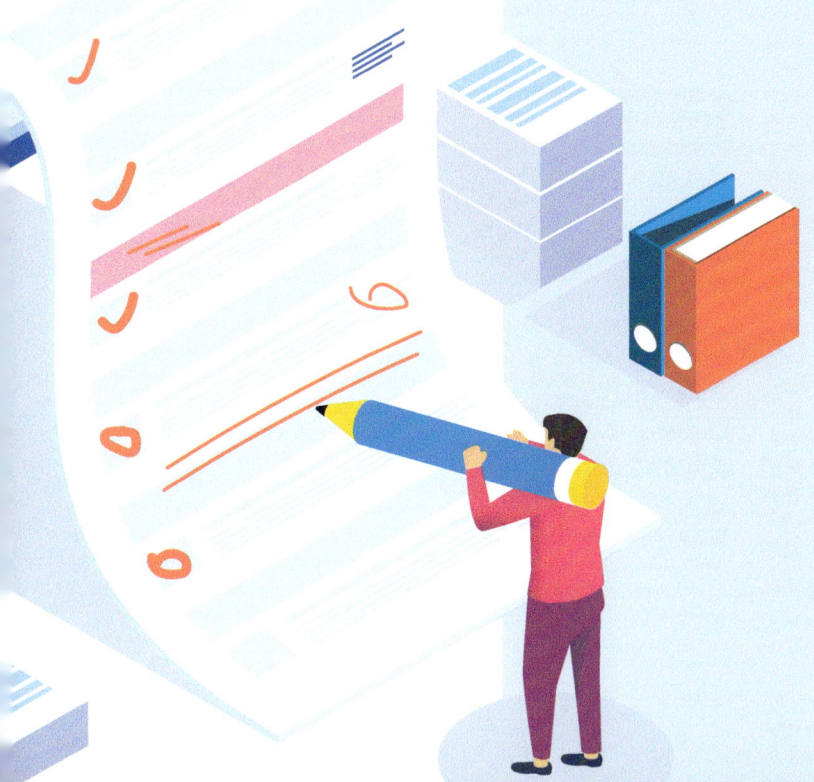

Background and antibacterial drug class

Infectious disease (ID) is caused by various pathogens and identifying the causative pathogen is essential in choosing the correct drug to treat the infection.

Bacterial organisms are identified using **gram staining** (see Table 7-1).[1]

- **Gram positive**—organism has a thick cell wall and appears dark purple from the crystal violet stain
- **Gram negative**—organism has a thin cell wall and appears pinkish from the safranin counterstain
- **Atypical organisms**—do not have a cell wall and do not stain well

A gram stain shows the shape of the organism and helps determine empiric therapy.

Cultures are taken to determine the exact organism and susceptibility testing is performed to determine antibiotic treatment.[1]

- **Minimum inhibitory concentration (MIC):** lowest antimicrobial concentration to prevent bacterial growth
- **Susceptibility breakpoint:** usual drug concentration that inhibits bacterial growth
- If MIC is ≤ breakpoint, bacteria is susceptible and can be used
  - If MIC is > breakpoint, bacteria is intermediate or resistant

Understanding the mechanism of action (see Figure 7-1) of antibiotics helps determine what types of organisms can be treated with certain antibiotics.[2-5]

Remember, the bugs *always win*—pathogen and drugs of choice are listed in Table 7-2.

Table 7-1	Common Gram-Stained Organisms[1]

COCCI — Cocci, Diplococci, Cocci chains, Cocci clusters

BACILLI — Bacilli, Diplobacilli, Coccobacilli, Spores

CURVED FORMS — Curved rod, Curved, Spirochete

G +	G −	G +	G −	G +	G −
Diplococci:	**Cocci:**	**Bacilli:**	**Bacilli:**	—	**Curved:**
Streptococcus pneumoniae	Neisseria spp	Listeria Corynebacterium Gardnerella	Pseudomonas spp Escherichia coli		Helicobacter pylori
Chains:	—	**Spore:**	**Chains:**	—	**Curved rod:**
Streptococci spp Enterococci spp		Actinomyces Clostridium Bacillus	Klebsiella spp Serratia spp Citrobacter spp Proteus spp		Vibrio cholerae
Clusters:	—	—	**Coccobacilli:**	—	**Spirochete:**
Staphylococci spp			Bordetella pertussis Haemophilus influenzae Moraxella catarrhalis		Campylobacter spp Treponema spp Borrelia spp

Abbreviations used: spp, species.

Figure 7-1 Mechanism of Action of Common Antibiotics[2-5]

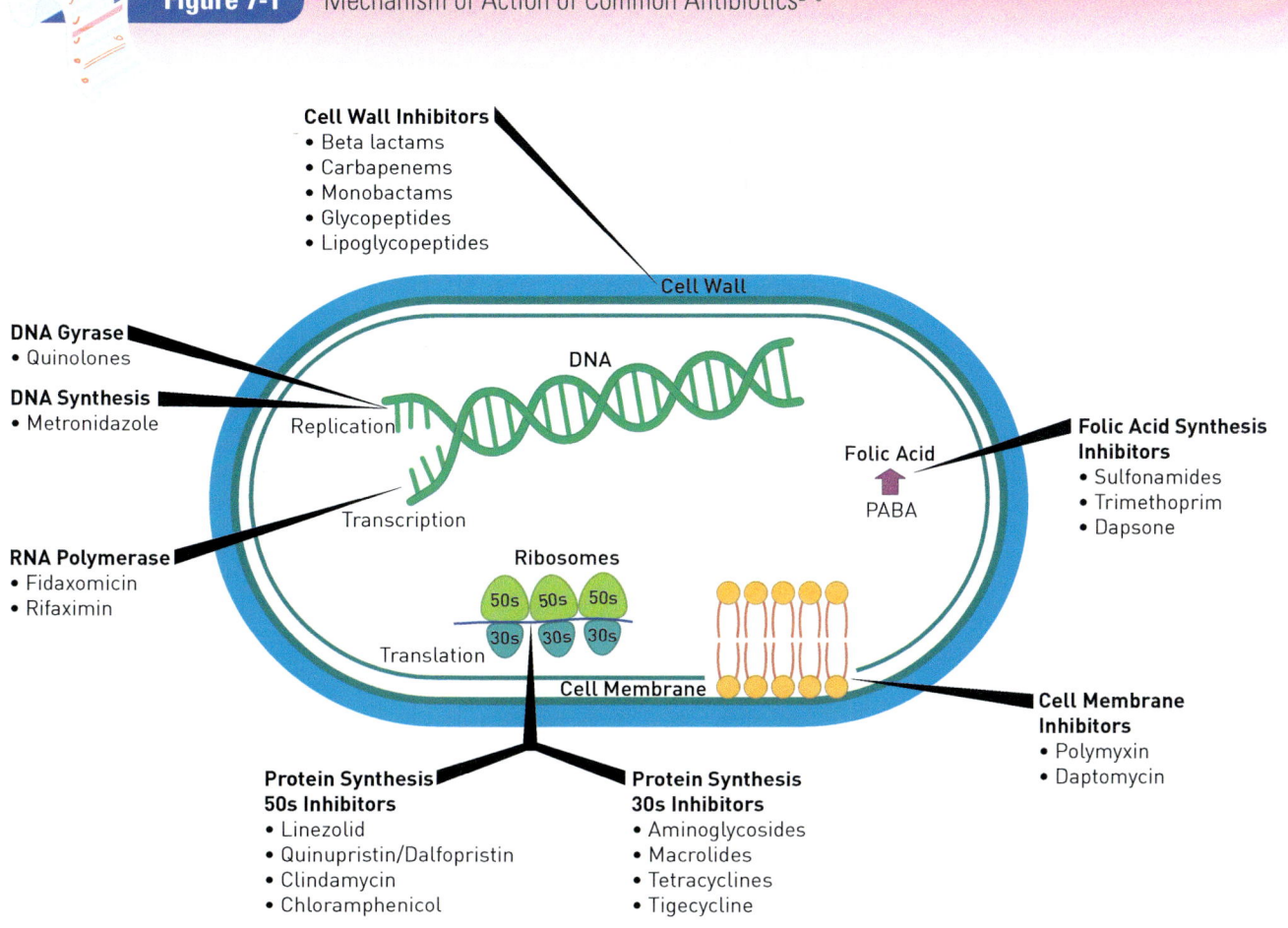

Abbreviations used: PABA, para-aminobenzoic acid.

Remember the following:

- Hydrophilic drugs—beta lactams, aminoglycosides, glycopeptides, daptomycin, polymyxin
- Lipophilic drugs—fluoroquinolones, macrolides, rifampin, linezolid, tetracyclines
- Penicillin G can NOT be given IV—cardiorespiratory arrest or death
- Ceftriaxone—hyperbilirubinemia, biliary sludging in neonates
- Aztreonam—used if penicillin allergy with gram-negative infections
- Vancomycin—red man syndrome, ototoxicity, nephrotoxicity
  - Trough: 10–15 and AUC/MIC >400 (infections)
  - Trough:[16] 15–20 and AUC/MIC: 400–600 (serious infections: bacteremia, endocarditis, meningitis, osteomyelitis, pneumonia)

- Aminoglycosides—ototoxicity, nephrotoxicity
- Macrolides—QT prolongation, drug–drug reaction: lovastatin, simvastatin
- Tetracyclines—ototoxicity, photosensitivity, discolored teeth in children, contraindicated with pregnancy
- Linezolid—bone marrow suppression, serotonin syndrome
- Daptomycin—increase CPK, myopathy
- Fluoroquinolones—tendon rupture, peripheral neuropathy, QT prolongation, photosensitivity, contraindicated in pregnancy
- Metronidazole—metallic taste, disulfiram reaction
- Sulfamethoxazole/Trimethoprim—photosensitivity, increase potassium

Table 7-2 Drug Regimens for Common Bacterial Infections[6,7]

INFECTION	PREFERRED DRUG	ALTERNATIVES
	GRAM POSITIVE	
Clostridioides difficile	Oral Vancomycin	Metronidazole
	Fidaxomicin	
Enterococcus faecalis		
Endocarditis, meningitis, pyelonephritis	Ampicillin + Gentamicin or Streptomycin	
Urinary tract infection	Ampicillin	Fosfomycin
	Amoxicillin	Nitrofurantoin
Enterococcus faecium		
Bacteremia	Daptomycin	Quinupristin/dalfopristin
	Linezolid	Tigecycline
Staphylococcus aureus		
MSSA	Nafcillin	SMZ-TMP
	Oxacillin	Clindamycin
MRSA	Vancomycin	Ceftaroline
		Daptomycin
		Linezolid
		Telavancin
		Tigecycline
		SMZ-TMP
		Quinupristin/dalfopristin
Streptococcus groups A, B, C, G, pyogenes		
Cellulitis	Cephalexin	Clindamycin
Pharyngitis	Penicillin G or V	Macrolides
	Ampicillin	
Streptococcus pneumoniae		
Acute otitis media	Amoxicillin	Cefdinir
Sinusitis	Amoxicillin/clavulanate	Ceftriaxone
MIC >1.0 mg/L	Vancomycin	Cefotaxime
		Ceftriaxone
		Fluoroquinolones
	GRAM NEGATIVE	
Acinetobacter		
Bacteremia, skin and soft tissue infection	Carbapenems	Ampicillin/sulbactam
		Polymyxin
		Tigecycline
Bacteroides fragilis		
Bacteremia, skin and soft tissue	Metronidazole	Clindamycin
		Carbapenems
Borrelia burgdorferi		
Lyme disease	Doxycycline	Cefotaxime
	Amoxicillin	
Chlamydia trachomatis		
Chlamydia	Azithromycin	Doxycycline

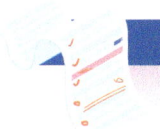

Infection	Preferred drug	Alternatives
Chlamydia trachomatis + neisseria gonorrhea		
Chlamydia and Gonorrhea	Azithromycin + Ceftriaxone	
Enterobacter		
Bacteremia	Carbapenems	Ciprofloxacin
	Cefepime	Levofloxacin
		Piperacillin/tazobactam
Escherichia coli		
Meningitis	Cefotaxime	
	Ceftriaxone	
	Meropenem	
Urinary tract infection	Nitrofurantoin	Fluoroquinolone
	SMZ-TMP	
	Fosfomycin	
Gardnerella vaginalis		
Vaginosis	Metronidazole	Clindamycin
Haemophilus influenzae		
Meningitis	Ceftriaxone	Meropenem
Other infections	Ampicillin	SMZ-TMP
	Amoxicillin	Azithromycin
		Clarithromycin
		Fluoroquinolone
Klebsiella pneumoniae		
Pneumonia	Ceftriaxone	Carbapenem
	Cefepime	Fluoroquinolone
Listeria monocytogenes		
Meningitis	Ampicillin + Cefotaxime	
Legionella		
Community acquired pneumonia	Azithromycin	SMZ-TMP
	Fluoroquinolone	Clarithromycin
		Doxycycline
Moraxella catarrhalis		
Acute otitis media	Amoxicillin/clavulanate	SMZ-TMP
	Ampicillin/sulbactam	Macrolides
Mycobacterium tuberculosis		
Latent tuberculosis	Isoniazid + Rifapentine weekly for 3 mo	Rifampin daily for 4 mo
Active tuberculosis "RIPE"	Rifampin + Isoniazid + Pyrazinamide + Ethambutol for 2 mo	Rifampin + Isoniazid + Pyrazinamide + Ethambutol for 2 mo
	Rifampin + Isoniazid for 4 mo	Rifampin + Isoniazid for 7 mo
Mycoplasma pneumoniae		
Community acquired pneumonia	Azithromycin	Doxycycline
	Fluoroquinolone	
Neisseria gonorrhoeae		
Gonorrhea	Ceftriaxone	

(*continued on next page*)

INFECTION	PREFERRED DRUG	ALTERNATIVES
Neisseria meningitis		
Meningitis	Penicillin G	Ceftriaxone
Pasteurella		
Soft tissue, bone and joint infections, animal bites	Penicillin G Ampicillin Amoxicillin	Doxycycline SMZ-TMP Ceftriaxone
Proteus mirabilis		
Urinary tract infection	Ampicillin	SMZ-TMP
Pseudomonas aeruginosa		
Urinary tract infection	Aminoglycoside	Ciprofloxacin Levofloxacin
Systemic infection	Cefepime Ceftazidime Carbapenem Piperacillin/tazobactam Aminoglycoside	Aztreonam Ciprofloxacin Levofloxacin Polymyxin
Rickettsia rickettsii		
Rocky Mountain Spotted Fever	Doxycycline	
Rickettsia typhi		
Typhus	Doxycycline	
Salmonella typhi		
Typhoid	Ciprofloxacin Ceftriaxone	SMZ-TMP Ampicillin
Serratia spp		
Hospital-acquired pneumonia, skin and soft tissue, urinary tract infections	Ceftriaxone Cefotaxime Cefepime Ciprofloxacin Levofloxacin	Aztreonam Carbapenem Piperacillin/tazobactam Aminoglycosides
Stenotrophomonas		
Pulmonary infection, bacteremia, endocarditis	SMZ-TMP	
Treponema pallidum		
Neurosyphilis	Penicillin G	Ceftriaxone
Syphilis	Penicillin G	Ceftriaxone Doxycycline
Trichomoniasis		
Vulvovaginitis	Metronidazole	

Abbreviations used: SMZ-TMP, sulfamethoxazole/trimethoprim.

Figure 7-2 Fungal Classifications[8]

Fungi		
Dimorphic fungi	Histoplasma capsulatum	
	Blastomyces dermatitidis	
	Coccidioides immitis	
Molds	Aspergillus spp	
	Zygomycetes	
Yeasts	Candida spp	
	Crypotcoccus neoformans	

Antifungals and antivirals

Fungi are eukaryotes with a nucleus enclosed by a nuclear membrane and a rigid cell wall.[8] Fungi can be classified as yeasts, molds, or dimorphic fungi (see Figure 7-2). Dimorphic fungi exist as mold in cold temperatures and as yeast in warm temperatures.[8]

Antifungals can be classified based on their site of action (see Table 7-3).

Prevention and treatment of invasive mycoses is particularly important for immunocompromised patients (see Table 7-4).

Viruses are obligate intracellular pathogens that replicate inside a host cell.[9] Treatment for viral

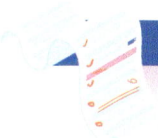

Table 7-3 Antifungal Classifications[8]

MECHANISM OF ACTION	ANTIFUNGALS	NOTES
Azoles: Inhibit synthesis of ergosterol and decrease cell membrane formation	Fluconazole Itraconazole Ketoconazole Posaconazole Voriconazole	SE: ↑ LFTs, QT prolongation Strong CYP3A4 inhibitors
Echinocandins: Inhibit synthesis of beta (1,3)-D-glucan in the fungal cell wall	Anidulafungin Caspofungin Micafungin	Injection-only formulations SE: ↑ LFTs, histamine-mediated symptoms
Amphotericin B: Binds ergosterol causing cell death	Amphotericin B Amphotericin B Lipid Complex Liposomal Amphotericin B	Broad-spectrum agents SE: infusion related: fever, chills, hypotension Lipid formulations have ↓ infusion reactions and nephrotoxicity
Flucytosine: Inhibits macromolecular synthesis	Flucytosine	Recommended in combination with Amphotericin B SE: ↑ SCr, ↑ BUN

Abbreviations used: BUN, blood urea nitrogen; LFTs, liver function tests; SCr, serum creatinine; SE, side effect.

Table 7-4 First-Line Treatment for Common Fungi Infections[8]

PATHOGEN	TREATMENT
Aspergilloma	Surgery then Voriconazole
Aspergillosis	Voriconazole
Blastomycosis prophylaxis	Itraconazole
Blastomycosis treatment	Liposomal Amphotericin B + Itraconazole
Candidiasis	Fluconazole
Candida albicans	Oropharyngeal: Clotrimazole, nystatin
	Esophageal: Fluconazole
Candida glabrata or Candida krusei	Echinocandins or Amphotericin B
Coccidioidomycosis	Fluconazole
Cryptococcus prophylaxis	Fluconazole
Cryptococcus treatment	Amphotericin B + Flucytosine
Dermatophytes	Nail infections: itraconazole, terbinafine
Histoplasmosis prophylaxis	Itraconazole
Histoplasmosis treatment	Liposomal Amphotericin B + Itraconazole
Zygomycetes (Rhizopus, Mucor)	Amphotericin B ± posaconazole

infections works by inhibiting viruses or enhancing host defenses. Antivirals target various stages of viral replication. Table 7-5 summarizes the common viral infections and their treatment options.[10–12]

Human immunodeficiency virus

Human immunodeficiency virus (HIV) is a single-stranded RNA retrovirus that attacks CD4 T helper cells and causes a progressive decrease in CD4 T cell count.[13] HIV is transmitted through high-risk fluids such as blood, semen, amniotic fluid, and breast milk. Once CD4 count falls below 200 cells/mm³ the person becomes more susceptible to opportunistic infection and certain malignancies due to loss of cell-mediated immunity.[13] HIV can eventually lead to acquired immunodeficiency syndrome (AIDS; see Table 7-6).[13]

Anti-retroviral therapy

Anti-retroviral therapy (ART) targets stages of replication in the HIV life cycle (see Table 7-7) to maintain the immune system and reduce the

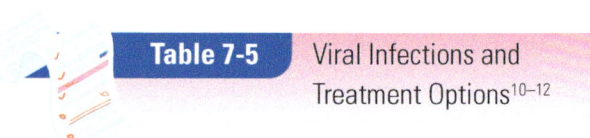

Table 7-5 Viral Infections and Treatment Options[10–12]

INFECTION	ANTIVIRAL
Influenza	Oseltamivir (oral)
	Peramivir (injection)
	Zanamivir (inhalation)
	Baloxavir marboxil (new, expensive)
Herpes simplex virus Varicella zoster virus	Acyclovir
	Famciclovir
	Valacyclovir
Herpes simplex labialis (cold sores)	Docosanol (OTC cream)
	Acyclovir
Cytomegalovirus	**First line:**
	Ganciclovir
	Valganciclovir
	Refractory:
	Cidofovir
	Foscarnet
Respiratory syncytial virus (RSV)	**Prophylaxis:** Palivizumab

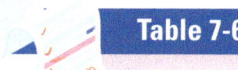

Table 7-6 HIV and AIDS Comparison[13]

HIV	AIDS
1. Positive HIV test	1. Positive HIV test
2. CD4 ≥200	2. CD4 <200
3. CD4 ≥14%	3. CD4 <14%
4. Absence of opportunistic illness	4. Diagnosis of opportunistic illness
5. Absence of AIDS–defining illness	5. Presence of an AIDS–defining illness

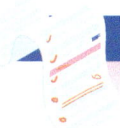

Table 7-7 HIV Replication Stages[13]

STAGE	HIV DRUG CLASS
Stage 1: Attachment HIV must attach to both CD4-receptor and co-receptors (CCR5/CXCR4)	CCR5 Antagonists
Stage 2: Fusion Fusion of the HIV envelope allows entry into the host cell ■ Uncoating ■ Release HIV-RNA into cytoplasm	Fusion inhibitors
Stage 3: Reverse transcriptase Single-stranded RNA converts to double-stranded DNA by reverse transcriptase	NRTIs and NNRTIs
Stage 4: Integration HIV DNA is transported into the nucleus and integrated into the host DNA	INSTIs
Stage 5: Transcription and translation HIV DNA is transcribed and translated into new HIV RNA and viral proteins	Not specified
Stage 6: Assembly New RNA and viral proteins migrate to host cell surface to form new immature HIV virus with protease enzyme	Not specified
Stage 7: Budding and maturation The newly formed HIV virus buds off from the cell to infect other CD4₊ cells	Protease inhibitors

progression of HIV.[13] Patients must have an adherence rate of 95% or higher for ART regimens to have long-term efficacy.

Initial valuation and monitoring[14]

- CD4 count—measured at baseline, every 3–6 months, and when clinical failure is suspected
  - Treatment goal is a normal CD4 count (800–1200)
- HIV viral load—measured at baseline, 2–8 weeks after ART initiation, and every 3–6 months
  - Treatment goal is an undetectable HIV viral load

Initial regimens

Triple therapy is recommended to reduce the incidence of opportunistic infections and improve survival. Preferred initial ART includes INSTI-based regimens with 2 NTRIs (see Table 7-8).[14]

ART is available as single agents (see Table 7-9), but combination products (see Table 7-10) increase adherence.[14]

Prophylaxis for HIV can be given in two forms—pre-exposure or post-exposure:[14]

- **Pre-exposure prophylaxis**
  - Emtricitabine + tenofovir DF (Truvada)—follow-up visit every 3 months

- Emtricitabine + tenofovir AF (Descovy), except those who have receptive vaginal sex → follow-up visit every 3 months
- **Occupational post-exposure prophylaxis**
  - Raltegravir + emtricitabine/tenofovir DF—given within 72 hours of exposure for duration of 4 weeks
- **Nonoccupational post-exposure prophylaxis**
  - Raltegravir OR dolutegravir + emtricitabine/tenofovir DF—given within 72 hours of exposure for duration of 28 days

Opportunistic infections

Opportunistic infections (OIs) occur when the immune system is unable to respond normally. OIs generally affect immunocompromised patients such as[15]

- HIV patients with CD4 T cells < 200 cells/mm^3
- Those with systemic steroid use for ≥14 days
- People with Asplenia
- Those taking immunosuppressant drugs (chemotherapy, transplant, autoimmune)

Patients with HIV are at risk for developing OIs. Chemoprophylaxis is recommended for the prevention of OIs in patients with HIV (see Table 7-11).[16]

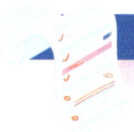

| **Table 7-8** | INSTI-Based Regimens[14] |

REGIMEN	BRAND NAME
Bictegravir/emtricitabine/tenofovir alafenamide fumarate (TAF)	Biktarvy
Dolutegravir/abacavir/lamivudine	Triumeq
Dolutegravir + lamivudine	Dovato
Dolutegravir + emtricitabine/tenofovir disoproxil fumarate (TDF)	Tivicay + Truvada
Dolutegravir + emtricitabine/tenofovir alafenamide fumarate	Tivicay + Descovy
Raltegravir + emtricitabine/tenofovir disoproxil fumarate	Isentress + Truvada
Raltegravir + emtricitabine/tenofovir alafenamide fumarate	Isentress + Descovy

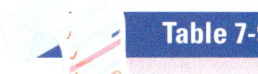

Table 7-9	Anti-Retroviral Therapy by Class[13]	

GENERIC NAME	BRAND NAME	COMMON ADVERSE EFFECT
INSTIs "tegravir"		**Class effect: Headache**
Bictegravir	—	HA
Dolutegravir	Tivicay	Increase SCr
Elvitegravir	—	HA, insomnia
Raltegravir	Isentress	Increase CPK, myopathy
NRTIs		**Class effect: Lactic acidosis**
Abacavir	Ziagen	Hypersensitivity
Didanosine	Videx	Pancreatitis, peripheral neuropathy
Emtricitabine	Emtriva	HA
Lamivudine	Epivir	HA
Stavudine	Zerit	Peripheral neuropathy, lipoatrophy
Tenofovir AF	Vemlidy	Increased lipids
Tenofovir DF	Viread	Renal toxicity, decrease bone mineral density
Zidovudine	Retrovir	Neutropenia, anemia, myopathy
NNRTIs "mid vir"		**Class effect: Rash**
Efavirenz	Sustiva	CNS effects
Etravirine	Intelence	Nausea
Nevirapine	Viramune	Hepatotoxicity, fatal rash
Rilpivirine	Edurant	Depression, insomnia
		Class effect: Metabolic abnormalities
PIs "navir"		Hyperlipidemia, hyperglycemia, lipohypertrophy
Atazanavir	Reyataz	Hyperbilirubinemia
Darunavir	Prezista	Hepatis, rash
Fosamprenavir	Lexiva	Rash
Indinavir	Crixivan	Nephrolithiasis
Lopinavir/ritonavir	Kaletra	Hyperlipidemia, GI intolerance
Nelfinavir	Viracept	Diarrhea
Saquinavir	Invirase	QT prolongation
Tipranavir	Aptivus	Intracranial hemorrhage, hepatotoxicity
Boosters		
Cobicistat	Tybost	
Ritonavir	Norvir	GI intolerance
Fusion inhibitor		
Enfuvirtide	Fuzeon	Injection site reaction
CCR-5 antagonist		
Maraviroc	Selzentry	Hepatitis, allergic reaction
CD4 Post-attachment inhibitor		
Ibalixumab-uiyk	Trogarzo	Diarrhea, nausea, rash

Abbreviations used: CNS, central nervous system; HA, headache; SCr, serum creatinine.
Adapted from Anderson PL, Yager J, Fletcher CV. Human immunodeficiency virus infection. In: DiPiro JT, Yee GC, Posey LM, Haines ST, Nolin TD, Ellingrod V, eds. *Pharmacotherapy: A Pathophysiologic Approach*. 11th ed. New York, NY: McGraw-Hill; 2020.

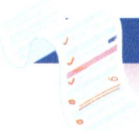

Table 7-10   HIV Combination Products[14]

GENERIC	BRAND
INSTI-BASED	
Bictegravir + emtricitabine + tenofovir AF	Biktarvy
Dolutegravir + abacavir + lamivudine	Triumeq
Dolutegravir + rilpivirine	Juluca
Dolutegravir + lamivudine	Dovato
Elvitegravir + cobicistat + emtricitabine + tenofovir AF	Genvoya
Elvitegravir + cobicistat + emtricitabine + tenofovir DF	Stribild
NRTI-BASED	
Abacavir + lamivudine	Epzicom
Abacavir + lamivudine + zidovudine	Trizivir
Emtricitabine + tenofovir AF	Descovy
Emtricitabine + tenofovir DF	Truvada
Lamivudine + zidovudine	Combivir
Lamivudine + tenofovir DF	Cimduo
NNRTI-BASED	
Efavirenz + emtricitabine + tenofovir DF	Atripla
Efavirenz + lamivudine + tenofovir DF	Symfi
Efavirenz + lamivudine + tenofovir DF	Symfi Lo
Rilpivirine + emtricitabine + tenofovir AF	Odefsey
Rilpivirine + emtricitabine + tenofovir DF	Complera
PI-BASED	
Atazanavir + cobicistat	Evotaz
Darunavir + cobicistat + emtricitabine + tenofovir AF	Symtuza
Darunavir + cobicistat	Prezcobix

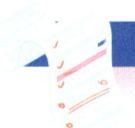

Table 7-11   Primary Prophylaxis of Opportunistic Infections in Patients with HIV[16]

INFECTION	PREFERRED DRUG	INDICATION FOR DISCONTINUATION
Pneumocystis jirovecii	Sulfamethoxazole/Trimethoprim DS daily	CD4 count ≥200 cells/mm³ for ≥3 mo on ART
Histoplasma capsulatum	Itraconazole 200 mg daily	CD4 count ≥150 cells/mm³ and undetectable HIV viral load for 6 mo and patients on ART
Toxoplasma gondii	Sulfamethoxazole/Trimethoprim DS daily	CD4 count ≥200 cells/mm³ for ≥ 3 mo on ART
Mycobacterium avium complex	Azithromycin 1200 mg weekly or Clarithromycin 500 mg BID	Initiation of ART

Abbreviations used: ART, antiretroviral therapy; BID, twice daily.

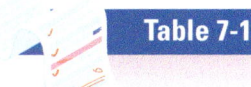

Table 7-12 Common Opportunistic Infections[13,15]

INFECTION	PREFERRED DRUG
FUNGI	
Candidiasis	Fluconazole for 7–14 d
Cryptococcal meningitis	Lipid Amphotericin B + Flucytosine for 14 d followed by fluconazole for 8 w
Coccidioidomycosis	Liposomal amphotericin B for 14 d
Histoplasmosis	Liposomal amphotericin B for 14 d, then Itraconazole for 12 mo
Pneumocystis jirovecii	Sulfamethoxazole/Trimethoprim for 21 d
PROTOZOA	
Toxoplasma gondii	Pyrimethamine daily + Sulfadiazine QID + Leucovorin daily for 6 w
BACTERIA	
Campylobacter enterocolitis	Ciprofloxacin BID for 7–10 d
Mycobacterium avium complex	Clarithromycin BID + ethambutol daily for 12 mo
Salmonella enterocolitis	Ciprofloxacin BID for 14 d
VIRUS	
Cytomegalovirus	Ganciclovir BID for 21–42 d, then switch to valganciclovir BID
Herpes simplex	Acyclovir Q8H until lesions regress

Abbreviations used: BID, twice daily; Q8H, every 8 h; QID, four times a day.
Adapted from Anderson PL, Yager J, Fletcher CV. Human immunodeficiency virus infection. In: DiPiro JT, Yee GC, Posey LM, Haines ST, Nolin TD, Ellingrod V, eds. *Pharmacotherapy: A Pathophysiologic Approach.* 11th ed. New York, NY: McGraw-Hill; 2020.

Table 7-12 outlines preferred treatment for common OIs in immunocompromised patients.[13,15]

ADDITIONAL RESOURCES

Infectious Disease Society of America. Guidelines. https://www.idsociety.org/practice-guideline/alphabetical-guidelines/.

Health and Human Services. Guidelines for the Use of Antiretroviral Agents in Adult and Adolescents with HIV. https://aidsinfo.nih.gov/guidelines/brief-html/1/adult-and-adolescent-arv/11/what-to-start--initial-combination-regimens-for-the-antiretroviral-naive-patient.

Health and Human Services. Adult and Adolescent Opportunistic Infection. https://aidsinfo.nih.gov/guidelines/brief-html/4/adult-and-adolescent-opportunistic-infection/318/introduction.

REFERENCES

1. Werth BJ, Barber KE, Smith JR, Rybak MJ. Laboratory tests to direct antimicrobial pharmacotherapy. In: DiPiro JT, Yee GC, Posey LM, Haines ST, Nolin TD, Ellingrod V, eds. *Pharmacotherapy: A Pathophysiologic Approach.* 11th ed. New York, NY: McGraw-Hill; 2020.

2. Beauduy CE, Winston LG. Tetracyclines, macrolides, clindamycin, chloramphenicol, streptogramins, & oxazolidinones. In: Katzung BG, ed. *Basic & Clinical Pharmacology.* 14th ed. New York, NY: McGraw-Hill; 2017.

3. Beauduy CE, Winston LG. Aminoglycosides & spectinomycin. In: Katzung BG, ed. *Basic & Clinical Pharmacology.* 14th ed. New York, NY: McGraw-Hill; 2017.

4. Beauduy CE, Winston LG. Sulfonamides, trimethoprim, & quinolones. In: Katzung BG, ed. *Basic & Clinical Pharmacology.* 14th ed. New York, NY: McGraw-Hill; 2017.

5. Beauduy CE, Winston LG. Beta-lactam and other cell wall and membrane-active antibiotics. In: Katzung BG, ed. *Basic & Clinical Pharmacology.* 14th ed. New York, NY: McGraw-Hill; 2017.

6. Lee GC, Burgess DS. Antimicrobial Regimen Selection. In: DiPiro JT, Yee GC, Posey LM, Haines ST, Nolin TD, Ellingrod V, eds. *Pharmacotherapy: A Pathophysiologic Approach.* 11th ed. New York, NY: McGraw-Hill; 2020.

7. Infectious Disease Society of America. Guidelines. Available at: https://www.idsociety.org/practice-guideline/alphabetical-guidelines/. Accessed June 22, 2020.

8. Carver PL. Invasive fungal infections. In: DiPiro JT, Yee GC, Posey LM, Haines ST, Nolin TD, Ellingrod V, eds. *Pharmacotherapy: A Pathophysiologic Approach.* 11th ed. New York, NY: McGraw-Hill; 2020.

9. Samji T. Influenza A: understanding the viral life cycle. *Yale J Biol Med.* 2009;82(4):153–159.

10. Centers for Disease Control and Prevention. Influenza antiviral medications: summary for clinicians. Available at: https://www.cdc.gov/flu/professionals/antivirals/summary-clinicians.htm. Updated June 17, 2020. Accessed June 22, 2020.

11. Tan BH. Cytomegalovirus treatment. *Curr Treat Options Infect Dis.* 2014;6(3):256–270.

12. World Health Organization. Treatment for genital herpes simplex virus. Available at: https://apps.who.int/iris/bitstream/handle/10665/250693/9789241549875-eng.pdf?sequence=11. Accessed June 22, 2020.

13. Anderson PL, Yager J, Fletcher CV. Human immunodeficiency virus infection. In: DiPiro JT, Yee GC, Posey LM, Haines ST, Nolin TD, Ellingrod V, eds. *Pharmacotherapy: A Pathophysiologic Approach.* 11th ed. New York, NY: McGraw-Hill; 2020.

14. Health and Human Services. Guidelines for the use of antiretroviral agents in adults and adolescents living with HIV. https://aidsinfo.nih.gov/guidelines/brief-html/1/adult-and-adolescent-arv/11/what-to-start--initial-combination-regimens-for-the-antiretroviral-naive-patient. Accessed June 21, 2020.

15. Mueller SW, Fish DN. Infections in immunocompromised patients. In: DiPiro JT, Yee GC, Posey LM, Haines ST, Nolin TD, Ellingrod V, eds. *Pharmacotherapy: A Pathophysiologic Approach.* 11th ed. New York, NY: McGraw-Hill; 2020.

16. Health and Human Services. Guidelines for the prevention and treatment of opportunistic infections in adults and adolescents with HIV. Available at: https://clinicalinfo.hiv.gov/en/guidelines/adult-and-adolescent-opportunistic-infection/introduction?view=brief. Accessed June 22, 2020.

CHAPTER 8

Renal and Hepatic Disease

With medical writing support provided by
Banner Medical LLC Writer: Miriam Opara

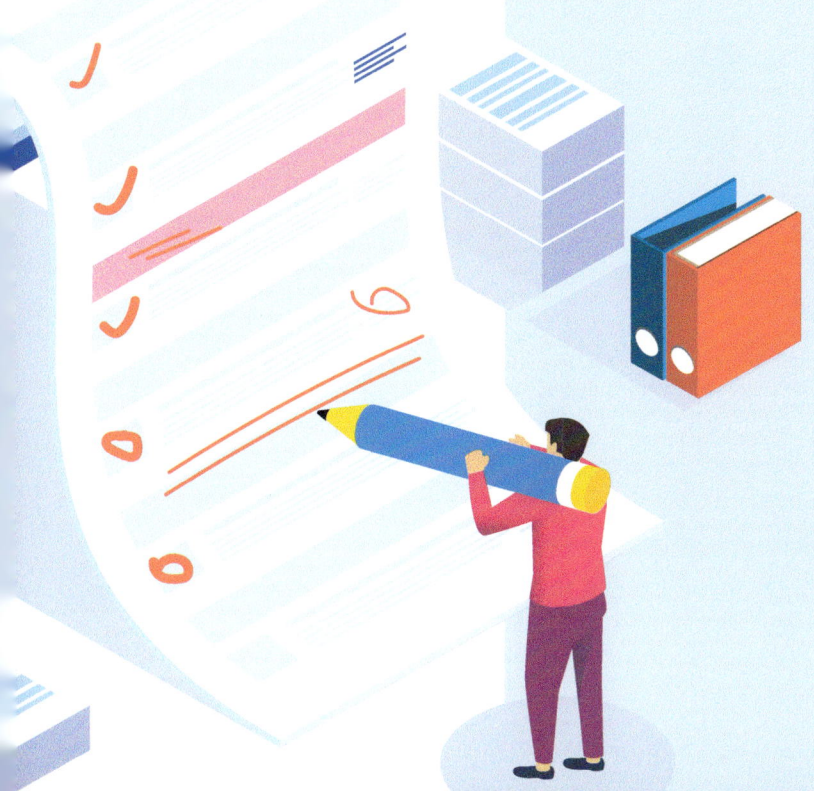

Renal disease

Renal function is essential for the regulation of blood volume and blood pressure.[1] The nephron is the functional unit of the kidney and its anatomy is outlined in Figure 8-1.[1]

- Albumin in the urine = damaged glomerulus
  - Glomerular filtration rate (GFR) is used to assess the severity of the damage[1]

- Remember the Cockcroft-Gault equation (see Table 8-1): the main equation used by pharmacists to estimate kidney function (creatinine clearance) when dosing medication[1]

Chronic kidney disease (CKD) is structural or functional damage of the kidney for ≥3 months.[2]

- KDIGO and KDOQI guidelines recommend evaluating the GFR, albuminuria, and cause of CKD to determine stage of renal failure.[2]

Figure 8-1	Anatomy of the Nephron

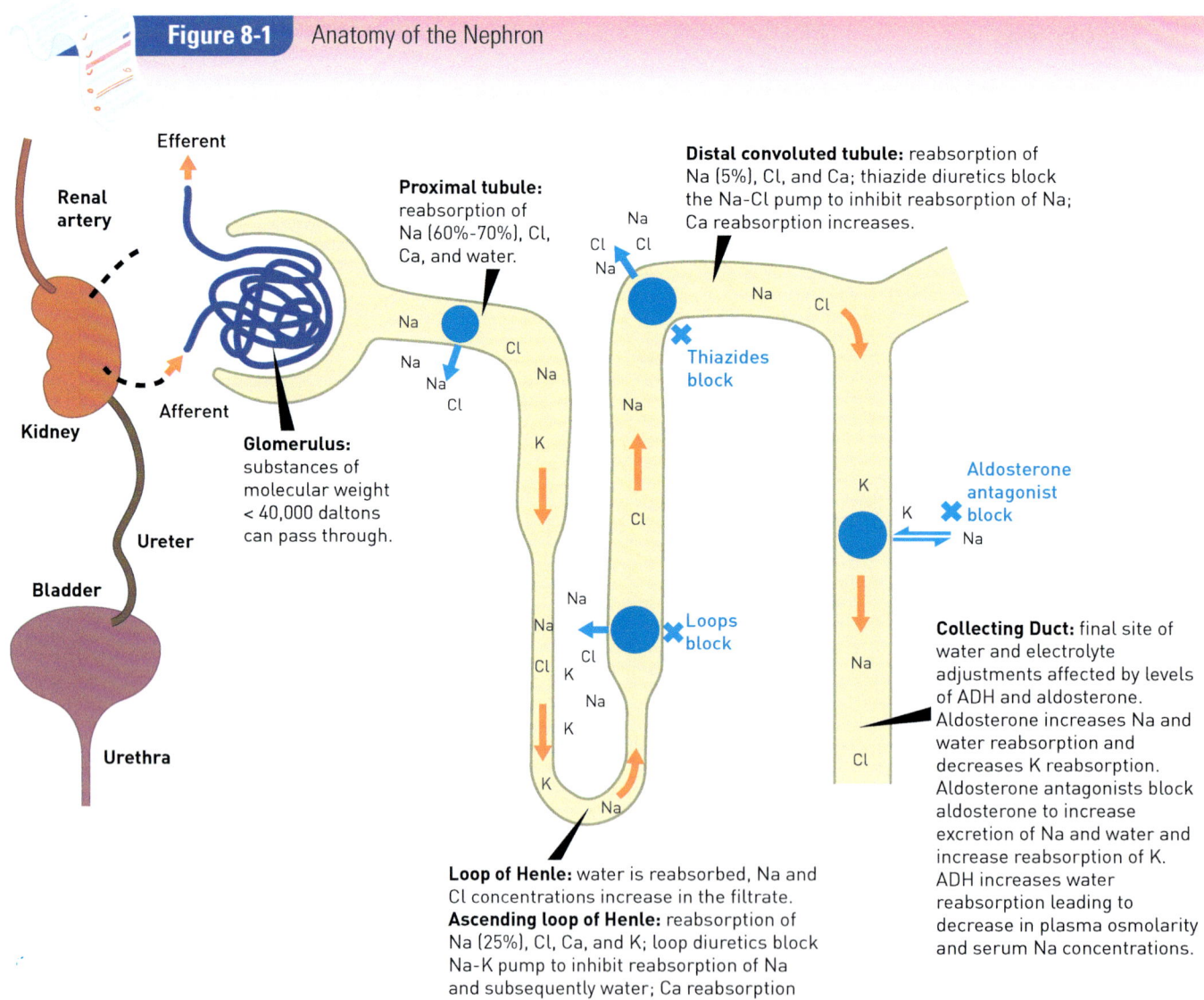

Proximal tubule: reabsorption of Na (60%-70%), Cl, Ca, and water.

Glomerulus: substances of molecular weight < 40,000 daltons can pass through.

Distal convoluted tubule: reabsorption of Na (5%), Cl, and Ca; thiazide diuretics block the Na-Cl pump to inhibit reabsorption of Na; Ca reabsorption increases.

Thiazides block

Aldosterone antagonist block

Loops block

Collecting Duct: final site of water and electrolyte adjustments affected by levels of ADH and aldosterone. Aldosterone increases Na and water reabsorption and decreases K reabsorption. Aldosterone antagonists block aldosterone to increase excretion of Na and water and increase reabsorption of K. ADH increases water reabsorption leading to decrease in plasma osmolarity and serum Na concentrations.

Loop of Henle: water is reabsorbed, Na and Cl concentrations increase in the filtrate.
Ascending loop of Henle: reabsorption of Na (25%), Cl, Ca, and K; loop diuretics block Na-K pump to inhibit reabsorption of Na and subsequently water; Ca reabsorption decreases.

Source: Adapted from Dowling TC. Evaluation of kidney function. In: DiPiro JT, Talbert RL, Yee GC, Matzke GR, Wells BG, Posey LM, eds. *Pharmacotherapy: A Pathophysiologic Approach*. 10th ed. New York, NY: McGraw-Hill; 2017.
Abbreviations used: ADH, antidiuretic hormone.

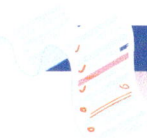

Table 8-1	Determining Kidney Function[1]

EQUATIONS	REMEMBER

COCKCROFT-GAULT CREATININE CLEARANCE

$$CrCl\left(\frac{mL}{min}\right) = \frac{140 - (patient\ age)}{72 \times SCr} \times weight\ (kg) \times 0.85\ (female)$$

- CrCl: ~120 mL/min
- BUN/SCr ↑ as renal function ↓
- Normal BUN 6–20 mg/dL
- Normal SCr 0.6–1.3 mg/dL
- Use AjBW when actual BW >30% IBW

or 201.?

IDEAL BODY WEIGHT

$$Male = 50\ kg + 2.3\ (inches\ over\ 5\ ft\ tall)$$

$$Female = 45.5\ kg + 2.3\ (inches\ over\ 5\ ft\ tall)$$

ADJUSTED BODY WEIGHT

$$AdjBW = [0.4 \times (Actual\ BW - IBW)] + IBW$$

Abbreviatons used: AjBW, adjusted body weight; BUN, blood urea nitrogen; BW, body weight; CrCl, creatinine clearance; IBW, ideal body weight; SCr, serum creatinine.

- **Remember:** GFR <60 mL/min/1.73m² and/or albuminuria (albumin to creatinine ratio ≥30 mg/g or albumin excretion rate ≥30 mg/24h) = CKD → treatment is necessary to prevent progression
- See Table 8-2 for target goals of CKD treatment.[2,3]
- **Remember:** first-line treatment to prevent the progression of CKD, diabetes, and HTN in the presence of albuminuria are angiotensin-converting enzyme (ACE) inhibitors or angiotensin receptor blockers (ARBs).[2] (See Ch. 10 for more information.)
- Consider the use of sodium-glucose cotransporter-2 inhibitors, canagliflozin, empagliflozin, or dapagliflozin in patients with diabetes and albuminuria >300mg/dL. (See Ch. 13 for more information.)

SGLT-2 inhibitors

Complications with CKD

Decreasing renal function inhibits regulatory functions of the kidney (see Figure 8-2). Common complications include:

- ↓ excretion of phosphate (PO₄) → no active 1,25-dihydroxy vitamin D
- ↓ active vitamin D → ↓ calcium (Ca⁺⁺) absorption in the gut
- ↓ erythropoietin production → anemia

activated by the kidneys Supplements must be in active form ↓ Calcitriol

*EPO

Mineral and bone disorder in CKD manifests with bone pain and skeletal fractures.[4] **Hyperphospha-temia** increases risk of mortality/vascular calcification.

Table 8-2	Goals for Managing Chronic Kidney Disease[2,3]

MEASURE	TARGET GOALS
Blood pressure	BP <130/80 mmHg
Glycemic control	A1C <7%
Sodium intake	Na⁺⁺ <2 g/d
Lifestyle	Physical activity: 30 m 5x week
	BMI: 20–25
	Smoking cessation

Abbreviations used: BP, blood pressure; BMI, body mass index; A1C, glycosylated hemoglobin; Na⁺⁺, sodium.

(Vitamin D analog) Zemplar for ↑ parathyroid gland (PTH level)

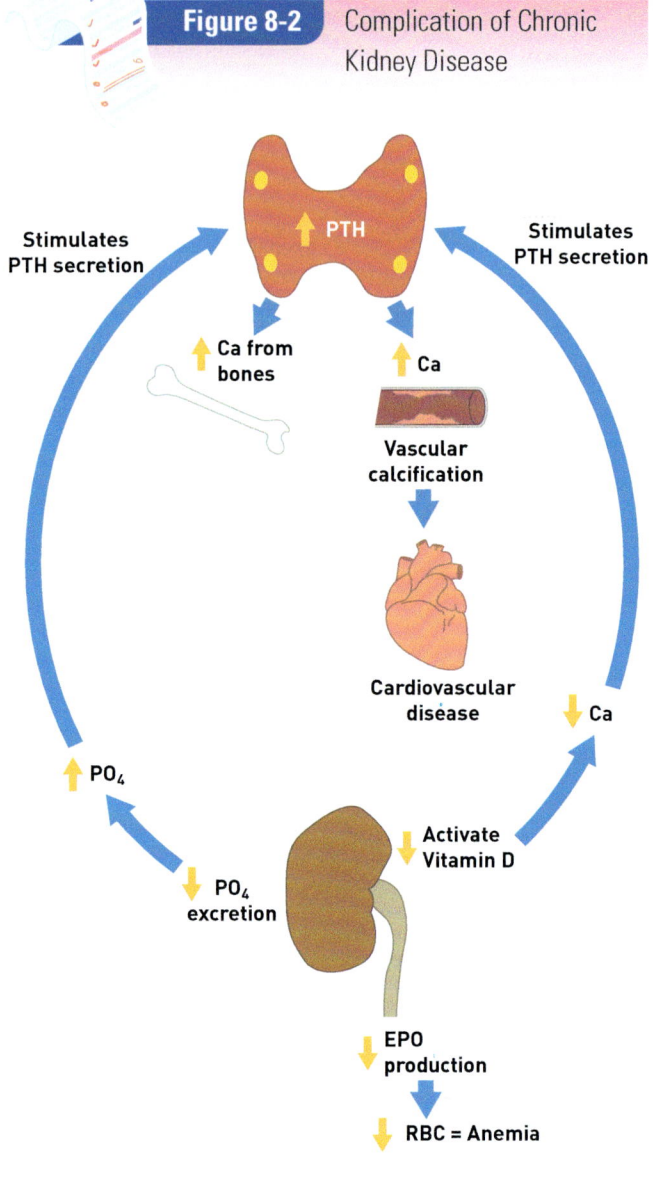

Figure 8-2 Complication of Chronic Kidney Disease

Stimulates PTH secretion

↑ PTH

Stimulates PTH secretion

↑ Ca from bones

↑ Ca

Vascular calcification

Cardiovascular disease

↓ Ca

↑ PO₄

↓ PO₄ excretion

Activate Vitamin D

↓ EPO production

↓ RBC = Anemia

Source: Adapted from Hudson JQ, Wazny LD. Chronic Kidney Disease. In: DiPiro JT, Talbert RL, Yee GC, Matzke GR, Wells BG, Posey LM, eds. *Pharmacotherapy: A Pathophysiologic Approach.* 10th ed. New York, NY: McGraw-Hill, 2017; Vangala C, Pan J, Cotton RT, Ramanathan V. Mineral and bone disorders after kidney transplantation. *Front Med (Lausanne).* 2018;5:211.

Phosphate binders (see Table 8-3) block the absorption of dietary phosphate.[4]

Remember the following:[3]

- ↓ serum concentrations of Ca^{++}/and ↑ PO_4 stimulate secretion of parathyroid hormone (PTH)
- PTH stimulates calcium absorption

- Increase frequency of monitoring Ca, PO_4, and PTH levels as kidney function declines
  - CKD stage 3 → monitor every 6–12 months
  - CKD stage 4 → monitor every 3–6 months
  - CKD stage 5 and end-stage renal disease → monitor every 1–3 months
- Chronic secretion of PTH draws calcium from the bones (↑ fractures) and deposits calcifications in the vasculature (↑ CVD)

Remember for all phosphate binders:

- Given 3 times a day with meals
- Side effects: constipation, diarrhea, nausea, vomiting, abdominal pain
- Separate administration from levothyroxine, quinolones, and tetracyclines by 1–2 hours before or 4–6 hours after

Vitamin D deficiency and secondary hyperparathyroidism must be addressed to decrease risk of CKD progression (see Table 8-4).[4]

- Vitamin D analogs: ↑ Ca^{++} absorption (gut), ↑ serum Ca^{++}, ↓ PTH secretion
- Calcimimetics: ↓ PTH, Ca^{++}, and PO_4

Anemia in CKD

- Low erythropoietin ↓ red blood cells → CKD associated anemia
- **Remember:** first-line treatment is IV iron (hemodialysis) and oral iron (non-hemodialysis)[3,4]
- Erythropoiesis-stimulating agents (ESA) → hemoglobin (Hgb) <10 g/dL[5]
  - Decrease or discontinue ESA → Hgb ≥11 g/dL (increased risk of death, serious cardiovascular events, and stroke)

Consult Ch. 11 for more information on iron therapy and ESA.

Hyperkalemia in CKD

- K^+ > 5 mEq/L
- ↓ renal function = impaired potassium (K^+) excretion = hyperkalemia

Table 8-3	Phosphate Binders for Treatment of Hyperphosphatemia in Adults[4]

BINDER	NOTES
Aluminum based* Aluminum hydroxide (AlternaGel) 300–600 mg TID with meals	**SE:** Constipation, hypophosphatemia **Remember:** Not first-line therapy, risk of aluminum toxicity, treatment duration limited to 4 w
Calcium based* Calcium acetate (PhosLo) 3–4 caps/tabs TID with meals Calcium carbonate (Tums) Maximum 2 g/day**	**SE:** Hypercalcemia, constipation, nausea **Remember:** Monitor Ca^{++} levels when given with vitamin D
Aluminum free, calcium free* Ferric citrate (Auryxia) 2 tabs TID (maximum 12 tabs/d) Sucroferric oxyhydroxide (Velphoro) 1 tab TID with meals (usual 3–4/d)	**SE:** N/V/D, constipation, black feces (with iron)
Aluminum free, calcium-free sevelamer* Sevelamer carbonate (Renvela) 800–1600 mg TID with meals Sevelamer hydrochloride (Renagel) 800–1600 mg TID with meals	**CI:** Bowel obstruction **SE:** Metabolic acidosis, diarrhea, dyspepsia, nausea **Remember:** Not systemically absorbed, ↓TC, LDL by 15%–30%

Abbreviations used: Ca^{++}, calcium; CI, contraindicated; LDL, low-density lipoproteins; N/V/D, nausea, vomiting, diarrhea; SE, side effects; TC, total cholesterol; TID, three times a day.
*All dosing is titrated based on individual patient serum PO_4 levels.
**total dose of elemental calcium (including dietary and calcium-based PO_4 binders).

- Medications used in CKD can also ↑ concentrations of K^+
  - Monitor more frequently (e.g., ACEI/ARBs, aldosterone antagonists[3])
- **Goals of therapy:** stabilize cardiac cellular membranes, shift extracellular potassium into cells, and eliminate potassium from the body[6]

Consult Ch. 20 for more information on treatment options for hyperkalemia.

End-stage renal disease requires dialysis or kidney transplant.[7] Avoidance or close monitoring of any drug that may further damage the kidneys is essential and requires an individualized approach. The following are some common offending agents (not all-inclusive):

- ACE inhibitors
- Aminoglycosides
- Diuretics
- Foscarnet
- Iodinated contrast dyes
- NSAIDs
- Vancomycin

There are two types of dialysis:

1. Hemodialysis (dialyzer machine)
2. Peritoneal dialysis (peritoneal membrane as a dialyzer)[8]

Medication considerations during dialysis:

- Multiple factors affect drug removal in dialysis (see Table 8-5)
- Medications and dosing/timing may need to be adjusted with dialysis[7,8]

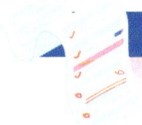

Table 8-4 Vitamin D Analogs and Calcimimetics[4]

DRUG/DOSE	NOTES
Vitamin D analogs*	**CI:** Hypercalcemia, vitamin D toxicity
Calcifediol (Rayaldee)	**SE:** Hypercalcemia, hyperphosphatemia, N/V/D
30–60 mcg daily	**Remember:** Take with food to decrease GI upset
Calcitriol (Rocaltrol)	▪ Doxercalciferol dosing for ESRD: 10 mcg TIW
0.25–0.5 mcg daily	▪ Paricalcitol dosing is based on PTH levels
Doxercalciferol (Hectorol)	
5–20 mcg daily	
Paricalcitol (Zemplar)	
1–4 mcg daily	
Calcimimetics*	
Cinacalcet (Sensipar)	**CI:** Hypocalcemia
30–180 mg daily	**Remember:** Take tablet by mouth whole daily with food
Etelcalcetide (Parsabiv)	**CI:** Hypocalcemia, worsening HF, GI bleeding
5–15 mg TIW	**Remember:** Only used in dialysis, administered IV 3x week, dosing based on PO_4, PTH, and corrected Ca^{++}

Abbreviations used: Ca^{++}, calcium; CI, contraindicated; ESRD, end-stage renal disease; GI, gastrointestinal; HF, heart failure; IV, intravenous, N/V/D, nausea, vomiting, diarrhea; PO_4, phosphorus; PTH, parathyroid hormone; SE, side effects; TIW, three times a week.
*All dosing is titrated based on individual patient needs.

Table 8-5 Factors Affecting Dialysis[8]

FACTOR	AFFECT
Dialysis membrane	large pore size and large surface area remove more substances
Dialysis blood flow rate	higher blood flow rates increase drug removal
Drug solute size	smaller molecules are easier to remove
Drug protein-binding	highly protein-bound drugs are less likely to be removed by dialysis

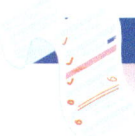

Table 8-6 Comparison of Viral Hepatitis[9]

Virus	Disease course	Transmission route	Vaccine	First-line treatment
Hepatitis A	Acute	Fecal/oral	Yes	Supportive
Hepatitis B	Acute or chronic	Blood or bodily fluids	Yes	PEG-INF or NRTI (tenofovir or entecavir)
Hepatitis C	Acute or chronic	Blood or bodily fluids	No	Treatment naïve: DAA combination

Abbreviations used: DAA, direct-acting antivirals; NRTI, nucleoside/tide reverse transcriptase inhibitors; PEG-INF, pegylated interferon.

Hepatic disease

Hepatitis is inflammation of the liver, most commonly caused by viral hepatitis A (HAV), hepatitis B (HBV), and hepatitis C (HCV) infection within the U.S. (see Table 8-6).[9]

HBV treatment

There are 8 HBV genotypes (A–H). **Remember:** first-line therapy includes interferons or nucleoside reverse transcriptase inhibitors (see Table 8-7).[10]

HCV treatment

There are 6 HCV genotypes (1–6) and treatment (see Table 8-8) is based on genotype, severity of liver damage, and comorbidities.[11]

Remember: preferred regimens for direct-acting antivirals (DAA) include 2–3 DAAs with different mechanisms of action (see Table 8-9).[11]

Cirrhosis is irreversible, progressive, fibrosis of the liver that impairs hepatic blood flow.[12]

- Management of complications is essential to decrease mortality and improve quality of life.

Table 8-7 First-Line Management of Viral Hepatitis B[10]

Treatment	Notes
Pegylated interferon alfa (PEG-INF-alfa) PEG-INF-alfa-2a (Pegasys) 180 mcg Sub-Q weekly for 48 w	**BBW:** Can cause neuropsychiatric, autoimmune, ischemic, or infectious disorders **Remember:** Monitor CBC, TSH
Nucleoside/tide reverse transcriptase inhibitors Entecavir (Baraclude) 0.5 mg daily for 48 w Tenofovir DF (Viread) 300 mg daily for 48 w Tenofovir AF (Vemlidy) 25 mg daily for 48 w	**BBW:** Lactic acidosis and severe hepatomegaly with steatosis **SE:** Headache, abdominal pain, renal impairment **Remember:** ■ Test for HIV prior to initiation for HBV

Abbreviations used: BBW, Black Box Warning; CBC, complete blood count; HBV, hepatitis B virus; HIV, human immunodeficiency virus; Sub-Q, subcutaneous; SE, side effects; TSH, thyroid-stimulating hormone.

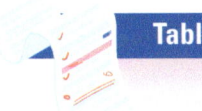

| Table 8-8 | Management of Hepatitis C in Treatment Naive Patients[11] |

GENOTYPE	TRADE NAME (GENERIC)	DURATION	NOTES
1–6	Epclusa* (sofosbuvir/velpatasvir)	12 w	**BBW:** Risk of reactivating HBV **Remember:**
1–6	Mavyret (glecaprevir/pibrentasvir)	8 w	■ DAAs ↑ statin concentrations and risk of myopathy ■ Separate from antacids by 4 h ■ Do not use amiodarone with sofosbuvir ■ Mavyret taken with food

Abbreviations used: BBW, black box warning; DAA, direct-acting antivirals; HBV, hepatitis B virus.
*Genotype 3 with compensated cirrhosis needs to test negative for NS5A RAS Y93H before initiating

■ Hepatic disease is evaluated with liver function tests (aspartate aminotransferase [AST], alanine aminotransferase, alkaline phosphatase, total bilirubin [TBL]), complete blood count with platelets, and prothrombin time test.[13]
  ● Hepatocellular injury → AST >3× upper limit of normal (UNL) and TBL >2× UNL
■ Treatment is dependent on the type of complication (see Table 8-10).

Hepatic disease may influence the pharmacokinetics of drug absorption, distribution, and clearance; dose and frequency adjustments may be necessary.[14] Monitoring or avoiding drugs that will further induce liver damage is essential. Common examples include the following (not all-inclusive):

■ Acarbose
■ Acetaminophen
■ Amiodarone
■ Augmentin
■ Carbamazepine
■ Cytotoxic drugs
■ Diclofenac
■ Fluoxetine
■ Furosemide
■ Isoniazid
■ Methotrexate
■ Losartan
■ Tetracycline

Pharmacodynamic changes may ↑ sensitivity of certain drugs such as opiates, benzodiazepines, and NSAIDs.

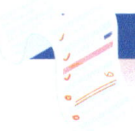

| Table 8-9 | Direct-Acting Antivirals' Mechanism of Action[11] |

MECHANISM	ENDING SUFFIX	EXAMPLES
NS3/4A Protease inhibitor	-previr	Gleca*previr* Voxila*previr*
NS5A Replication complex inhibitor	-asvir	Pibrent*asvir* Velpat*asvir*
NS5B Polymerase inhibitor	-buvir	Dasa*buvir* Sofos*buvir*

Table 8-10 | Cirrhosis Complications

Portal hypertension is increased blood pressure in the portal vein as a result of hepatic fibrosis impeding the blood flow. Portal hypertension backs up the blood flow into smaller blood vessels, leading to **esophageal varices**. If the blood flow is too much, variceal bleeding occurs and can be fatal.[16,17]

Treatment for variceal bleeding:

- Octreotide infusion

Prophylaxis for variceal bleeding recurrence:

- Nadalol

Hepatic encephalopathy is characterized by impaired mental status and decreased levels of consciousness due to the accumulation of ammonia. The goal of treatment for hepatic encephalopathy is to decrease blood ammonia levels or excreting ammonia buildup.[18]

Treatment:

- Protein restriction
- Lactulose: ↓ ammonia and ammonia precursors in from intestine
  - Side effects: flatulence, diarrhea, dyspepsia, dehydration, electrolyte imbalance

Ascites is the accumulation of fluid in the peritoneal space that can lead to spontaneous bacterial peritonitis, shortness of breath, and respiratory failure.[12]

Treatment:

- Dietary salt restriction (<2000 mg/d)
- Fluid restriction
- Furosemide (40–160 mg/d) + spironolactone (100–400 mg/d)

Drug-induced liver disease results from a hepatotoxic drug that elevates liver function tests 3 times the upper limit of normal.[19]

Treatment:

- Stop offending agent
- Re-challenge can be considered
- Antidote if necessary

Alcohol-induced liver disease results from increased duration, frequency, and amount of alcohol consumption. Chronic alcohol consumption can lead to hepatitis and cirrhosis.

Treatment:

- Alcohol cessation

Withdrawal treatment:

- Thiamine and benzodiazepines or anticonvulsants

Relapse prevention:

- Naltrexone, Acamprosate or disulfiram

ADDITIONAL RESOURCES

Kidney Disease Improving Global Outcomes. KDIGO 2012 Clinical Practice Guideline for the Evaluation and Management of Chronic Kidney Disease. *International Society of Nephrology.* 2013;3(1).

Kidney Disease Improving Global Outcomes. KDIGO 2017 Clinical Practice Guideline Update for the Diagnosis, Evaluation, Prevention, and Treatment of Chronic Kidney Disease–Mineral and Bone Disorder (CKD-MBD). *International Society of Nephrology.* 2017;7(1):1–59.

Infectious Diseases Society of America. HCV guidance: recommendations for testing, managing, and treating hepatitis C. Available at: https://www.hcvguidelines.org/.

Simonetto DA, Singal AK, Garcia-Tsao G, Caldwell SH, Ahn J, Kamath PS. ACG clinical guideline: disorders of the hepatic and mesenteric circulation. *Am J Gastroenterology.* 2020;115(1):18–40.

REFERENCES

1. Dowling TC. Evaluation of Kidney Function. In: DiPiro JT, Talbert RL, Yee GC, Matzke GR, Wells BG, Posey LM, eds. *Pharmacotherapy: A Pathophysiologic Approach, 10e.* New York, NY: McGraw-Hill Education; 2017.

2. Kidney Disease Improving Global Outcomes. KDIGO 2012 Clinical Practice Guideline for the Evaluation and Management of Chronic Kidney Disease. *International Society of Nephrology.* 2013;3(1).

3. Hudson JQ, Wazny LD. Chronic Kidney Disease. In: DiPiro JT, Talbert RL, Yee GC, Matzke GR, Wells BG, Posey LM, eds. *Pharmacotherapy: A Pathophysiologic Approach, 10e.* New York, NY: McGraw-Hill Education; 2017.

4. Kidney Disease Improving Global Outcomes. KDIGO 2017 Clinical Practice Guideline Update for the Diagnosis, Evaluation, Prevention, and Treatment of Chronic Kidney Disease–Mineral and Bone Disorder (CKD-MBD). *International Society of Nephrology.* 2017;7(1):1–59.

5. Kidney Disease Improving Global Outcomes. KDIGO Clinical Practice Guideline for Anemia in Chronic Kidney Disease. *International Society of Nephrology.* 2012;2(4).

6. Hunter RW, Bailey MA. Hyperkalemia: pathophysiology, risk factors and consequences. *Nephrology Dialysis Transplantation.* 2019;34:iii2–iii11.

7. Foundation NK. KDOQI Clinical Practice Guideline for Hemodialysis Adequacy: 2015 update. *Am J Kidney Dis.* 2015; 66(5):884–930.

8. Sowinski KM, Churchwell MD, Decker BS. Hemodialysis and Peritoneal Dialysis. In: DiPiro JT, Talbert RL, Yee GC, Matzke GR, Wells BG, Posey LM, eds. *Pharmacotherapy: A Pathophysiologic Approach, 10e.* New York, NY: McGraw-Hill Education; 2017.

9. Daniels D, Grytdal S, Wasley A, (CDC) CfDCaP. Surveillance for acute viral hepatitis - United States, 2007. *MMWR Surveill Summ.* 2009;58(3):1–27.

10. Terrault NA, Lok ASF, McMahon BJ, et al. Update on Prevention, Diagnosis, and Treatment of Chronic Hepatitis B: AASLD 2018 Hepatitis B Guidance. *Clin Liver Dis (Hoboken).* 2018;12(1):33–34.

11. Panel A-IHG. Hepatitis C Guidance 2018 Update: AASLD-IDSA Recommendations for Testing, Managing, and Treating Hepatitis C Virus Infection. *Clin Infect Dis.* 2018;67(10):1477–1492.

12. Runyon BA. Management of Adult Patients with Ascites Due to Cirrhosis: Update 2012. In: American Association for the Study of Liver Disease 2012.

13. Smith A, Baumgartner K, Bositis C. Cirrhosis: Diagnosis and Management. *Am Fam Physician.* 2019;100:759–770.

14. Kirchain W, Allen RE. Drug-Induced Liver Disease. In: DiPiro JT, Yee GC, Posey LM, Haines ST, Nolin TD, Ellingrod V, eds. *Pharmacotherapy: A Pathophysiologic Approach, 11e.* New York, NY: McGraw-Hill Education; 2020.

15. Vangala C, Pan J, Cotton RT, Ramanathan V. Mineral and Bone Disorders After Kidney Transplantation. *Front Med (Lausanne).* 2018;5:211.

16. Garcia-Tsao G, Abraldes JG, Berzigotti A, Bosch J. Portal hypertensive bleeding in cirrhosis: Risk stratification, diagnosis, and management: 2016 practice guidance by the American Association for the study of liver diseases. *Hepatology.* 2017;65(1):310–335.

17. Sease JM, Clements JN. Portal Hypertension and Cirrhosis. In: DiPiro JT, Talbert RL, Yee GC, Matzke GR, Wells BG, Posey LM, eds. *Pharmacotherapy: A Pathophysiologic Approach, 10e.* New York, NY: McGraw-Hill Education; 2017.

18. Vilstrup H, Amodio P, Bajaj J, et al. Hepatic encephalopathy in chronic liver disease: 2014 Practice Guideline by the American Association for the Study Of Liver Diseases and the European Association for the Study of the Liver. *Hepatology.* 2014;60(2): 715–735.

19. Kirchain WR, Allen RE. Drug-Induced Liver Disease. In: DiPiro JT, Talbert RL, Yee GC, Matzke GR, Wells BG, Posey LM, eds. *Pharmacotherapy: A Pathophysiologic Approach, 10e.* New York, NY: McGraw-Hill Education; 2017.

20. Crabb DW, Im GY, Szabo G, Mellinger JL, Lucey MR. Diagnosis and Treatment of Alcohol-Associated Liver Diseases: 2019 Practice Guidance From the American Association for the Study of Liver Diseases. *Hepatology.* 2020;71(1):306–333.

CHAPTER 9

Eyes, Ears, Nose, and Skin

With medical writing support provided by
Banner Medical LLC Writer: Miriam Opara

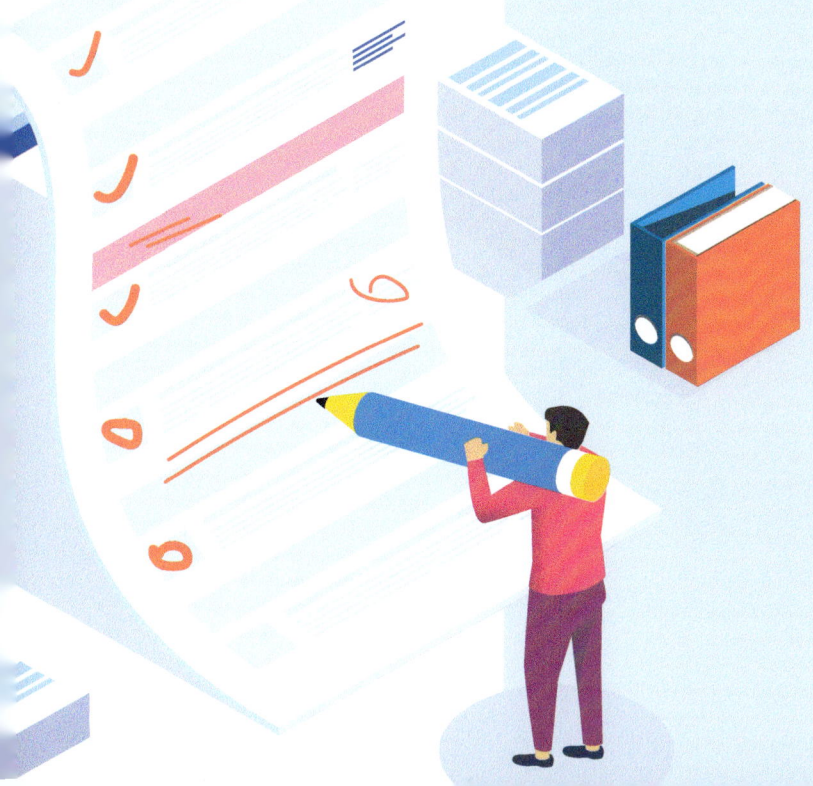

Allergic rhinitis and common cold

Allergic rhinitis is caused by exposure to allergens (e.g., pollen, molds, dust, pet dander).[1,2] The common cold is caused by upper respiratory viral infection.[1,2] Symptomatology frequently overlaps (see Table 9-1).[1,2]

Treatment for allergic rhinitis is based on the severity and frequency of symptoms.[1]

- Intranasal steroids (e.g., fluticasone, budesonide, triamcinolone) are first line for moderate to severe symptoms.
- Oral antihistamines (e.g., levocetirizine, fexofenadine, loratadine, cetirizine) are used for patients complaining of sneezing and itching.
- Intranasal antihistamines (e.g., olopatadine, azelastine) may also be considered and have the advantage of quick onset of action (15–30 minutes).

Treatment for cough and cold is based on the presentation of symptoms.[2,3] The goal of treatment is to decrease the frequency/duration of symptoms affecting quality of life. Table 9-2 lists the common treatment options for cough and cold symptoms.

Common eye and ear conditions

Glaucoma is a disease of the eye that results in damage to the optic nerve and loss of the visual field.[5] Glaucoma causes intraocular pressure (IOP)

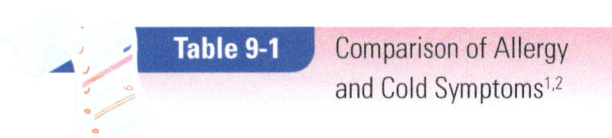

Table 9-1   Comparison of Allergy and Cold Symptoms[1,2]

Allergy	Cold
Sneezing	Sneezing
Runny nose	Runny nose
Thin, clear mucus	Thick, dark mucus
Wheezing	Sore throat
Red, watery eyes	Coughing
Symptoms can last for days or months after contact with an allergen	Symptoms can last 7–10 d (referral for symptoms >10 d)

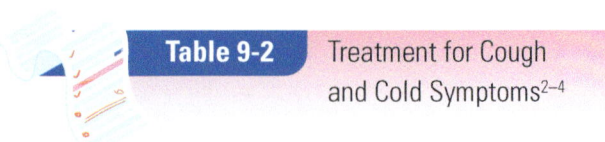

Table 9-2   Treatment for Cough and Cold Symptoms[2-4]

Treatment	Notes
DECONGESTANTS	
Systemic oral Phenylephrine Pseudoephedrine **Intranasal** Naphazoline Oxymetazoline Phenylephrine Tetrahydrozoline	**CI:** MAO inhibitors within 14 days **Side effects:** increased BP, palpitations, insomnia, anxiety, dizziness **Remember:** - Do not use oxymetazoline for longer than 3 days; can cause rebound congestion. - Use with caution in patients with CV disease, uncontrolled HTN, glaucoma, BPH, and thyroid disease. - Combat Methamphetamine Epidemic Act
EXPECTORANTS	
Guaifenesin	**Maximum dose:** 2.4 g/d
COUGH SUPPRESSANTS	
Dextromethorphan Benzonatate	**CI:** dextromethorphan with MAO inhibitors within 14 days; children <10 years old **Remember:** Dextromethorphan increases serotonin syndrome risk.
COMBINATION PRODUCTS	
Brompheniramine/ PSE/DM Chlorpheniramine/ hydrocodone DM/promethazine Guaifenesin/ codeine Guaifenesin/ codeine/PSE Promethazine/ codeine Promethazine/PE/ codeine	If product ends with - **DM:** contains dextromethorphan - **D:** decongestant - **AC:** contains codeine - **PE:** contains phenylephrine

Abbreviations used: BP, blood pressure; BPH, benign prostatic hyperplasia; CI, contraindicated; CV, cardiovascular; DM, dextromethorphan; HTN, hypertension; MAO, monoamine oxidase; PE, phenylephrine; PSE, pseudoephedrine.

>12–22 mm Hg. Treatment of open-angle glaucoma decreases intraocular pressure by targeting the aqueous humor (see Table 9-3[5]), whereas closed-angle glaucoma may be a medical emergency and may require surgery.

Conjunctivitis is caused by a virus, bacteria, allergen, or ocular irritants (such as a chemical or contact lenses). Symptoms include swelling, itching, burning, and redness. Table 9-4 describes the treatment options for conjunctivitis based on the etiology and symptomatology.[6]

Ear conditions include pain from outer ear infection (otitis externa) and ear wax (cerumen) impaction. Chronic ear wax impaction can be prevented with ear wax removal medication used every 4–8 weeks.[7]

Table 9-3	Glaucoma Treatment[5]

MOVE FLUID OUT—INCREASE AQUEOUS OUTFLOW
Prostaglandin analogs
Bimatoprost
Latanoprost
Travoprost
Tafluprost
Cholinergic (miotics)
Carbachol
Pilocarpine
Rho kinase inhibitors
Netarsudil
Combination
Netarsudil + latanoprost

MAKE LESS FLUID—REDUCE AQUEOUS HUMOR PRODUCTION
Beta-blockers
Cartelol
Levobunolol
Timolol ± Dorzolamide
Carbonic anhydrase inhibitors
Brinzolamide
Dorzolamide

BOTH—INCREASE AQUEOUS OUTFLOW AND REDUCE AQUEOUS HUMOR PRODUCTION
Adrenergic alpha-2 agonists
Apraclonidine
Brimonidine
Combination
Brimonidine + Brinzolamide
Brimonidine + Timolol

Table 9-5 discusses the treatment options for common ear conditions.[7,8]

Common skin conditions

Acne consists of lesions on the skin that are classified as whiteheads, blackheads, small bumps, cysts, or nodules.[9]

The primary cause is androgens, *P. acnes,* and sebum present in the sebaceous glands.

First-line treatment and topical/oral options are outlined in Table 9-6.[9]

Alopecia is hair loss caused by age, hormonal factors, medical conditions, or medications.[10] Treatment includes corticosteroids (e.g., triamcinolone acetonide, desoximetasone), minoxidil topical, and finasteride.

Burns are classified as first degree (red, minor swelling), second degree (thicker, painful, blisters), and third degree (damage to all layers of skin, white or charred).[17] Treatment is dependent on burn severity and risk of infection.

- Bacitracin/Neomycin/Polymyxin B/Hydrocortisone
- Mupirocin: covers staph and strep including MRSA
- Polymyxin/Bacitracin/Neomycin ointment
- Silver sulfadiazine

Cold sores result from the herpes simplex labialis virus. Sore eruption is preceded by prodromal symptoms, including tingling, itching, and soreness. Triggers include fatigue, stress, sun exposure, and dental work.[11]

Treatment includes docosanol (OTC), acyclovir topical cream/ointment, and penciclovir topical cream.

Dandruff is caused by itchy scalp when small pieces of dry skin flake off.[12] Treatment includes selenium sulfide, pyrithione zinc, and ketoconazole shampoo.

Diaper rash is caused by friction and tender skin being exposed to urine and feces.[13] Treatment includes skin protectants (e.g., petrolatum ± zinc oxide, miconazole ± zince oxide and petrolatum).

Table 9-4   Topical Conjunctivitis Treatment[6]

ETIOLOGY OR SYMPTOMATOLOGY	TREATMENTS

Bacterial infection
   Staphylococcus aureus
   Streptococcus pneumoniae
   Haemophilus influenzae
   Moraxella catarrhalis
	Antibiotic eye drops or ointments
	Azithromycin
	Ciprofloxacin
	Erythromycin
	Gentamicin
	Moxifloxacin
	Ofloxacin
	Sulfacetamide
	Tobramycin
	Neomycin/Bacitracin/Polymyxin B
	Neomycin/Polymyxin B/Dexamethasone
	Trimethoprim/Polymyxin B
	Tobramycin/Dexamethasone

Allergic causes
   Dust mites
   Mold
   Pet dander
   Pollen
	Mast cell stabilizers
	Alcaftadine
	Cromolyn
	Ketotifen
	Lodoxamide
	Nedocromil
	Olopatadine
	
	Antihistamines
	Azelastine

Inflammation	**Steroids** Dexamethasone Fluorometholone Loteprednol Prednisolone **NSAIDs** Bromfenac Diclofenac Ketorolac
Dry eye disease	**Artificial tears** Liquifilm Refresh Systane **Immunosuppressive** Cyclosporine
Redness	**LFA-1 antagonist** Lifitegrast (Xiidra) Brimonidine (Lumify) Naphazoline (Clear eyes redness relief) Tetrahydrozoline (Visine)

Abbreviation used: LFA-1, lymphocyte function-associated antigen-1 antagonist.

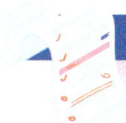

Table 9-5　Treatment for Otitis Externa and Ear Wax Impaction[7,8]

CONDITION	TREATMENT	NOTES
Otitis externa	**Nonpharmacologic guidance:** ■ Stay out of water (swimming pool, lakes, bathtub) ■ Avoid flying due to pressure differences ■ Avoid using headphones and earplugs **Antimicrobials:** ■ Acetic acid ■ Ciprofloxacin/Dexamethasone ■ Neomycin/Polymyxin/Hydrocortisone ■ Ofloxacin	**Ear drop administration:** ■ For adults, gently pull the earlobe **up and back**. ■ For children under 3, gently pull the earlobe **down and back**. ■ Do not touch tip of applicator to the ear.
Ear wax impaction	Carbamide peroxide Docusate sodium Triethanolamine polypeptideoleate	

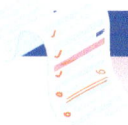

Table 9-6　Treatment for Acne[9]

	MILD	MODERATE	SEVERE
First-line treatment	BPO Topical retinoid Topical combo therapy	Topical combo therapy Oral antibiotic + BPO + topical retinoid	Topical combo therapy + oral antibiotic Oral isotretinoin
Treatment options	**Topical** **Retinoids** ■ Adapalene ■ Adapalene + BPO Tazarotene ■ Tretinoin	**Oral** **Isotretinoin** ■ Requires 2 negative pregnancy tests before treatment ■ Requires 2 forms of birth control ■ REMS (IPLEDGE) program required ■ Maximum fill of 30 d ■ Must fill within 7 d with yellow sticker	
	Antibiotics/combo ■ Clindamycin + BPO ■ Dapsone gel ■ Erythromycin + BPO	**Antibiotics** ■ Doxycycline ■ Minocycline ■ Sulfamethoxazole/Trimethoprim	

Abbreviations used: BPO, benzoyl peroxide; topical combo (combination) therapy = BPO + topical antibiotics, BPO + retinoid, BPO + retinoid + topical antibiotic.
Source: Adapted from Zaenglein AL, Pathy AL, Schlosser BJ, et al. Guidelines of care for the management of acne vulgaris. *J Am Acad Dermatol*. 2016;74(5): 945–973.e933.

Eczema (atopic dermatitis) is inflammation of the skin, causing it to be dry, red, itchy, and sore. Common triggers include irritants, allergens, hormones, stress, or weather change.[14] Treatment includes monotherapy or a combination of moisturizers, topical steroids, or antihistamines (for itching).

Fungal skin infections are generally caused by fungi *Tinea* or *Candida* and are transmitted by human-to-human contact, animal-to-human contact, or soil-to-human contact.[23,24] Table 9-7 differentiates the various fungal skin infections and the treatment options available.[23,24]

Genital warts are caused by human papillomavirus (HPV) and are a common sexually transmitted infection. The HPV vaccine is recommended as preventative therapy.[18]

Treatment for HPV commonly includes imiquimod cream, podofilox, and antivirals (e.g., acyclovir, valacyclovir).

Hemorrhoids are caused by constipation and straining to have a bowel movement, causing pruritus, burning, and rectal bleeding (blood is usually bright red).[19] Treatment may include dietary fiber or psyllium, phenylephrine or hydrocortisone (cream, ointment, suppositories), witch hazel pads (astringent), and topical lidocaine (pain reliever).

Inflammation can occur anywhere on the body.[16]

Treatment commonly includes Hydrocortisone 0.5% or 1% (potency from highest to weakest: ointment > creams > lotions > gels > foams).

Lice are parasitic insects that survive by feeding on human blood. Common symptoms include itching, sleeplessness, and sores on the head.[21] Treatment may include permethrin 1% (watch out for 5% prescribed in error), pyrethrin/piperonyl butoxide, ivermectin lotion, or malathion lotion.

Pinworm is caused by a thin, small roundworm called *Enterobius vermicularis* that causes anal itching.[22] Treatment may include pyrantel pamoate, mebendazole, or albendazole.

Poison ivy is an allergic reaction from the sap of plants that contain the toxin urushiol.[15] Treatment includes

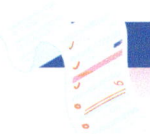

Table 9-7	Treatment for Fungal Skin Infections[23,24]

FUNGAL INFECTION	TREATMENT
Athletes foot (*Tinea pedis*): fungal infection of the foot	Betamethasone/Clotrimazole
Jock itch (*Tinea cruris*): fungal infection around the genitals, inner thighs, and buttocks	Butenafine Clotrimazole Ketoconazole
Ringworm (*Tinea corporis, Tinea capitis*): fungal infection appears in a circular shape with red, flat sore	Miconazole Terbinafine Tolnaftate *Duration:* based on selected agent + 7 d with first fungal infection
Onychomycosis (*Tinea unguium*): fungal infection of the nail	Itraconazole for up to 12 w Terbinafine oral for up to 6 w
Vaginal fungal infections (*Candida* or *Trichomoniasis*)	Butoconazole Clotrimazole Fluconazole Miconazole Terconazole *Duration:* 1, 3, or 7 d

aluminum acetate solution, colloidal oatmeal, and calamine lotion + pramoxine.

Scabies is caused by an infestation of mites that burrow into the skin. Common symptoms include intense itching and pimple-like rash.[20] Treatment includes permethrin 5% (watch out for 1% prescribed in error) or ivermectin.

REFERENCES

1. Seidman MD, Gurgel RK, Lin SY, et al. Clinical practice guideline: allergic rhinitis. *Otolaryngol Head Neck Surg.* 2015; 152(suppl 5):S1–43.
2. DeGeorge KC, Ring DJ, Dalrymple SN. Treatment of the common cold. *Am Fam Physician.* 2019;100(5):281–289.
3. Fashner J, Ericson K, Werner S. Treatment of the common cold in children and adults. *Am Fam Physician.* 2012;86(2):153–159.
4. Malesker MA, Callahan-Lyon P, Ireland B, Irwin RS, Panel CEC. Pharmacologic and nonpharmacologic treatment for acute cough associated with the common cold: CHEST Expert Panel Report. *Chest.* 2017;152(5):1021–1037.
5. American Optometric Association. *Care of the Patient With Open Angle Glaucoma.* St. Louis, MO: AOA; 2011.
6. American Optometric Association. *Care of the Patient With Conjunctivitis.* St. Louis, MO: AOA; 2002.
7. Michaudet C, Malaty J. Cerumen impaction: diagnosis and management. *Am Fam Physician.* 2018;98(8):525–529.
8. Schaefer P, Baugh RF. Acute otitis externa: an update. *Am Fam Physician.* 2012;86(11):1055–1061.
9. Zaenglein AL, Pathy AL, Schlosser BJ, et al. Guidelines of care for the management of acne vulgaris. *J Am Acad Dermatol.* 2016;74(5):945–973.e933.
10. Strazzulla LC, Wang EHC, Avila L, et al. Alopecia areata: an appraisal of new treatment approaches and overview of current therapies. *J Am Acad Dermatol.* 2018;78(1):15–24.
11. American Academy of Dermatology. Cold sores: diagnosis and treatment. Available at: https://www.aad.org/public/diseases/a-z/cold-sores-treatment. Accessed April 10, 2020.
12. American Academy of Dermatology. How to treat dandruff. Available at: https://www.aad.org/public/everyday-care/hair-scalp-care/scalp/treat-dandruff. Accessed April 10, 2020.
13. The Society for Pediatric Dermatology. What is diaper rash? Patient Perspectives. Available at: https://pedsderm.net/site/assets/files/1028/spd_diaper_care_color_web.pdf.
14. National Eczema Association. Atopic dermatitis. Available at: https://nationaleczema.org/eczema/types-of-eczema/atopic-dermatitis/. Accessed April 10, 2020.
15. American Academy of Dermatology. Poison ivy, oak, and sumac: how to treat the rash. Available at: https://www.aad.org/public/everyday-care/itchy-skin/poison-ivy/treat-rash. Accessed April 10, 2020.
16. Gabros S, Zito P. Topical corticosteroids. StatPearls. Available at: https://www.ncbi.nlm.nih.gov/books/NBK532940/. Accessed April 11, 2020.
17. National Institute of General Medical Sciences. Burns. Available at https://www.nigms.nih.gov/education/fact-sheets/Pages/burns.aspx.
18. Kodner CM, Nasraty S. Management of genital warts. *Am Fam Physician.* 2004;70(12):2335–2342.
19. National Institute of Diabetes and Digestive and Kidney Diseases Health Information Center. Hemorrhoids. Available at: https://www.niddk.nih.gov/health-information/digestive-diseases/hemorrhoids/all-content. Accessed April 10, 2020.
20. Centers for Disease Control and Prevention. Scabies. Available at: https://www.cdc.gov/parasites/scabies/index.html. Accessed April 10, 2020.
21. Centers for Disease Control and Prevention. Head lice. Available at: https://www.cdc.gov/parasites/lice/head/index.html. Accessed April 10, 2020.
22. Centers for Disease Control and Prevention. Pinworm infection. Available at: https://www.cdc.gov/parasites/pinworm/. Accessed April 10, 2020.
23. Centers for Disease Control and Prevention. Vulvovaginal candidiasis - 2015 STD treatment guidelines. Available at: https://www.cdc.gov/std/tg2015/candidiasis.htm. Accessed April 11, 2020.
24. Centers for Disease Control and Prevention. Treatment for ringworm. Available at: https://www.cdc.gov/fungal/diseases/ringworm/treatment.html. Accessed April 10, 2020.

CHAPTER 10

Cardiology

With medical writing support provided by Banner Medical LLC Writers: Jennifer Miller and Miriam Opara

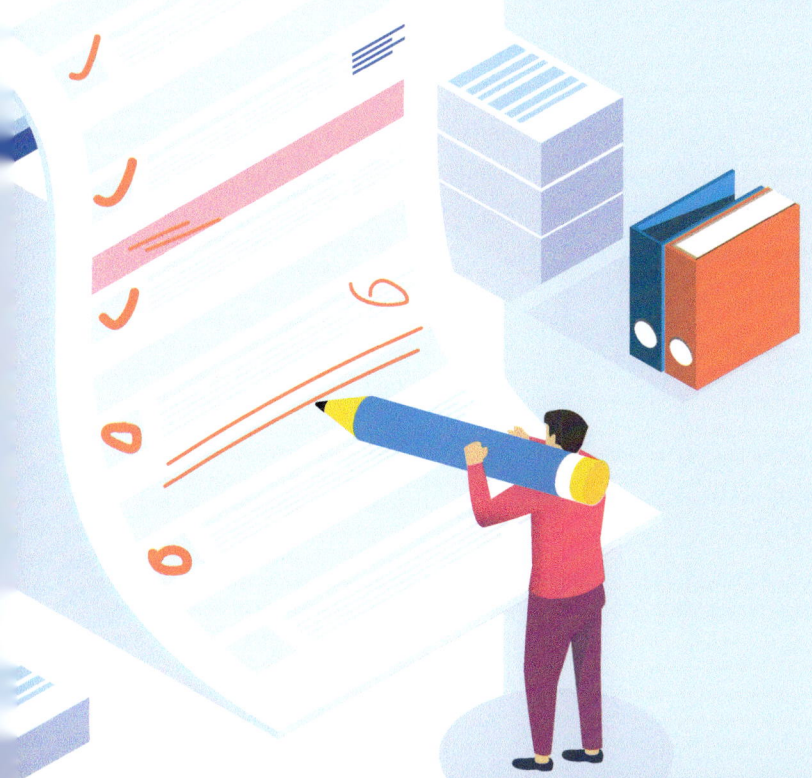

Hypertension

Hypertension (HTN) is defined as primary or secondary and is generally asymptomatic. Risk factors include the following:

- Obesity
- Sedentary lifestyle
- Excessive salt intake
- Excessive alcohol intake
- Family history
- Comorbidities (e.g., diabetes, dyslipidemia)

Uncontrolled hypertension increases the risk of myocardial infarction, stroke, and renal failure. Blood pressure (BP) is categorized as normal, elevated, stage 1, or stage 2 hypertension (see Table 10-1).

Factors that influence blood pressure include the autonomic nervous system, cardiac system, vascular smooth muscle, plasma volume, hormones, and blood movement (see Figure 10-1).[1]

Goals of therapy are to maintain BP and decrease the risk of complications.[2]

Remember:

- BP goal for all patients per the 2017 American College of Cardiology (ACC)/American Heart Association (AHA) Hypertension Guideline is <130/80 mmHg
  - Per the American Diabetes Association, goal BP for patients with diabetes, HTN, and 10-year atherosclerotic cardiovascular disease (ASCVD) risk is as follows:[3]
    - Diabetes + HTN + ASCVD risk <15%: <140/90 mmHg
    - Diabetes + HTN + ASCVD risk ≥15%: <130/80 mmHg
- Lifestyle interventions are vital for all patients with HTN (regardless of drug therapy):
  - Weight loss (1 kg of weight loss lowers BP by 1 mmHg)
  - Dietary Approaches to Stop Hypertension (DASH) diet
  - Moderate alcohol intake (men: ≤2 drinks per day, women: ≤1 drink per day)
  - Reduced sodium intake (<1500 mg/day)
  - Adequate potassium intake (3500–5000 mg/day)
  - Aerobic exercise (90–150 min/week)

Pharmacologic treatment

- The preferred antihypertensive medications (see Table 10-2) for initial HTN treatment

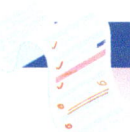

Table 10-1 Blood Pressure Categories and Recommended Treatment[2]

CATEGORIES	SBP VALUE	DBP VALUE	INITIAL PREVENTION/TREATMENT OPTIONS
Normal (both must be met)	<120 mmHg	<80 mmHg	Promote optimal lifestyle habits as a preventive strategy
Elevated (both must be met)	120–129 mmHg	<80 mmHg	Lifestyle modifications
HYPERTENSION			
Stage 1 (SBP or DBP must be met)	130–139 mmHg	80–89 mmHg	▪ CCBs* ▪ ACEIs or ARBs ▪ Thiazide diuretics*
Stage 2 (SBP or DBP must be met)	≥140 mmHg	≥90 mmHg	Consider initiating 2 first-line agents of different classes

Abbreviations used: ACEI, angiotensin-converting enzyme inhibitor; ARB, angiotensin receptor blocker; CCB, calcium channel blocker; DBP, diastolic blood pressure; SBP, systolic blood pressure.
*Preferred drug class if African American.
Adapted from Whelton PK, Carey RM, Aronow WS, et al. 2017 ACC/AHA/AAPA/ABC/ACPM/AGS/APhA/ASH/ASPC/NMA/PCNA Guideline for the Prevention, Detection, Evaluation, and Management of High Blood Pressure in Adults: A Report of the American College of Cardiology/American Heart Association Task Force on Clinical Practice Guidelines. *Hypertension*. 2018;71(6):e13–e115.

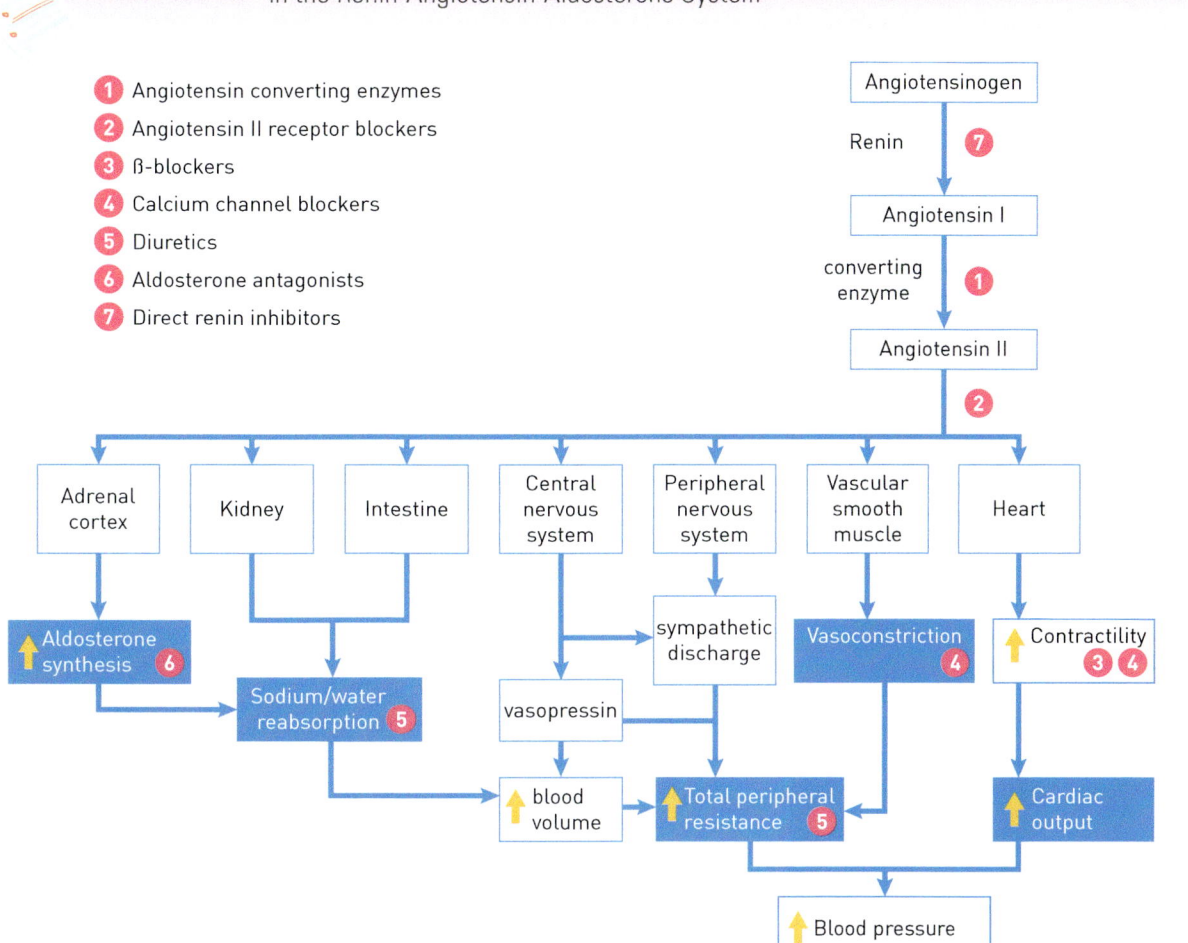

Adapted from: DiPiro J, Talbert R, Yee G, Matzke G, Wells B, Posey L. Hypertension. In: *Pharmacotherapy: A Pathophysiologic Approach*. McGraw-Hill; 2011:101–135.

include angiotensin-converting enzyme inhibitors (ACEIs), angiotensin receptor blockers (ARBs), calcium channel blockers (CCBs), and thiazide diuretics.

■ If still not at goal BP after initial treatment options, maximize first medication or add a new medication class not previously selected (thiazide diuretic, ACEI, ARB, CCB).[4]

■ Adding an aldosterone antagonist or beta-blocker are additive options if goal BP is not achieved.[4]

　● Aldosterone antagonists are a preferred fourth-line agent in the absence of contraindications and if no compelling indication exists for a beta-blocker

Hypertensive urgencies and emergencies[2]

■ Hypertensive urgency: BP >180/120 mmHg **without** target organ damage
■ Hypertensive emergency: BP >180/120 mmHg **with** target organ damage
　● Reduce BP by no more than 25% over 1st hour, then to 160/100–110 mmHg over next 2–6 hours, then to normal over next 24–48 hours with parenteral agents

Ischemic heart disease

Ischemic heart disease (IHD) is caused by plaque buildup (atherosclerosis) in coronary arteries, which can block the flow of blood in large arteries of the heart,

Table 10-2 Pharmacologic Treatment for Hypertension[1,2]

DRUG AGENT	NOTES
ANGIOTENSIN-CONVERTING ENZYME INHIBITORS	
Benazepril (Lotensin)	**SE:** cough, angioedema, hyperkalemia, acute renal failure
Captopril (Capoten)	**CI:** Do not use in combination with ARBs; history of angioedema with ACEI
Enalapril (Vasotec)	**Remember:** Avoid in pregnancy; dry cough from bradykinin
Lisinopril (Zestril)	
Perindopril (Coversyl)	
Quinapril (Accupril)	
Ramipril (Altace)	
ANGIOTENSIN RECEPTOR BLOCKERS	
Candesartan (Atacand)	**SE:** cough, angioedema, hyperkalemia, acute renal failure
Irbesartan (Avapro)	**CI:** Do not use in combination with ACEIs; history of angioedema with ACEI
Losartan (Cozaar)	**Remember:** Avoid in pregnancy; can give ARB 6 wk after ACEI discontinued
Olmesartan (Benicar)	
Telmisartan (Micardis)	
Valsartan (Diovan)	
ALDOSTERONE ANTAGONISTS	
Eplerenone (Inspra)	**SE:** hyperkalemia, gynecomastia
Spironolactone (Aldactone)	**Remember:** Preferred add-on therapy in resistant hypertension
ALPHA 1 BLOCKERS	
Doxazosin (Cardura)	**SE:** orthostatic hypotension
Prazosin (Minipress)	Consider in patients with benign prostatic hyperplasia
Terazosin (Hytrin)	
ALPHA 2 AGONISTS	
Clonidine (Catapres)	**SE:** rebound hypertension, CNS symptoms, erectile dysfunction
Methyldopa (Aldomet)	**Remember:** Avoid abrupt discontinuation; methyldopa may be used in pregnancy
Guanfacine (Tenex, Intuniv)	
BETA-BLOCKERS	
Cardioselective	**SE:** bradycardia, fatigue, depression, heart block, bronchospasm, sweating with
Atenolol (Tenormin)	hypoglycemia
Bisoprolol (Zebeta)	■ Useful in bronchospastic airway disease
Metoprolol (Toprol XL, Lopressor)	
Cardioselective & vasodilatory	**SE:** Induces nitric oxide-induced vasodilation
Nebivolol (Bystolic)	
Non-cardioselective	■ Avoid in patients with reactive airway disease
Nadolol (Corgard)	■ Avoid abrupt discontinuation
Propranolol (Inderal)	
Intrinsic sympathomimetic activity	Generally, avoid, especially in ischemic heart disease or HF
Acebutolol (Sectral)	
Pindolol (Visken)	

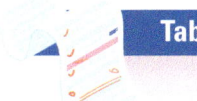

Table 10-2 Pharmacologic Treatment for Hypertension[1,2] (*Continued*)

DRUG AGENT	NOTES
ALPHA AND BETA RECEPTORS	
Carvedilol (Coreg) Labetalol (Normodyne)	■ Carvedilol preferred in HFrEF ■ Labetalol may be used in pregnancy
CALCIUM CHANNEL BLOCKERS	
Dihydropyridines Amlodipine (Norvasc) Nicardipine SR/LA (Cardene) Nifedipine (Procardia XL, Adalat CC) Nisoldipine (Sular)	**SE:** reflex tachycardia, lower extremity edema, headaches **CI:** Avoid in HF with reduced ejection fraction Nifedipine may be used in pregnancy
Non-dihydropyridines Diltiazem ER (Cardizem) Verapamil IR, SR/ER (Calan, Isoptin, Verelan)	**SE:** constipation (most with verapamil), bradycardia, can worsen HF **Remember:** Major substrates and moderate inhibitors of CYP3A4
DIRECT RENIN INHIBITOR	
Aliskiren (Tekturna)	**CI:** With ACEI or ARB **Remember:** Avoid in pregnancy
LOOP DIURETICS	
Bumetanide (Bumex) Furosemide (Lasix) Torsemide (Demadex)	**SE:** hypokalemia, hypocalcemia, hypomagnesemia ■ Preferred diuretic class in symptomatic HF ■ Preferred over thiazides in GFR <30 mL/min
POTASSIUM SPARING DIURETICS	
Amiloride (Midamor) Triamterene (Dyrenium)	**SE:** hyperkalemia Avoid in chronic kidney disease
THIAZIDE DIURETICS	
Chlorthalidone (Thalitone) HCTZ (Hydrodiuril) Indapamide (Lozol) Metolazone (Zaroxolyn)	**SE:** hypokalemia, hyperglycemia, hyperuricemia, hyponatremia, hypercalcemia ■ Chlorthalidone preferred (long half-life and reduction of CVD) ■ Use with caution in gout
VASODILATORS	
Hydralazine (Apresoline)	**SE:** sodium and water retention, reflex tachycardia

Abbreviations used: ACEI, angiotensin-converting enzyme inhibitor; ARB, angiotensin receptor blocker; BID, twice daily; CI, contraindication; CNS, central nervous system; CVD, cardiovascular disease; DHP, dihydropyridine; ER, extended release; GI, gastrointestinal; GFR, glomerular filtration rate; HCTZ, hydrochlorothiazide; HF, heart failure; HFrEF, heart failure with reduced ejection fraction; IR, immediate release; LA, Long-acting; NDHP, non-dihydropyridine; SE, side effects; SR, sustained release; TID, 3 times daily.
*Intrinsic sympathomimetic activity
Adapted from Whelton PK, Carey RM, Aronow WS, et al. 2017 ACC/AHA/AAPA/ABC/ACPM/AGS/APhA/ASH/ASPC/NMA/PCNA Guideline for the Prevention, Detection, Evaluation, and Management of High Blood Pressure in Adults: A Report of the American College of Cardiology/American Heart Association Task Force on Clinical Practice Guidelines. *Hypertension.* 2018;71(6):e13-e115; DiPiro J, Talbert R, Yee G, Matzke G, Wells B, Posey L. Hypertension. In: *Pharmacotherapy: A Pathophysiologic Approach.* 8th ed. New York, NY: McGraw-Hill; 2011:101–135.

CLASS	DESCRIPTION
I	Angina caused by strenuous, rapid, or prolonged exertion, either at work or recreation
II	Angina caused by rapidly walking/climbing stairs or walking/climbing stairs after meals, in cold or windy weather, or under emotional distress; by walking uphill
III	Obvious limitations during normal physical activity; angina caused by walking 1–2 blocks on level ground and climbing a single flight of stairs in normal conditions
IV	Angina may be present at rest; angina occurs frequently where it causes inability to perform any physical activity without experiencing discomfort

Adapted from Campeau L. Letter: Grading of Angina Pectoris. *Circulation.* 1976;54(3):522–523.

causing an inadequate supply of blood to the heart.[5] IHD may present as acute coronary syndromes, angina pectoris, and ischemia without clinical symptoms.[6] Angina is graded into four classes (see Table 10-3).

- Diagnostic tests used in IHD evaluate the myocardial oxygen demand and monitor changes in heart rate, BP, and heart rhythm. An electrocardiogram is generally used with an exercise.
- Percutaneous coronary intervention or coronary artery bypass grafting are used when revascularization is required.

Optimal management includes a comprehensive approach to prevent cardiovascular disease:[7]

- Anti-anginal therapy (see Table 10-4) used to improve function and reduce the risk of death
- Antiplatelet therapy (see Acute Coronary Syndromes section)
- Lipid-lowering therapy (see Dyslipidemia section)
- Risk factor reduction (smoking cessation, weight reduction, at goal BP, A1C)

Acute coronary syndromes

Acute coronary syndromes (ACS) encompass both unstable angina and myocardial infarction (MI); MI is further broken down into ST-segment elevation MI (STEMI) and non-ST-segment elevation MI (non-STEMI).[8]

- ACS is caused by erosion of atherosclerotic plaques with platelet adherence and ultimate activation of the clotting cascade; components of clot include fibrin and platelets
- Lab markers of cell death: creatine kinase myocardial band and troponin

Treatment for ACS (see Table 10-5) must be administered immediately and continued long term.[8–10]

Heart failure

Heart failure (HF) is a complex clinical condition associated with a structural or functional abnormality that affects or impairs the ability of the heart to relax and/or to contract.[11,12]

- Functional impairment of ventricle to fill with blood—heart failure with **preserved** ejection fraction (HFpEF)
- Functional impairment of ventricle to contract and eject blood—heart failure with **reduced** EF (HFrEF)

There are four compensatory mechanisms to maintain acceptable cardiac output:

1. Tachycardia and increased contractility
2. Fluid/sodium retention and increased preload

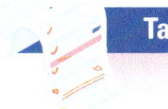

Table 10-4 Therapies Used in Angina[6,7]

Drug therapy class	Effect on myocardial oxygen demand	Notes
Beta-blockers	Heart rate: **Decrease** Myocardial contractility: **Decrease** Systolic pressure: **Decrease** LV volume: **Increase**	▪ Recommended 1st line ▪ Improves survival in patients with myocardial infarction
Calcium channel blockers (preferred agents: long-acting diltiazem, verapamil; amlodipine)	Heart rate: **Decrease** (non-DHP CCBs) Myocardial contractility: **No Effect or Decrease** Systolic pressure: **Decrease** LV volume: **No Effect or Decrease**	▪ Recommended in vasospastic/prinzmetal angina, peripheral vascular disease, hypertension
Long-acting nitrates Isosorbide mononitrate/dinitrate Short-acting nitrates Nitroglycerin	Heart rate: **Increase** Myocardial contractility: **No Effect** Systolic pressure: **Decrease** LV volume: **Decrease**	MOA: Venodilation and reduction in wall stress ▪ Used for acute management Remember: patch-free period of 10–12 h; call 911 if pain not resolved after 1st SL tab
Ranolazine	No effect on heart rate, inotropic state, hemodynamic state; does not increase coronary blood flow	MOA: Inhibits late sodium current; reducing calcium overload in the ischemic myocyte

Abbreviations used: CCB, calcium channel blockers; DHP, dihydropyridine; IV, intravenous; LV, left ventricular; MOA, mechanism of action; SL, sublingual.
Adapted from[6,7] DiPiro J, Talbert R, Yee G, Matzke G, Wells B, Posey L. Ischemic Heart Disease. In: *Pharmacotherapy: A Pathophysiologic Approach.* 8th ed. New York, NY: McGraw-Hill; 2011:209–240; Fihn SD, Gardin JM, Abrams J, et al. 2012 ACCF/AHA/ACP/AATS/PCNA/SCAI/STS Guideline for the Diagnosis and Management of Patients With Stable Ischemic Heart Disease: Executive Summary: A report of the American College of Cardiology Foundation/American Heart Association Task Force on Practice Guidelines, and the American College of Physicians, American Association for Thoracic Surgery, Preventive Cardiovascular Nurses Association, Society for Cardiovascular Angiography and Interventions, and Society of Thoracic Surgeons. *Circulation.* 2012;126(25):3097–3137.

3. Vasoconstriction and increased afterload
4. Ventricular hypertrophy and cardiac remodeling

Key clinical presentation findings[11]

- Peripheral edema (cardinal finding)
- Pulmonary rales/edema
- Hepatomegaly
- Dyspnea
- Fatigue
- Paroxysmal nocturnal dyspnea
- Hemoptysis
- Brain natriuretic peptide >100 pg/mL

Treatment of HF is dependent on the New York Heart Association Heart Failure Functional Classi-fication (see Table 10-6) and the AHA/ACC Heart Failure Stages (see Table 10-7).

Arrhythmias

Normal cardiac conduction involves initiation of electrical activity by the sinoatrial node and moves through the heart via a treelike conduction system.[13,14] Arrhythmias (see Table 10-8) are abnormal heart rates or rhythms caused by changes in the normal sequence of cardiac electrical impulses secondary to structural and/or electrophysiological abnormalities (abnormal impulse generation or abnormal impulse conduction).

Antiarrhythmic medications (see Table 10-9) have different mechanisms to alter conduction activity and

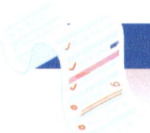

Table 10-5 Summary of Acute Coronary Syndrome Management[8-10]

ACUTE MANAGEMENT (MONA-GAP-BA)	
Possible reperfusion	PCI or CABG
Fibrinolytics in STEMI only	Alteplase, tenecteplase, reteplase
ADMINISTER IMMEDIATELY	
Morphine*	Provides pain relief
Oxygen	Administer when oxygen saturation is <90%
Nitrates	Dilates coronary arteries to improve blood flow
Aspirin	Inhibits platelet aggregation
ADMINISTER NEXT	
Glycoprotein IIb/IIIa inhibitors if undergoing PCI	Abciximab, eptifibatide, tirofiban
Anticoagulant	UFH, enoxaparin, bivalirudin
P2Y12 Inhibitor	Clopidogrel, prasugrel, ticagrelor
GIVE WITHIN 24 HOURS	
Beta-Blockers	Decrease oxygen demand
ACE Inhibitors	ARBs used if ACEIs are contraindicated
POST-ACS MANAGEMENT	
Aspirin 81 mg daily	Continued indefinitely
P2Y12 inhibitor	Continued for 12 mo
Beta-blocker	Continued for at least 3 y
Nitroglycerin SL PRN	Continued indefinitely
ACE inhibitor	Indicated in patients with heart failure, LVEF <40%, diabetes, or CKD; continued indefinitely
Aldosterone antagonist	Indicated in patients with LVEF ≤40% + either heart failure or diabetes who are already receiving an ACEI + beta-blocker; continued indefinitely
Statins	■ See secondary prevention algorithm in Dyslipidemia section ■ Moderate or high-intensity statin initiated as appropriate

Abbreviations used: ARB, angiotensin receptor blocker; ACE, angiotensin-converting enzyme; ACEI, angiotensin-converting enzyme inhibitor; CABG, coronary artery bypass graft; CKD, chronic kidney disease; LVEF, left ventricular ejection fraction; PCI, percutaneous coronary intervention; PRN, as needed; SL, sublingual; UFH, unfractionated heparin.

*Morphine administration occurs after nitrates only if pain is not adequately controlled and deemed appropriate.

Adapted from DiPiro J, Talbert R, Yee G, Matzke G, Wells B, Posey L. Acute Coronary Syndromes. In: *Pharmacotherapy: A Pathophysiologic Approach*. 8th ed. New York, NY: McGraw-Hill; 2011:241–271; Amsterdam EA, Wenger NK, Brindis RG, et al. 2014 AHA/ACC Guideline for the Management of Patients With Non-ST-Elevation Acute Coronary Syndromes. *Circulation*. 2014;130(25):e344–e426; O'Gara PT, Kushner FG, Ascheim DD, et al. 2013 ACCF/AHA Guideline for the Management of ST-Elevation Myocardial Infarction. *Circulation*. 2013;127(4):e362–e425.

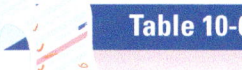

Table 10-6	NYHA Heart Failure Functional Classification[11,24]

Class I	Ordinary physical activity does NOT cause palpitations, dyspnea, or fatigue—no limitations of physical activity
Class II	Ordinary physical activity does result in palpitations, angina, dyspnea, or fatigue—slight limitations of physical activity
Class III	Comfortable at rest—less than ordinary activity results in symptoms
Class IV	Symptoms present at rest—increased discomfort upon any activity

Adapted from DiPiro J, Talbert R, Yee G, Matzke G, Wells B, Posey L. Systolic Heart Failure. In: *Pharmacotherapy: A Pathophysiologic Approach*. 8th ed. New York, NY: McGraw-Hill; 2011:137–172; Heart.Org. Classes of Heart Failure. 2020. Available at: https://www.heart.org/en/health-topics/heart-failure/what-is-heart-failure/classes-of-heart-failure. Accessed April 8, 2020.

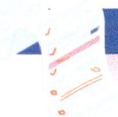

Table 10-7	American Heart Association/American College of Cardiology Heart Failure Stages and Corresponding Management[11,12,25,26]

STAGE	DESCRIPTION	MANAGEMENT
A	High risk of developing HF; **NO** structural heart disease present	Control CV risk factors (smoking cessation, obesity) Treatment of HTN, DM, dyslipidemia, and vascular risk If vascular risk/atherosclerotic disease can initiate ACEI/ARB
B	Presence of structural heart disease; **NO** signs or symptoms of HF	ACEI/ARB + BB ▪ ACEI/ARB + BB should be initiated and titrated in those w/LVEF <40% with or without history of MI ▪ Morbidity/mortality benefit in HFrEF BBs of choice and target dose in HFrEF (BCCM): ▪ Bisoprolol*: 10 mg/day ▪ Carvedilol: 25 mg BID (goal dose if ≤85 kg); 50 mg BID (goal dose if >85 kg) ▪ Carvedilol CR: 80 mg/day ▪ Metoprolol succinate CR/XL: 200 mg/day

C	Presence of structural heart disease + current **OR** previous symptoms of HF	Diuretics in those with fluid retention (furosemide)
		Aldosterone antagonist if EF ≤35%; GFR ≥30 mL/min; K <5 mEq/L
		▪ Morbidity/mortality benefit
		Other agents:
		▪ Hydralazine + ISDN: recommended in African Americans
		▪ Digoxin (cardiac glycoside)—Target range: 0.5–1 ng/mL
		▪ Ivabradine
		▪ Sacubitril/valsartan—Target maintenance dose: sacubitril 97 mg/valsartan 103 mg BID
		  ● Requires 36-h washout period when switching from or to an ACEI
		  ● Contraindications: Concomitant use of ACEI, angioedema

(*continued on next page*)

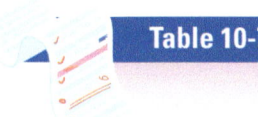

Table 10-7 American Heart Association/American College of Cardiology Heart Failure Stages and Corresponding Management[11,12,25,26] *(Continued)*

STAGE	DESCRIPTION	MANAGEMENT

D	Refractory/end-stage disease necessitating dedicated interventions, cardiac support, or hospice	Mechanical circulatory support
		Continuous positive inotropic therapy
		  ▪ Adrenergic agonists: dopamine, dobutamine
		  ▪ PDE inhibitor: milrinone
		Palliative care and cardiac transplant

Acute decompensated HF	Classified into 4 categories: 1. Warm and Dry 2. Warm and Wet 3. Cold and Dry 4. Cold and Wet	Diuretics for fluid overload Inotropes for symptom relief and end-organ dysfunction Vasodilators (nitroprusside, nitroglycerin) for acute pulmonary edema, severe HTN, or refractory to diuretics

Abbreviations used: ACEI, angiotensin-converting enzyme inhibitor; ACS, acute coronary syndrome; ARB, angiotensin receptor blocker; BB, beta-blocker; BCCM, bisoprolol, carvedilol, carvedilol CR, metoprolol XL; BID, twice daily; CCB, calcium channel blockers; CR, controlled release; CV, cardiovascular; DM, diabetes mellitus; EF, ejection fraction; HF, heart failure; HFrEF, heart failure with reduced ejection fraction; HTN, hypertension; ISDN, isosorbide dinitrate; LVEF, left ventricular ejection fraction; MI, myocardial infarction; NDHP, non-dihydropyridine; PDE, phosphodiesterase; XL, extended release.
*Bisoprolol is a BB of choice and used off-label for the treatment of stage B HFrEF.
Adapted from DiPiro J, Talbert R, Yee G, Matzke G, Wells B, Posey L. Systolic Heart Failure. In: *Pharmacotherapy: A Pathophysiologic Approach.* 8th ed. New York, NY: McGraw-Hill; 2011:137–172; Yancy CW, Jessup M, Bozkurt B, et al. 2013 ACCF/AHA Guideline for the Management of Heart Failure. *Circulation.* 2013;128(16):e240–e327; Yancy CW, Jessup M, Bozkurt B, et al. 2017 ACC/AHA/HFSA Focused Update of the 2013 ACCF/AHA Guideline for the Management of Heart Failure: A Report of the American College of Cardiology/American Heart Association Task Force on Clinical Practice Guidelines and the Heart Failure Society of America. *J Am Coll Cardiol.* 2017;70(6):776–803; DiPiro J, Talbert R, Yee G, Matzke G, Wells B, Posey L. Acute Decompensated Heart Failure. In: *Pharmacotherapy: A Pathophysiologic Approach.* 8th ed. New York, NY: McGraw-Hill; 2011:191–207.

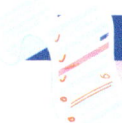

Table 10-8 Various Types and Origins of Arrhythmias[13]

TYPE/ORIGIN	ARRHYTHMIAS

Supraventricular arrhythmias	▪ Atrial fibrillation (most common)
	  ● Long-standing
	  ● Paroxysmal
	  ● Persistent
	  ● Permanent
	  ● Non-valvular
	▪ Atrial flutter
	▪ Paroxysmal supraventricular tachycardia

Ventricular arrhythmias	▪ Premature ventricular contractions ▪ Ventricular tachycardia ● Torsades de Pointes ▪ Ventricular fibrillation ▪ Ventricular proarrythmia
Bradyarrhythmias	▪ Sinus node dysfunction ▪ Atrioventricular block

Adapted from DiPiro J, Talbert R, Yee G, Matzke G, Wells B, Posey L. The Arrhythmias. In: *Pharmacotherapy: A Pathophysiologic Approach.* 8th ed. New York, NY: McGraw-Hill; 2011:273–309.

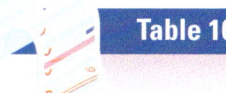

Table 10-9 Classification of Antiarrhythmic Medications[13,27]

CLASS	DRUG AGENT
0: Sodium and potassium channel blocker	Ivabradine
I: Sodium channel blockers	
Ia	Disopyramide
	Procainamide
	Quinidine
Ib	Lidocaine
	Mexiletine
Ic	Flecainide
	Propafenone
Id	Ranolazine (Ca and Na)
II: Indirectly block calcium channels	Beta-blockers
III: Potassium channel blockers	Amiodarone*
	Dofetilide
	Dronedarone
	Ibutilide
	Sotalol
IV: Calcium channel blockers	Diltiazem
	Verapamil

*Amiodarone monitoring: pulmonary fibrosis, hypo/hyperthyroidism, neuropathy, hepatotoxicity, optic neuritis, tremor, ataxia, peripheral neuropathy, bradycardia, photosensitivity.

Adapted from DiPiro J, Talbert R, Yee G, Matzke G, Wells B, Posey L. The Arrhythmias. In: *Pharmacotherapy: A Pathophysiologic Approach*. 8th ed. New York, NY: McGraw-Hill; 2011:273–309; Lei M, Wu L, Terrar DA, Huang CL. Modernized Classification of Cardiac Antiarrhythmic Drugs. *Circulation*. 2018;138(17):1879–1896.

are associated with pharmacokinetic drug interactions and prolongation of QT interval.[13–15]

Atrial fibrillation (AF) treatment approach includes rate and rhythm control (see Table 10-10). Patients with AF must be started on stroke prophylaxis and treated for thromboembolism risk. The CHA$_2$DS$_2$-VASc score is used to determine stroke risk in non-valvular AF.

Stroke

Stroke is a focal neurologic deficit that has an abrupt onset, lasts ≥24 hours, and is presumed to be of vascular origin.[16] The two types of strokes are ischemic (blood clot) and hemorrhagic (bleeding). Signs and symptoms (see Table 10-11) of stroke are essential to recognize and respond to in a timely manner to minimize damage.

Stroke management[17–19]

- First, determine the type of stroke (ischemic vs. hemorrhagic) via computed tomography (CT) scan
- Nonpharmacologic and pharmacologic therapies for ischemic and hemorrhagic stroke are approached differently (see Table 10-12)

Dyslipidemia

Cholesterol, triglycerides, and phospholipids are transported throughout the body as lipoproteins (complexes

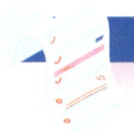

| **Table 10-10** | Management of Atrial Fibrillation[13–15] |

GOAL	MANAGEMENT

Thromboembolic risk and treatment	CHA₂DS₂-VASc ≥2 (males) or CHA₂DS₂-VASc ≥3 (females) with end-stage CKD/hemodialysis
	◾ Warfarin: vitamin K antagonist
	   ● INR goal of 2.5–3.5 in patients with AF and a mechanical heart valve
	   ● Apixaban: Direct oral anticoagulant
	AF or flutter + prior stroke, TIA, or CHA₂DS₂-VASc score ≥2 (males) or CHA₂DS₂-VASc ≥3 (females)
	◾ Oral anticoagulants

Rate control	Beta-blocker or NDHP-CCB recommended in paroxysmal, permanent, or persistent AF Alternative agents (off-label): amiodarone and digoxin; digoxin typically reserved for patients with AF + HFrEF Cardioversion indicated if hemodynamically unstable
Rhythm control	Direct-current cardioversion Pharmacologic cardioversion: flecainide, dofetilide, propafenone, amiodarone, ibutilide Maintenance of sinus rhythm with amiodarone, dofetilide, dronedarone, flecainide, propafenone, or sotalol Anticoagulation therapy must be started at least 3 wk BEFORE cardioversion and continued for at least 4 wk AFTER successful cardioversion to NSR ◾ If AF/flutter for ≥48 h or unknown duration; anticoagulation with warfarin, factor Xa inhibitor or direct thrombin inhibitor ◾ If AF/flutter <48 h + high stroke risk—anticoagulation with heparin/LMWH, factor Xa or direct thrombin inhibitor

Abbreviations used: AF, atrial fibrillation; CCB, calcium channel blocker; CKD, chronic kidney disease; HFrEF, heart failure with reduced ejection fraction; INR, international normalized ratio; IV, intravenous; LMWH, low molecular weight heparin; NDHP, non-dihydropyridine; NSR, normal sinus rhythm; TIA, transient ischemic attack.

Adapted from DiPiro J, Talbert R, Yee G, Matzke G, Wells B, Posey L. The Arrhythmias. In: *Pharmacotherapy: A Pathophysiologic Approach*. 8th ed. New York, NY: McGraw-Hill; 2011:273–309; January CT, Wann LS, Alpert JS, et al. 2014 AHA/ACC/HRS Guideline for the Management of Patients With Atrial Fibrillation. *Circulation*. 2014;130(23):e199–e267; January CT, Wann LS, Calkins H, et al. 2019 AHA/ACC/HRS Focused Update of the 2014 AHA/ACC/HRS Guideline for the Management of Patients With Atrial Fibrillation: A Report of the American College of Cardiology/American Heart Association Task Force on Clinical Practice Guidelines and the Heart Rhythm Society in Collaboration With the Society of Thoracic Surgeons. *Circulation*. 2019;140(2):e125–e151.

| **Table 10-11** | Signs and Symptoms of Stroke[17,28] |

THINK "FAST"

Face—Is one side droopy/uneven/numb?	**H**emorrhagic stroke = **h**eadache
Arms—Can person lift both arms; does one arm drift down?	
Speech—Is person's speech slurred or incomprehensible?	
Time—Time to call 911; goal to reperfusion therapy <4.5 h	

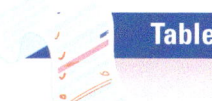

Table 10-12 Management for Ischemic and Hemorrhagic Stroke[17–19]

STROKE TYPE	MANAGEMENT
Hemorrhagic	▪ DHP CCB: nimodipine 60 mg Q 4 h x 21 d recommended for reduction of the incidence and severity of deficits ▪ Clipping or coiling vascular abnormality, external ventricular drain ▪ Surgical evacuation of intracerebral hemorrhage
Ischemic	**Acute management:** ▪ Blood pressure goal ≤185/110 prior to thrombolytic therapy ● IV clevidipine, labetalol, nicardipine ▪ If within 3 h of symptom onset (off label: up to 4.5 h): Alteplase (t-PA) ● Dose: 0.9 mg/kg (maximum 90 mg) IV over 1 h ● 10% given as bolus over 1 min ▪ ASA 160–325 mg PO within 48 h of symptom onset ● Administration generally delayed 24 h if t-PA given ▪ If minor stroke: Dual antiplatelet therapy should be started within 24 h symptom onset and continued for up to 90 d **Secondary prevention:** ▪ Antiplatelet therapy ● ASA ● ASA + ER dipyridamole ● Clopidogrel ● Warfarin ▪ Antihypertensive therapy (even if not hypertensive prior to stroke) ● ACEI/ARB ● Diuretic ▪ Lipid management ● High-intensity statins ▪ Glycemic control if diabetic ▪ Lifestyle modification

Abbreviations used; ACEI, angiotensin-converting enzyme inhibitor; ARB, angiotensin receptor blocker; ASA, aspirin; CCB, calcium channel blocker; DHP, dihydropyridine; ER, extended release; t-PA, tissue plasminogen activator; PO, by mouth; IV, intravenous.

of lipids and proteins).[20] Dyslipidemia is an elevation of total cholesterol, low-density lipoprotein (LDL), or triglycerides; low high-density lipoprotein (HDL); or a combination of these abnormalities.

▪ Cholesterol levels are classified as ideal, borderline high, and high (see Table 10-13).[20]
▪ Therapeutic Lifestyle Changes (TLC) diet[20–22]
 ● Saturated fats <7% total calories and dietary cholesterol <200 mg/day

▪ Lipid-lowering agents are the mainstay to treat dyslipidemia (see Table 10-14).
▪ Statin intensity classification is outlined in Table 10-15.

Primary prevention of ASCVD and subsequent management based on risk is summarized in Table 10-16.

Risk enhancers:[22]
▪ Family history of premature ASCVD
▪ LDL persistently ≥160 mg/dL

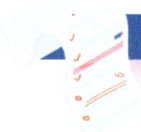

Table 10-13 Total Cholesterol, Low-Density Lipoprotein, High-Density Lipoprotein, and Triglyceride Classification[20]

PARAMETER	VALUE	CLASSIFICATION
Total cholesterol	<200 mg/dL	Desirable
	200–239 mg/dL	Borderline high
	≥240 mg/dL	High
LDL cholesterol	<100 mg/dL	Ideal
	100–129 mg/dL	Near/above ideal
	130–159 mg/dL	Borderline high
	160–189 mg/dL	High
	≥190 mg/dL	Very high
HDL cholesterol	<40 mg/dL	Low
	≥60 mg/dL	High
Triglycerides	<150 mg/dL	Normal
	150–199 mg/dL	Borderline high
	200–499 mg/dL	High
	≥500 mg/dL	Very high

Abbreviations used: HDL, high-density lipoprotein; LDL, low-density lipoprotein.
Adapted from DiPiro J, Talbert R, Yee G, Matzke G, Wells B, Posey L. Dyslipidemia. In: *Pharmacotherapy: A Pathophysiologic Approach*. 8th ed. New York, NY: McGraw-Hill; 2011:365–388.

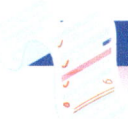

Table 10-14 Lipid-Lowering Agents[20]

DRUG AGENT	MECHANISM OF ACTION	NOTES
HMG COA REDUCTASE INHIBITORS (STATINS)		
Atorvastatin (Lipitor) Fluvastatin (Lescol) Lovastatin (Mevacor) Pitavastatin Pravastatin (Pravachol) Rosuvastatin (Crestor) Simvastatin (Zocor)	Inhibits HMG CoA reductase; decreases intracellular cholesterol production	**SE:** increases liver enzymes, myopathy, and rhabdomyolysis **Common interactions with statins:** grapefruit juice, gemfibrozil, azoles, erythromycin, clarithromycin, diltiazem, verapamil, amiodarone
PCSK9 INHIBITORS		
Alirocumab (Praluent) Evolocumab (Repatha)	Prevents degradation of LDL-receptor on hepatic surface	Subcutaneous administration
BILE ACID SEQUESTRANTS		
Cholestyramine (Questran, Prevalite, Questran Light) Colesevelam (WelChol) Colestipol (Colestif)	Inhibits reabsorption and enterohepatic cycling by binding to bile acids in the GI tract; fecal cholesterol excretion	**SE:** GI adverse effects common, may cause transient increase in enzymes

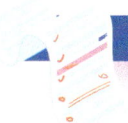

Table 10-14   Lipid-Lowering Agents[20] (*Continued*)

DRUG AGENT	MECHANISM OF ACTION	NOTES
CHOLESTEROL ABSORPTION/NPC1L1 INHIBITOR		
Ezetimibe (Zetia)	Inhibits intestinal absorption of cholesterol by blocking NPC1L1 peptide on the enterocyte luminal surface within the small intestine; decreases intra-hepatocellular concentrations	▪ Best as add-on therapy; may be used as monotherapy (no mortality benefit) ▪ Converted to glucuronide metabolite via UGT1A1, 1A3, 2B15
NICOTINIC ACID DERIVATIVES		
ER Niacin (Rx) (Niaspan) IR Niacin (OTC) (Niacor) Slo-Niacin (OTC)	Decreases hepatic synthesis of TG and secretion of VLDL by inhibiting mobilization of free fatty acids from peripheral tissues; conversion of VLDL; LDL may also be inhibited	▪ Start low, go slow ▪ Flushing common; use ASA ▪ May cause gout (increase in uric acid) and blurry vision
OMEGA-3-ACID ETHYL ESTERS (FISH OIL)		
Omega-3 fish oils (Lovaza)	Reduced hepatic production of TG-rich VLDL	**SE**: bleeding ▪ Consider as adjunct to a maximally tolerated statin for cardiovascular risk reduction in those with mild hypertriglyceridemia ▪ Monitor TGs and LDL, liver enzymes, signs/symptoms of bleeding
Icosapent ethyl (Vascepa)	▪ Multifactorial ▪ Reduced hepatic VLDL TGs synthesis and/or secretion ▪ Enhances TG clearance ▪ Mechanism of action for cardiovascular event reduction is not fully understood	**SE**: musculoskeletal pain, peripheral edema, constipation, gout, atrial fibrillation, arthralgia, oropharyngeal pain ▪ Consider as adjunct to a maximally tolerated statin for cardiovascular risk reduction ▪ Consider as adjunct to diet to lower TGs in severe hypertriglyceridemia ▪ Fish allergy ▪ Monitor for risk of bleeding with anticoagulants and antiplatelets
FIBRIC ACID DERIVATIVES		
Fenofibrate (TriCor)	Down regulates apoprotein C-III; up regulates apolipoprotein A-I synthesis, fatty-acid transport protein, and lipoprotein lipase; increase in VLDL catabolism and elimination of TG-rich particles	**SE:** Increases liver enzymes (fenofibrate); dyspepsia (both agents, more common with gemfibrozil) ▪ Combination of fenofibrate with statins may lead to myopathy and rhabdomyolysis ▪ Administer gemfibrozil 30 min prior to meals
Gemfibrozil (Lopid)	Theorized to inhibit lipolysis and decrease hepatic fatty-acid uptake as well as inhibit hepatic secretion of VLDL	

Abbreviations used: ASA, aspirin; LDL, low-density lipoprotein; ER, extended release; GI, gastrointestinal; HDL, high-density lipoprotein; IR, immediate release; NPC1L1: Niemann-Pick C1 like 1; OTC, over the counter; PCSK9: proprotein convertase subtilisin/kexin type 9; Rx, prescription; SE, side effects; TG, triglycerides; UGT, UDP glucuronosyltransferase family 1 member A1; VLDL, very low-density lipoprotein.
Adapted from DiPiro J, Talbert R, Yee G, Matzke G, Wells B, Posey L. Dyslipidemia. In: *Pharmacotherapy: A Pathophysiologic Approach.* 8th ed. New York, NY: McGraw-Hill; 2011:365–388.

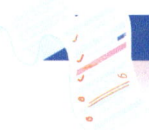

Table 10-15 Statin Intensity Classifications[20]

INTENSITY LEVEL	PERCENT REDUCTION IN LDL	STATIN
High	>50%	Atorvastatin 40–80 mg Rosuvastatin 20–40 mg
Moderate	30%–49%	Atorvastatin 10–20 mg Fluvastatin XL 80 mg Fluvastatin 40 mg BID Lovastatin 40–80 mg Pitavastatin 1–4 mg Pravastatin 40–80 mg Rosuvastatin 5–10 mg Simvastatin 20–40 mg
Low	<30%	Fluvastatin 20–40 mg Lovastatin 20 mg Pravastatin 10–20 mg Simvastatin 10 mg

Abbreviations used: LDL, low-density lipoprotein.

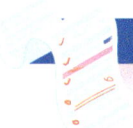

Table 10-16 Primary Prevention of Atherosclerotic Cardiovascular Disease[21,22]

PATIENT POPULATION	MANAGEMENT
Age 0–19	▪ Assess ASCVD risk ▪ Lifestyle changes to prevent or reduce ASCVD risk
Age 20–29	▪ Assess ASCVD risk ▪ Lifestyle changes to prevent or reduce ASCVD risk ▪ Consider statin if all 3 present: family history + premature ASCVD + LDL ≥160 mg/dL
Age 40–75 + LDL ≥70 to <190 mg/dL without DM	Calculate 10-y ASCVD risk and treat based on risk
LDL-C ≥190 mg/dL	No risk assessment necessary; start high-intensity statin
DM + Age 40–75	▪ Moderate-intensity statin (preferred) ▪ May perform ASCVD risk assessment to consider high-intensity statin
Age >75	Risk discussion + clinical assessment

RISK CATEGORY	MANAGEMENT
<5% = Low risk	Lifestyle changes to reduce risk factors
5–7.5% = Borderline risk	If risk enhancers present (see below)—discussion regarding moderate-intensity statin
≥7.5% to <20% = Intermediate risk	Risk discussion—if statin is favored due to risk estimate + risk enhancers, start moderate-intensity statin; decrease LDL by 30%–49%
≥20% = High risk	Start statin to decrease LDL ≥50%

Abbreviations used: ASCVD, atherosclerotic cardiovascular disease; DM, diabetes mellitus; LDL, low-density lipoprotein.
Adapted from Arnett DK, Blumenthal RS, Albert MA, et al. 2019 ACC/AHA Guideline on the Primary Prevention of Cardiovascular Disease: Executive Summary: A Report of the American College of Cardiology/American Heart Association Task Force on Clinical Practice Guidelines. *Circulation.* 2019;140(11):e563–e595; Grundy SM, Stone NJ, Bailey AL, et al. 2018 AHA/ACC/AACVPR/AAPA/ABC/ACPM/ADA/AGS/APhA/ASPC/NLA/PCNA Guideline on the Management of Blood Cholesterol: A Report of the American College of Cardiology/American Heart Association Task Force on Clinical Practice Guidelines. *J Am Coll Cardiol.* 2019;73(24):e285–e350.

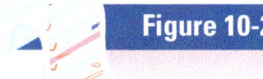
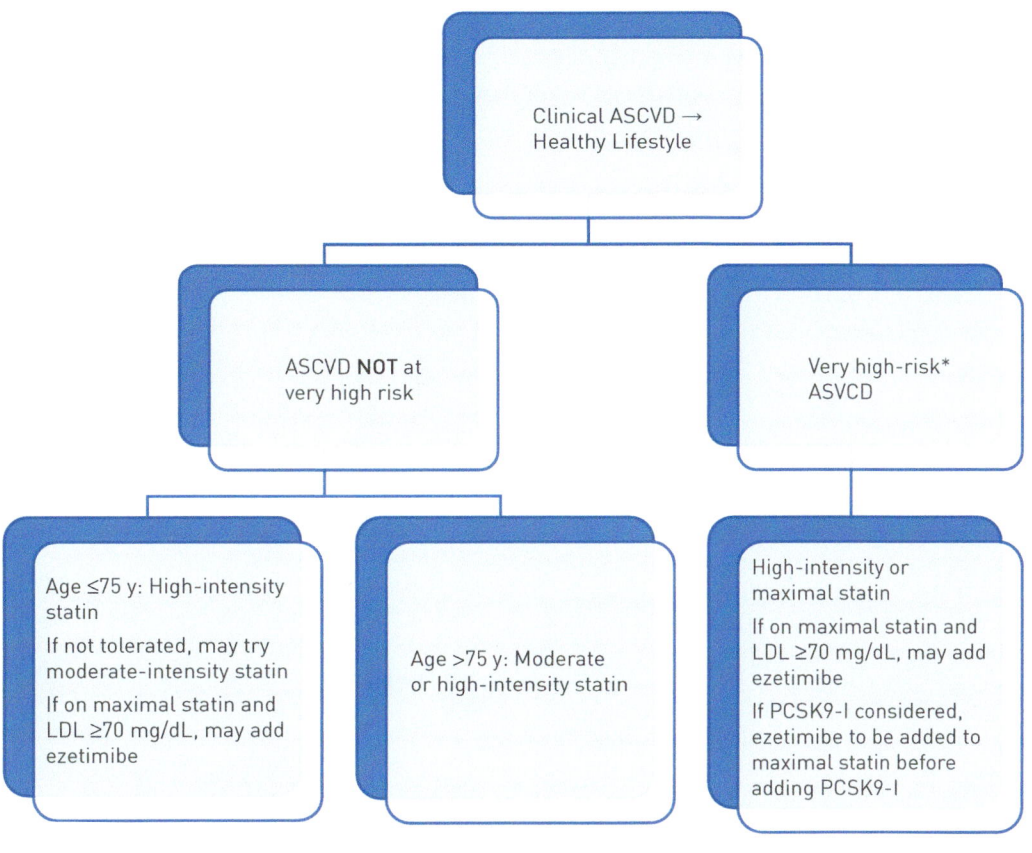

Abbreviations used: ASCVD, atherosclerotic cardiovascular disease; LDL, low-density lipoprotein, PCSK9: proprotein convertase subtilisin/kexin type 9.
*Very high-risk = History of multiple major ASCVD events OR 1 major ASCVD event + multiple high-risk conditions.

- Chronic kidney disease
- Metabolic syndrome
- Preeclampsia or premature menopause
- Inflammatory diseases (e.g., rheumatoid arthritis, HIV)
- South Asian ancestry
- Triglycerides persistently >175 mg/mL

Secondary prevention algorithm is depicted in Figure 10-2.

- Major ASCVD events:
  - ACS in the past 12 months
  - History of MI (other than ACS listed above)
  - History of ischemic stroke
  - Symptomatic peripheral artery disease

ADDITIONAL RESOURCES

Whelton PK, Carey RM, Aronow WS, et al. 2017 ACC/AHA/AAPA/ABC/ACPM/AGS/APhA/ASH/ASPC/NMA/PCNA guideline for the prevention, detection, evaluation, and management of high blood pressure in adults: a report of the American College of Cardiology/American Heart Association task force on clinical practice guidelines. *Hypertension.* 2018;71(6):e13–e115.

Yancy CW, Jessup M, Bozkurt B, et al. 2017 ACC/AHA/HFSA focused update of the 2013 ACCF/AHA guideline for the management of heart failure: a report of the American College of Cardiology/American Heart Association task force on clinical practice guidelines and the Heart Failure Society of America. *J Am Coll Cardiol.* 2017;70(6):776–803.

Powers WJ, Rabinstein AA, Ackerson T, et al. Guidelines for the early management of patients with acute ischemic stroke: 2019 update to the 2018 guidelines for the early management of acute ischemic stroke: a guideline for healthcare professionals from the American Heart Association/American Stroke Association. *Stroke.* 2019;50(12):e344–e418.

Arnett DK, Blumenthal RS, Albert MA, et al. 2019 ACC/AHA guideline on the primary prevention of cardiovascular disease: executive summary: a report of the American College of Cardiology/American Heart Association task force on clinical practice guidelines. *Circulation*. 2019;140(11):e563–e595.

Grundy SM, Stone NJ, Bailey AL, et al. 2018 AHA/ACC/AACVPR/AAPA/ABC/ACPM/ADA/AGS/APhA/ASPC/NLA/PCNA guideline on the management of blood cholesterol: a Report of the American College of Cardiology/American Heart Association task force on clinical practice guidelines. *J Am Coll Cardiol*. 2019;73(24):e285–e350.

REFERENCES

1. DiPiro J, Talbert R, Yee G, Matzke G, Wells B, Posey L. Hypertension. In: *Pharmacotherapy: A Pathophysiologic Approach*. McGraw-Hill; 2011:101–135.

2. Whelton PK, Carey RM, Aronow WS, et al. 2017 ACC/AHA/AAPA/ABC/ACPM/AGS/APhA/ASH/ASPC/NMA/PCNA Guideline for the Prevention, Detection, Evaluation, and Management of High Blood Pressure in Adults: A Report of the American College of Cardiology/American Heart Association Task Force on Clinical Practice Guidelines. *Hypertension*. 2018;71(6):e13–e115.

3. American Diabetes Association. Cardiovascular Disease and Risk Management: Standards of Medical Care in Diabetes-2020. *Diabetes Care*. 2020;43(Suppl 1):S111–S134.

4. James PA, Oparil S, Carter BL, et al. 2014 evidence-based guideline for the management of high blood pressure in adults: report from the panel members appointed to the Eighth Joint National Committee (JNC 8). *JAMA*. 2014;311(5):507–520.

5. National Heart Lung and Blood Institute. Coronary Heart Disease. https://www.nhlbi.nih.gov/health-topics/coronary-heart-disease. Published 2020. Accessed April 5, 2020.

6. DiPiro J, Talbert R, Yee G, Matzke G, Wells B, Posey L. Ischemic Heart Disease. In: *Pharmacotherapy: A Pathophysiologic Approach*. McGraw-Hill; 2011:209–240.

7. Fihn SD, Gardin JM, Abrams J, et al. 2012 ACCF/AHA/ACP/AATS/PCNA/SCAI/STS guideline for the diagnosis and management of patients with stable ischemic heart disease: executive summary: a report of the American College of Cardiology Foundation/American Heart Association task force on practice guidelines, and the American College of Physicians, American Association for Thoracic Surgery, Preventive Cardiovascular Nurses Association, Society for Cardiovascular Angiography and Interventions, and Society of Thoracic Surgeons. *Circulation*. 2012;126(25):3097–3137.

8. DiPiro J, Talbert R, Yee G, Matzke G, Wells B, Posey L. Acute Coronary Syndromes. In: *Pharmacotherapy: A Pathophysiologic Approach*. McGraw-Hill; 2011:241–271.

9. Amsterdam EA, Wenger NK, Brindis RG, et al. 2014 AHA/ACC Guideline for the Management of Patients With Non-ST-Elevation Acute Coronary Syndromes. *Circulation*. 2014;130(25):e344–e426.

10. O'Gara PT, Kushner FG, Ascheim DD, et al. 2013 ACCF/AHA Guideline for the Management of ST-Elevation Myocardial Infarction. *Circulation*. 2013;127(4):e362–e425.

11. DiPiro J, Talbert R, Yee G, Matzke G, Wells B, Posey L. Systolic Heart Failure. In: *Pharmacotherapy: A Pathophysiologic Approach*. McGraw-Hill; 2011:137–172.

12. Yancy CW, Jessup M, Bozkurt B, et al. 2013 ACCF/AHA Guideline for the Management of Heart Failure. *Circulation*. 2013;128(16):e240–e327.

13. DiPiro J, Talbert R, Yee G, Matzke G, Wells B, Posey L. The Arrhythmias. In: *Pharmacotherapy: A Pathophysiologic Approach*. McGraw-Hill; 2011:273–309.

14. January CT, Wann LS, Alpert JS, et al. 2014 AHA/ACC/HRS Guideline for the Management of Patients With Atrial Fibrillation. *Circulation*. 2014;130(23):e199–e267.

15. January CT, Wann LS, Calkins H, et al. 2019 AHA/ACC/HRS Focused Update of the 2014 AHA/ACC/HRS Guideline for the Management of Patients With Atrial Fibrillation: A Report of the American College of Cardiology/American Heart Association Task Force on Clinical Practice Guidelines and the Heart Rhythm Society in Collaboration With the Society of Thoracic Surgeons. *Circulation*. 2019;140(2):e125–e151.

16. Centers for Disease Control and Prevention. Stroke Facts. https://www.cdc.gov/stroke/facts.htm. Published 2020. Accessed April 9, 2020.

17. DiPiro J, Talbert R, Yee G, Matzke G, Wells B, Posey L. Stroke. In: *Pharmacotherapy: A Pathophysiologic Approach*. McGraw-Hill; 2011:353–364.

18. Powers WJ, Rabinstein AA, Ackerson T, et al. Guidelines for the Early Management of Patients With Acute Ischemic Stroke: 2019 Update to the 2018 Guidelines for the Early Management of Acute Ischemic Stroke: A Guideline for Healthcare Professionals From the American Heart Association/American Stroke Association. *Stroke*. 2019;50(12):e344–e418.

19. Powers WJ, Rabinstein AA, Ackerson T, et al. 2018 Guidelines for the Early Management of Patients With Acute Ischemic Stroke: A Guideline for Healthcare Professionals From the American Heart Association/American Stroke Association. *Stroke*. 2018;49(3):e46–e99.

20. DiPiro J, Talbert R, Yee G, Matzke G, Wells B, Posey L. Dyslipidemia. In: *Pharmacotherapy: A Pathophysiologic Approach*. McGraw-Hill; 2011:365–388.

21. Arnett DK, Blumenthal RS, Albert MA, et al. 2019 ACC/AHA Guideline on the Primary Prevention of Cardiovascular Disease: Executive Summary: A Report of the American College of Cardiology/American Heart Association Task Force on Clinical Practice Guidelines. *Circulation*. 2019;140(11):e563–e595.

22. Grundy SM, Stone NJ, Bailey AL, et al. 2018 AHA/ACC/AACVPR/AAPA/ABC/ACPM/ADA/AGS/APhA/ASPC/NLA/PCNA Guideline on the Management of Blood Cholesterol: A Report of the American College of Cardiology/American Heart Association Task Force on Clinical Practice Guidelines. *J Am Coll Cardiol*. 2019;73(24):e285–e350.

23. Campeau L. Letter: Grading of angina pectoris. *Circulation*. 1976;54(3):522–523.

24. Heart.Org. Classes of Heart Failure. https://www.heart.org/en/health-topics/heart-failure/what-is-heart-failure/classes-of-heart-failure. Published 2020. Accessed April 8, 2020.

25. Yancy CW, Jessup M, Bozkurt B, et al. 2017 ACC/AHA/HFSA Focused Update of the 2013 ACCF/AHA Guideline for the Management of Heart Failure: A Report of the American College of Cardiology/American Heart Association Task Force on Clinical Practice Guidelines and the Heart Failure Society of America. *J Am Coll Cardiol*. 2017;70(6):776–803.

26. DiPiro J, Talbert R, Yee G, Matzke G, Wells B, Posey L. Acute Decompensated Heart Failure. In: *Pharmacotherapy: A Pathophysiologic Approach*. McGraw-Hill; 2011:191–207.

27. Lei M, Wu L, Terrar DA, Huang CL. Modernized Classification of Cardiac Antiarrhythmic Drugs. *Circulation*. 2018;138(17):1879–1896.

28. Stroke.org. Stroke Symptoms. https://www.stroke.org/en/about-stroke/stroke-symptoms. Published 2020. Accessed April 9, 2020.

CHAPTER 11

Anticoagulation and Blood Disorders

With medical writing support provided by Banner Medical LLC Writers: Jennifer Miller and Miriam Opara

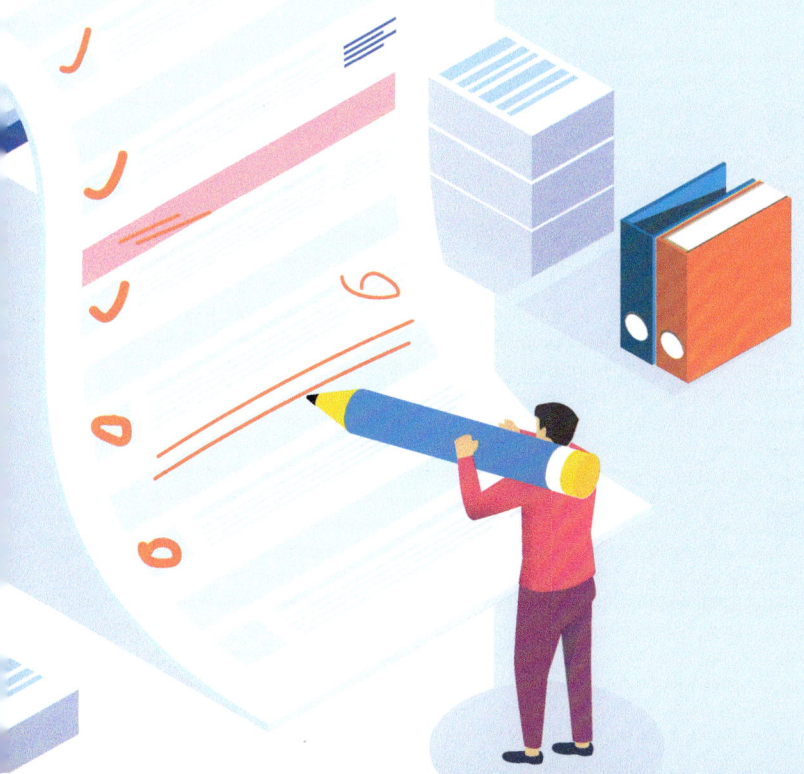

Anticoagulation

Anticoagulants are used to treat and prevent blood clots from forming and to keep existing clots from becoming larger.[1]

- Venous thromboembolism (VTE) is a blood clot that originates in a vein and can be classified as either
  - **Pulmonary embolism (PE):** a blood clot that travels through circulation to the arteries of the lungs
  - **Deep vein thrombosis (DVT):** a blood clot in a deep vein, typically in the legs, arms, or groin
- Coronary thrombosis is a blood clot inside the blood vessel of the heart that restricts blood flow within the heart (see Ch. 10 for more information).
- Anticoagulation is also used for stroke prevention with atrial fibrillation (see Ch. 10 for more information).

Coagulation is the process by which blood clots form. Virchow's Triad (stasis of the blood flow, hypercoagulability, endothelial injury) are the main factors that lead to the activation of the coagulation process.[1] The coagulation process involves the activation of platelets and the clotting cascade until fibrin is formed (see Figure 11-1).

Anticoagulants used for treatment and prophylaxis of VTE, blood clots in the heart, and stroke prophylaxis in patients with Afib are summarized in Tables 11-1 and 11-2.[1-4] Anticoagulation therapy is generally contraindicated in patients with active bleeding or a high risk of bleeding.

Interactions with warfarin:

- CYP **IN**hibitors can **IN**crease INR (e.g., rifampin)
- CYP In**DU**cers can **DE**crease INR (e.g., amiodarone)
- Antibiotics (e.g., macrolides, quinolones, penicillins, cephalosporins) can increase anticoagulant effect of warfarin

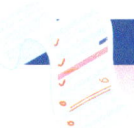

Figure 11-1 Coagulation Cascade[1]

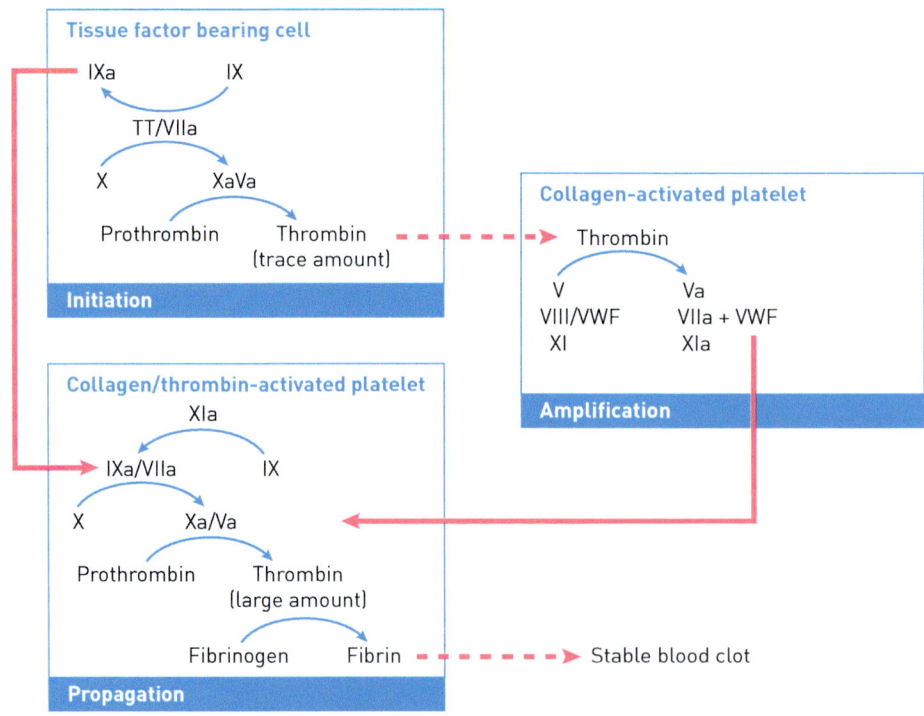

Adapted from: DiPiro J, Talbert R, Yee G, Matzke G, Wells B, Posey L. Venous thromboembolism. In: *Pharmacotherapy: A Pathophysiologic Approach.* 8th ed. New York, NY: McGraw-Hill; 2011:311–352.

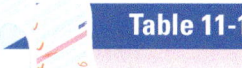

Table 11-1 Anticoagulant Agents: Indications and Dosing[1]

Drug agent	VTE prophylaxis dose	VTE treatment dose	ACS dose	Stroke prophylaxis with afib	Renal adjustment (CrCl in mL/min)
Unfractionated heparin					
Heparin IV Sub-Q	5000 units Q 8–12H	18 units/kg/hr	12–15 units/kg/hr	—	None
Low-molecular weight heparin					
Dalteparin (Fragmin) Sub-Q	2500–5000 units Q 24H	100 units/kg Q 12H or 200 units/kg Q 24H	—	—	None
Enoxaparin (Lovenox) Sub-Q	40 mg Q 24H or 30 mg Q 12H	1 mg/kg Q 12H or 1.5 mg/kg Q 24H	1 mg/kg Q 12H + aspirin		CrCl <30: 30 mg/day, 1 mg/kg/day
Direct thrombin inhibitor					
Dabigatran (Pradaxa) PO	150 mg BID	150 mg BID	—	150 mg BID	CrCl 15–30: 75 mg BID CrCl <15: avoid
Factor Xa inhibitors					
Apixaban (Eliquis) PO	2.5 mg BID	10 mg BID × 7 days, then 5 mg BID	—	5 mg BID ↓ dose to 2.5 mg if ≥ 2 below is present: ▪ SCr ≥ 1.5 mg/dL ▪ Weight ≤60 kg ▪ Age ≥ 80 y	None
Edoxaban (Savaysa) PO	—	<60 kg: 30 mg daily >60 kg: 60 mg daily	—	60 mg daily	CrCl <50: 30 mg/day CrCl <15: avoid CrCl >95: avoid
Fondaparinux (Arixtra) Sub-Q	2.5 mg Q 24H	50–100 kg: 7.5 mg daily >100 kg: 10 mg daily	—	—	CrCl <30: avoid
Rivaroxaban (Xarelto) PO	20 mg daily	15 mg BID × 21 days, then 20 mg daily	—	20 mg daily	VTE: CrCl < 30: avoid Afib: CrCl 15–50: 15 mg/day
Vitamin K antagonist					
Warfarin (Coumadin) PO	Based on INR; initiate 5–10 mg daily	Based on INR	Based on INR	Based on INR	None

Abbreviations used: ACS, acute coronary syndrome; Afib, atrial fibrillation; BID, twice daily; CrCl, creatinine clearance; INR, international normalized ratio; IV, intravenous; Sub-Q, subcutaneous; SCr, serum creatinine; VTE, venous thromboembolism.

Table 11-2   Anticoagulant Agents: Clinical Considerations[1]

DRUG AGENT	LAB MONITOR	DDI	ANTIDOTE	NOTES
UNFRACTIONATED HEPARIN				
Heparin IV Sub-Q	Monitor PLT for HIT Monitor aPTT Q 6h	—	Protamine	**SE:** increased bleeding, necrosis, hyperkalemia
LOW-MOLECULAR WEIGHT HEPARIN				
Dalteparin (Fragmin) Sub-Q	Monitor PLT for HIT	—	Protamine	**SE:** increased bleeding, necrosis
Enoxaparin (Lovenox) Sub-Q	Monitor PLT for HIT	Caution with P-gp inhibitors and inducers	Protamine	Do not expel air bubbles **SE:** increased bleeding, necrosis
DIRECT THROMBIN INHIBITOR				
Dabigatran (Pradaxa) PO	None	Avoid with P-gp inducers	Idarucizumab	Do not chew, break, or open capsules
FACTOR Xa INHIBITORS				
Apixaban (Eliquis) PO	None	Caution with P-gp and 3A4 inhibitors	Andexanet, PCC	Not recommended with liver impairment
Edoxaban (Savaysa) PO	None	Avoid with P-gp inhibitors	Andexanet, PCC	Take with or without food
Fondaparinux (Arixtra) Sub-Q	None	—	Andexanet, PCC	May be used in HIT **SE:** increased bleeding, necrosis
Rivaroxaban (Xarelto) PO	None	Avoid with strong P-gp and 3A4 inhibitors	Andexanet, PCC	▪ Take with food ▪ If missed dose: take immediately ▪ May crush tablets
VITAMIN K ANTAGONIST				
Warfarin (Coumadin) PO	Monitor INR	See below	Vitamin K	▪ Goal INR 2–3 or 2.5–3.5 with mechanical heart valve ▪ Inhibits factors II, VII, IX, X (factor II has the longest half-life). ▪ Can use with prosthetic heart valve

Abbreviations used: DDI, drug–drug interaction; HIT, heparin-induced thrombocytopenia; INR, international normalized ratio; IV, intravenous; PCC, prothrombin complex concentrate; PLT, platelets; SE: side effect; Sub-Q, subcutaneous; VTE, venous thromboembolism

- Increased bleeding risk: antacids, cold and allergy medication, NSAIDs, anticoagulants, antiplatelet agents
- Food interactions (not all-inclusive): alcohol, high vitamin K, garlic, ginseng, gingko, grapefruit, green leafy vegetables, green tea

Initiating warfarin requires INR monitoring every 1–3 days until patient is stable. Afterward, INR monitoring interval may be gradually increased to weekly, biweekly, and then monthly if stable. If patients begin new medications, change diet habits, or develop conditions that alter INR, additional monitoring is necessary until resolution of the problem or a new warfarin dose is found to provide stability. The likelihood of bleeding increases with higher INR levels; therefore, maintaining INR within the target range is important to reduce the risk of bleeding.

Adjusting warfarin doses in patients who are not actively bleeding, based on INR levels:[5]

- INR outside of range by ≤0.3: recheck in 1–2 weeks (adjust if persistent)
- INR 4.5–10: withhold dose and measure INR again
- INR >10: 2.5 mg of oral vitamin K

Conversion from warfarin to another oral anticoagulant: stop warfarin and convert to (**READ**)[5]

Rivaroxaban when INR is <3
Edoxaban when INR is ≤2.5
Apixaban when INR is <2
Dabigatran when INR is <2

Patients at high risk of thromboembolism (e.g., DVT or PE in last month, atrial fibrillation, and mechanical heart valve) may require bridge therapy. Bridge therapy has been associated with increased risk of bleeding, so the decision to bridge should be individualized based on risk factors. Bridge therapy with a parenteral anticoagulant is required to allow time for warfarin to reach steady state. Combination anticoagulation is continued for a minimum of 5 days, and INR is therapeutic for 2 consecutive INRs.[5]

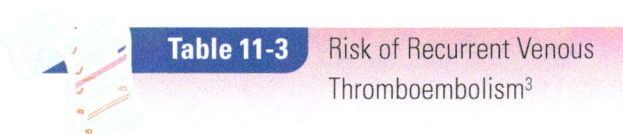

Table 11-3	Risk of Recurrent Venous Thromboembolism[3]	
HIGH	**MODERATE**	**LOW**
VTE within past 3 mo	VTE within previous 3–12 mo	Previous VTE >12 mo prior + no other risk factors
Deficiency of protein C or S or antithrombin	Heterozygous factor V Leiden	
Antiphospholipid antibody syndrome	Prothrombin 20210 mutation	
Multiple thrombophilic abnormalities	Recurrent VTE	
	Active cancer	

Abbreviations used: VTE, venous thromboembolism.
Adapted from Witt DM, Nieuwlaat R, Clark NP, et al. American Society of Hematology 2018 guidelines for management of venous thromboembolism: optimal management of anticoagulation therapy. *Blood Advances.* 2018; 2(22):3257–3291.

If low-to-moderate risk (based on Table 11-3) plus invasive procedure where vitamin K antagonist (VKA) therapy interruption is required, there is no need to bridge peri-procedurally; interruption of VKA is adequate.[1-4] Risk of recurrent VTE when prophylaxis treatment is interrupted for invasive procedures is categorized in Table 11-3.

Management summary/key points[1-4]

- Duration of anticoagulants for VTE treatment, bioprosthetic valve replacement—3 months
- Duration of anticoagulants for unprovoked or recurrent VTE, mechanical valve replacement, atrial fibrillation—indefinite

Anemia

Anemia is characterized by the decreased oxygen-carrying capacity of the blood, typically caused by a

| **Table 11-4** | Lab Findings Seen in Various Types of Anemia[6] |

PARAMETER	B[12] DEFICIENCY	FOLIC ACID DEFICIENCY	IRON DEFICIENCY	CHRONIC DISEASE
Hemoglobin	Decreased	Decreased	Decreased	Decreased
Mean cell volume	Increased	Increased	Decreased	Decreased or no change
Reticulocyte count	Decreased	Decreased	Decreased	Decreased
Red blood cell size	Macrocytic	Macrocytic	Microcytic	Normocytic

Adapted from DiPiro J, Talbert R, Yee G, Matzke G, Wells B, Posey L. Anemias. In: *Pharmacotherapy: A Pathophysiologic Approach*. 8th ed. New York, NY: McGraw-Hill; 2011:1717–1740.

decrease in hemoglobin (Hgb) or volume of red blood cells (RBCs).[6,7]

- Anemia is defined by the World Health Organization as
  - Hgb <12 g/dL in women
  - Hgb <13 g/dL in men

Pertinent lab tests when evaluating anemia include complete blood count, RBC indices, iron studies, and tests such as folic acid and vitamin B[12]. Mean corpuscular volume[8] reflects the size or average volume of RBCs and can help determine the type of anemia and the possible underlying cause, which is essential for choosing the appropriate treatment. The common types of anemia are diagnosed based on lab values (see Table 11-4).

Clinical presentation may be asymptomatic, but lack of oxygen leads to fatigue, dizziness, weakness, and tachycardia. Neurological symptoms can be present with vitamin B[12] deficiency.[6] The management of anemia is dependent on the etiology and presentation (see Table 11-5).

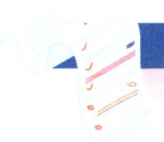

| **Table 11-5** | Management of Various Types of Anemias[6,9] |

ANEMIA	MANAGEMENT
Cyanocobalamin (B[12]) deficiency	Oral, parenteral (intramuscular), nasal administrations of B[12] formulations
	▪ Oral: 1000–2000 mcg daily for 1–2 w; 1000 mcg daily for maintenance
	▪ Intramuscular (cyanocobalamin): 100 mcg daily × 1 w; alternate days × 7 doses every 3–4 d × 2–3 w monthly for maintenance
	▪ Intranasal: 500 mcg in 1 nostril once weekly
	▪ Dietary sources
	Note: B[12] and folic acid supplementation commonly given together
Folic acid deficiency	Exogenous oral administration of folic acid
	▪ Folic acid 1–5 mg daily
Iron deficiency	Iron replacement with oral or parenteral administration of iron products (see Table 11-6)
Chronic kidney disease	Oral/parenteral iron replacement and erythropoietin stimulating agents (see Table 11-7)

Adapted from DiPiro J, Talbert R, Yee G, Matzke G, Wells B, Posey L. Anemias. In: *Pharmacotherapy: A Pathophysiologic Approach*. 8th ed. New York, NY: McGraw-Hill; 2011:1717–1740; Short MW, Domagalski M. Iron deficiency anemia: evaluation and management. *Am Fam Physician*. 2013;87(2):98–104.

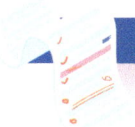

Table 11-6 — Oral and Parenteral Iron Preparations[6,9–14]

Iron product	Notes
Oral preparations	
Ferrous fumarate 33% elemental iron	324 mg (106 mg elemental iron) tablets in up to 3 divided doses
Ferrous gluconate 12% elemental iron	324 mg (38 mg elemental iron) or 240 mg (27 mg elemental iron) } in up to 3 divided doses
Ferrous sulfate 20% elemental iron	325 mg (65 mg elemental iron) in up to 3 divided doses
Parenteral preparations	
Ferric carboxymaltose (Injectafer)	Treatment course: 2 doses of 750 mg
Ferric gluconate (Ferrlecit)	Treatment course: typically 8 doses for total dose of 1000 mg
Ferumoxytol (Feraheme)	▪ Test dose required ▪ Treatment course: typically 2 doses of 510 mg
Iron dextran (Infed)	▪ Black box warning for anaphylactic-type reactions ▪ Test dose required
Iron sucrose (Venofer)	▪ Treatment course: typically up to 10 doses in dialysis patients ▪ Treatment is divided into 3 doses in nondialysis patients

Adapted from DiPiro J, Talbert R, Yee G, Matzke G, Wells B, Posey L. Anemias. In: *Pharmacotherapy: A Pathophysiologic Approach.* 8th ed. New York, NY: McGraw-Hill; 2011:1717–1740; Short MW, Domagalski M. Iron Deficiency Anemia: Evaluation and Management. *Am Fam Physician.* 2013;87(2):98–104; Injectafer [package insert]. Shirley, NY: American Regent; 2020; Feraheme [package insert]. Waltham, MA: AMAG Pharmaceuticals, Inc.; 2018; Infed [package insert]. Madison, NJ: Allergan USA, Inc.; 2018; Venofer [package insert]. Shirley, NY: American Regent, Inc.; 2000; Ferrlecit [package insert]. Bridgewater, NJ: Sanofi-Aventis, LLC.; 2011.

Table 11-7 — Erythropoietic Stimulating Agents for Anemia of Chronic Disease[6,15–17]

ESA agent	Notes
Darbepoetin alfa (Aranesp)	▪ CKD HD: 0.45 mcg/kg IV or Sub-Q weekly ▪ CKD non-HD: 0.45 mcg/kg IV or Sub-Q Q4W ▪ IV route preferred in dialysis patients ▪ Half-life is 3-fold longer than epoetin alfa
Epoetin alfa (Epogen, Procrit)	▪ CKD: 50–100 units/kg IV or Sub-Q 3x/w ▪ Titrate dose up or down based on Hgb levels; do NOT increase dose more frequently than once Q4W

Abbreviations used: CKD, chronic kidney disease; HD, hemodialysis; Hgb, hemoglobin; IV, intravenous; Sub-Q, subcutaneously; Q4W, every 4 weeks.
Adapted from DiPiro J, Talbert R, Yee G, Matzke G, Wells B, Posey L. Anemias. In: *Pharmacotherapy: A Pathophysiologic Approach.* 8th ed. New York, NY: McGraw-Hill; 2011:1717–1740; Short MW, Domagalski M. Iron Deficiency Anemia: Evaluation and Management. *Am Fam Physician.* 2013;87(2):98–104.

Table 11-6 outlines oral and intravenous iron preparations.

Remember:

- Oral preparations are available OTC or with a prescription
- Common side effects of iron products include constipation, dark stools, and stomach pain
- Iron absorption may decrease with food; iron absorption is best if taken 1 hour before or 2 hours after meals

Table 11-7 outlines ESA agents for treatment of anemia of chronic disease.

Remember:

- Contraindications: uncontrolled hypertension, pure red cell aplasia after initiating erythropoiesis-stimulating agent
- Side effects: bone pain, fever, headache, rash, dyspnea, dizziness

- Monitor: hemoglobin monthly, TStat and ferritin every 3 months
- Dosing recommendations for CKD anemia:
  - Initiate if Hgb <10 g/dL and decrease dose or stop if Hgb ≥11 g/dL
  - If 1 g/dL increase in Hgb not seen after 4 weeks, increase dose by 25%
  - If Hgb increases by >1 g/dL in a 2-week period, decrease dose by ≥25%

Sickle cell disease

Sickle cell disease (SCD) is an autosomal recessive disorder caused by the hemoglobin gene defect in one of the hemoglobin beta chains.[18] Sickle cell hemoglobin has a 20-day life cycle, and the sickled blood cells impair circulation and cause stasis of blood flow. Hemolysis and vaso-occlusive disease are clinical hallmark manifestations of SCD; complications include fever, infection, neurologic symptoms, acute chest syndrome, and priapism.[18]

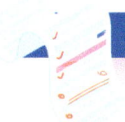

Table 11-8	Sickle Cell Management[18,19]	

INTERVENTION	TREATMENT	PLACE IN THERAPY
Immunizations	Pneumococcal (PCV13 or PPSV23) Hib Meningococcal	Disease prevention
Antibiotic	Penicillin prophylaxis BID until age 5	Reduces risk of death from pneumococcal infection
Analgesics	NSAIDs and APAP	Mild-to-moderate pain
	Opioids (PCA)	Severe pain and vaso-occlusive crisis
Disease-modifying agent	Hydroxyurea	Increases HgbF levels
		Reduces frequency of acute pain crisis
		Clinical response may take 3–6 mo
Amino acid	L-Glutamine	Reduces acute complications of SCD

Abbreviations used: APAP, acetaminophen; BID, twice daily; HgbF, hemoglobin F; Hib, *Haemophilus Influenzae* type B; NSAID, nonsteroidal anti-inflammatory drug; PCA, patient-controlled analgesia; PCV, pneumococcal conjugate vaccine; PPSV, pneumococcal polysaccharide vaccine; RBC, red blood cell; SCD, sickle cell disease.
Adapted from[1] DiPiro J, Talbert R, Yee G, Matzke G, Wells B, Posey L. Sickle Cell Disease. In: *Pharmacotherapy: A Pathophysiologic Approach.* 8th ed. New York, NY: McGraw-Hill; 2011:1765–1780; Yawn BP, Buchanan GR, Afenyi-Annan AN, et al. Management of Sickle Cell Disease: Summary of the 2014 Evidence-Based Report by Expert Panel Members. *Jama.* 2014;312(10):1033–1048.

Management of SCD involves multiple components for health maintenance, pain management, and management of acute and chronic complications (e.g., increased risk of fever, infection, stroke, acute chest syndrome). Table 11-8 describes the key therapies for SCD.

ADDITIONAL RESOURCES

DiPiro J, Talbert R, Yee G, Matzke G, Wells B, Posey L. Venous thromboembolism. In: *Pharmacotherapy: A Pathophysiologic Approach*. 8th ed. McGraw-Hill; 2011:311–352.

Kearon C, Akl EA, Ornelas J, et al. Antithrombotic therapy for VTE disease: CHEST guideline and expert panel report. *Chest*. 2016;149(2):315–352.

DiPiro J, Talbert R, Yee G, Matzke G, Wells B, Posey L. Anemias. In: *Pharmacotherapy: A Pathophysiologic Approach*. 8th ed. McGraw-Hill; 2011:1717–1740.

DiPiro J, Talbert R, Yee G, Matzke G, Wells B, Posey L. Sickle Cell Disease. In: *Pharmacotherapy: A Pathophysiologic Approach*. 8th ed. McGraw-Hill; 2011:1765–1780.

REFERENCES

1. DiPiro J, Talbert R, Yee G, Matzke G, Wells B, Posey L. Venous thromboembolism. In: *Pharmacotherapy: A Pathophysiologic Approach*. 8th ed. New York, NY: McGraw-Hill; 2011:311–352.

2. Kearon C, Akl EA, Ornelas J, et al. Antithrombotic therapy for VTE disease: CHEST guideline and expert panel report. *Chest*. 2016;149(2):315–352.

3. Witt DM, Nieuwlaat R, Clark NP, et al. American Society of Hematology 2018 guidelines for management of venous thromboembolism: optimal management of anticoagulation therapy. *Blood Advances*. 2018;2(22):3257–3291.

4. Kearon C, Akl EA, Comerota AJ, et al. Antithrombotic therapy for VTE disease: antithrombotic therapy and prevention of thrombosis, 9th ed: American College of Chest Physicians evidence-based clinical practice guidelines. *Chest*. 2012;141(suppl 2): e419S–e496S.

5. Witt DM, Clark NP, Kaatz S, Schnurr T, Ansell JE. Guidance for the practical management of warfarin therapy in the treatment of venous thromboembolism. *J Thromb Thrombolysis*. 2016; 41(1):187–205.

6. DiPiro J, Talbert R, Yee G, Matzke G, Wells B, Posey L. Anemias. In: *Pharmacotherapy: A Pathophysiologic Approach*. 8th ed. New York, NY: McGraw-Hill; 2011:1717–1740.

7. World Health Organization. Worldwide prevalence of Anaemia 1993–2005. Available at: https://apps.who.int/iris/bitstream/handle/10665/43894/9789241596657_eng.

8. Burnett AL, Nehra A, Breau RH, et al. Erectile dysfunction: AUA guideline. *J Urol*. 2018;200(3):633–641.

9. Short MW, Domagalski M. Iron deficiency anemia: evaluation and management. *Am Fam Physician*. 2013;87(2):98–104.

10. Injectafer [package insert]. Shirley, NY: American Regent; 2020.

11. Feraheme [package insert]. Waltham, MA: AMAG Pharmaceuticals, Inc.; 2018.

12. Infed [package insert]. Madison, NJ: Allergan USA, Inc.; 2018.

13. Venofer [package insert]. Shirley, NY: American Regent, Inc.; 2000.

14. Ferrlecit [package insert]. Bridgewater, NJ: Sanofi-Aventis, LLC.; 2011.

15. Aranesp [package insert]. Thousand Oaks, CA: Amgen, Inc.; 2011.

16. Epogen [package insert]. Thousand Oaks, CA: Amgen, Inc.; 2018.

17. DiPiro J, Talbert R, Yee G, Matzke G, Wells B, Posey L. Chronic kidney disease: management of complications. In: *Pharmacotherapy: A Pathophysiologic Approach*. 8th ed. New York, NY: McGraw-Hill; 2011:787–816.

18. DiPiro J, Talbert R, Yee G, Matzke G, Wells B, Posey L. Sickle cell disease. In: *Pharmacotherapy: A Pathophysiologic Approach*. 8th ed. New York, NY: McGraw-Hill; 2011:1765–1780.

19. Yawn BP, Buchanan GR, Afenyi-Annan AN, et al. Management of sickle cell disease: summary of the 2014 evidence-based report by expert panel members. *Jama*. 2014;312(10):1033–1048.

CHAPTER 12

Respiratory Conditions

With medical writing support provided by
Banner Medical LLC Writer: Miriam Opara
and Tomasz Jurga

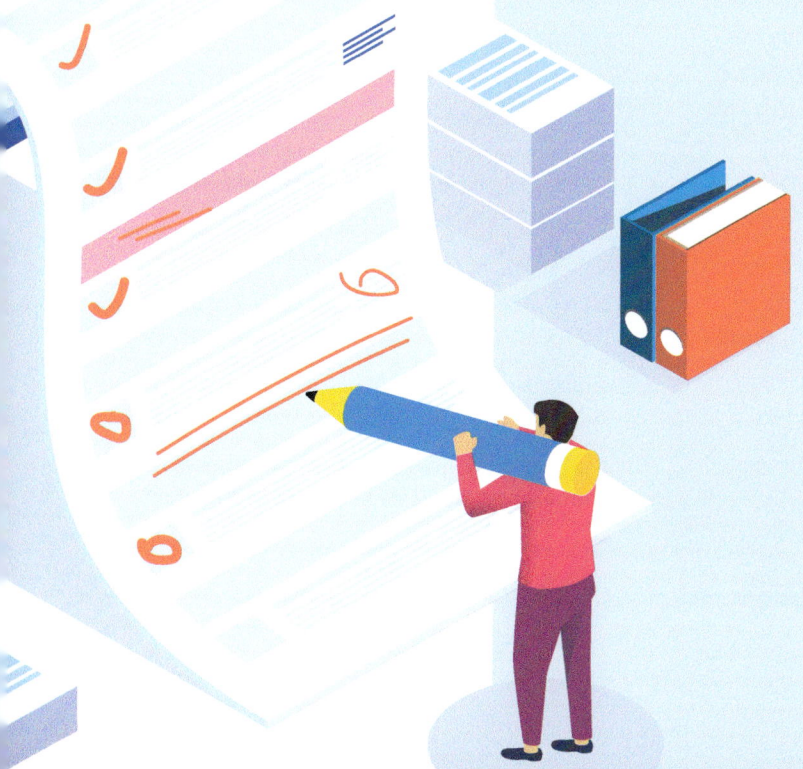

Pulmonary arterial hypertension

Pulmonary arterial hypertension (PAH) is mean pulmonary arterial pressure of ≥25 mmHg at rest.[1] PAH is due to a progressive narrowing of distal pulmonary arteries, which increases pulmonary arterial pressure and strains the right ventricle walls. Symptoms include fatigue, dyspnea, chest pain, edema, and tachycardia.[1]

Presentation of symptoms—begin treatment with calcium channel blockers (see Table 12-1)[1,2]

- If no response to calcium channel blockers—add vasodilating drugs to reduce symptoms and increase exercise tolerance
- If on a sodium-restricted diet (<2.4 grams/day)—manage volume, routine influenza and pneumococcal immunizations, and oxygen (as needed) to maintain saturation above 90%[1,2]

Asthma

Asthma is a clinical syndrome related to underlying inflammation of the airway, lumen wall thickening, increased mucus, bronchoconstriction, and airway hyperresponsiveness. It is classified as an obstructive disease in which there may be little to no interference with inspiration and resulting in decreased expiration.[3,4]

- Symptomatology may include wheezing, shortness of breath, chest tightness, and cough
- Common triggers: viral infections, allergens (e.g., dust mites), tobacco smoke, noxious chemicals, exercise, stress, and medications

Diagnosis requires a detailed medical history, physical exam, and is confirmed with spirometry. Other tests may be used as indicated to guide therapy (e.g., blood eosinophilia, serum IgE).[3,4] Asthma is reversible but may become irreversible if damage to the lung tissue occurs as a result of remodeling.

Remember: 12% reversibility rule—forced expiratory volume in 1 second (FEV1) increases by >200 mL and >12% of baseline (children: FEV1 increases from

Table 12-1 Treatment for Pulmonary Arterial Hypertension[1,2]

TREATMENT	DRUG AGENT	NOTES
Calcium channel blockers	Amlodipine (Norvasc) Diltiazem (Cardizem) Nifedipine (Procardia)	**SE:** Tachycardia, edema, headache, constipation **Remember:** Avoid with HFrEF
Prostacyclin analogs and receptor agonists	Epoprostenol (Flolan) Iloprost (Ventavis) Selexipag (Uptravi) Treprostinil (Tyvaso)	**SE:** Vasodilation reaction, edema, tachycardia **Remember:** ■ Avoid interruption of therapy (short half-life) ■ Decrease dose gradually if SE occur
Endothelin receptor antagonists	Ambrisentran (Letairis) Bosentan (Tracleer) Macitentan (Opsumit)	**CI:** Pregnancy **Remember:** Available through REMS program
Phosphodiesterase-5 inhibitors	Sildenafil (Revatio) Tadalafil (Adcirca)	**CI:** Used with nitrates or riociguat **SE:** Headache, flushing, N/D, priapism, hypotension
Soluble guanylate cyclase stimulator	Riociguat (Adempas)	**CI:** Pregnancy, use with nitrates or PDE-5 inhibitors **Remember:** Available through REMS program

Abbreviations used: CI, contraindicated; HFrEF, heart failure with reduced ejection fraction; N/D, nausea, diarrhea; PDE-5, phosphodiesterase-5; REMS, risk evaluation and mitigation strategies; SE, side effects.

baseline by 12% of the predicted value) after bronchodilator inhalation.[5]

Classification of asthma severity determines the initial treatment (or stepwise approach) for asthma management. Table 12-2 outlines the severity components assessed when classifying asthma severity for individuals ≥12 years of age recommended by the National Heart, Lung, and Blood Institute Expert Panel-3 (NHLBI EPR-3) guidelines.[4]

Follow up is recommended 2–6 weeks after initial evaluation. At this time an assessment of asthma control should be performed.

The NHLBI EPR-3 and the Global Institute for Asthma (GINA) guidelines drive recommendations for the treatment of asthma.[4,5] Both guidelines are very similar with slight differences in the classification of asthma. The treatment of asthma should be personalized; however, general principles include reducing impairment (e.g., frequency of symptoms and short-acting beta-2 agonist [SABA] use, activity limitations) and risk of exacerbations, hospitalizations, medication side effects, and loss of lung function.[4,5]

Personalized management of asthma is based on three components:[5]

- **Assess** symptom control and modifiable risk factors (including lung function), inhaler technique and adherence, comorbidities, and patient preference
- **Adjust** step-up or step-down therapy, treat modifiable risk factors, use of nonpharmacologic strategies, education, and skills training
- **Review** symptoms, exacerbations, side effects, lung function, and patient satisfaction

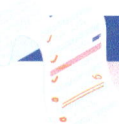

Table 12-2 National Heart, Lung, and Blood Institute Expert Panel-3 Classification of Asthma Severity and Treatment Initiation in Individuals ≥12 Years[13]

		CLASSIFICATION OF ASTHMA SEVERITY		
		PERSISTENT		
COMPONENTS OF SEVERITY	INTERMITTENT	MILD	MODERATE	SEVERE
IMPAIRMENT				
Symptoms	≤2 d/wk	>2 d/wk, but not daily	Daily	Throughout the day
Nighttime awakenings	≤2x/mo	3-4x/mo	>1x/wk but not nightly	Often (7x/wk)
SABA use	≤2 d/wk	>2 d/wk, but not daily and not >1x/day	Daily	Several times per day
Activity limitations	None	Minor	Some	Extreme
FEV1	>80%	>80%	60%–80%	<60%
FEV1/FVC	Normal	Normal	Reduced 5%	Reduced 5%
RISK				
Exacerbations requiring oral systemic corticosteroids*	0–1/y	≥2/y	≥2/y	≥2/y
STEPS FOR INITIATING THERAPY				
(Table 12-4 outlines stepwise approach algorithm)	Step 1	Step 2	Step 3	Step 4 or 5
				Consider short course oral-systemic steroid
	In 2–6 wk, depending on severity, assess the level of asthma control and adjust therapy as needed.			

Abbreviations used: FEV1, forced expiratory volume in 1 second; FVC, forced vital capacity; SABA, short-acting beta-2 agonist.
*Consider severity and interval since last exacerbation; frequency and severity may fluctuate over time.
Adapted from National Asthma Education and Prevention Program. Expert Panel Report 3 (EPR-3): Guidelines for the Diagnosis and Management of Asthma - Summary Report 2007. *J Allergy Clin Immunol.* 2007;120(suppl 5):s94-s138. doi:10.1016/j.jaci.2007.09.043. Published correction appears in *J Allergy Clin Immunol.* 2007;121(6):1330; National Asthma Education and Prevention Program: Expert Panel Report 3 (EPR-3): Guidelines for the Diagnosis and Management of Asthma - Summary Report 2007. *J Allergy Clin Immunol.* 2007;120(suppl 5):s94–s138.

Drug therapy consists of rescue and maintenance therapies. Although agents come in oral, injectable, and inhaled formulations, inhaled therapies are preferred because they work directly at the site of action and reduce the risk of toxicity.

Remember:

- All patients should have a rescue inhaler for as-needed relief of breakthrough symptoms and prevention of exercise-induced bronchoconstriction.
  - Use of rescue inhaler >2 days a week for symptom relief indicates inadequate control.

- Both NHLBI EPR-3 and GINA recommend a step approach for management of asthma and the use of a rescue inhaler (e.g., albuterol or levalbuterol) for intermittent or exercise-induced asthma symptoms.[4,5]
  - GINA guidelines recommend the use of an as-needed low-dose inhaled corticosteroid (ICS) plus formoterol as an alternative to a SABA for rescue therapy.

Table 12-3 compares the stepwise approach of NHLBI EPR-3 and GINA for the treatment of individuals ≥12 years of age and older.[4–6]

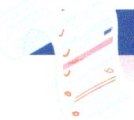

Table 12-3 Comparison of National Heart, Lung, and Blood Institute Expert Panel-3 and Global Initiative for Asthma Stepwise Approach for Treatment of Asthma in Individuals ≥12 Years[5,6,13,14]

PURPOSE	GUIDELINE	STEP 1[a]	STEP 2[b]	STEP 3[b]	STEP 4[b]	STEP 5[b]	STEP 6[b]
Rescue	EPR-3	SABA prn					
	GINA	Low-dose ICS + FOR[c] prn OR SABA prn					
Controller	EPR-3	None	Low-dose ICS[d]	Low-dose ICS + LABA OR Med-dose ICS[e]	Med-dose ICS + LABA[f]	High-dose ICS + LABA AND OMAL[g]	High-dose ICS + LABA + oral STER AND OMAL[g]
	GINA	None	Low-dose ICS	Low-dose ICS + LABA	Med-dose ICS + LABA; High-dose ICS + LABA; Add TIOT	Consider OMAL; Consider MEPO; Add TIOT; Add low-dose oral STER	

Abbreviations used: EPR-3, National Heart, Lung, and Blood Institute Expert Panel-3; FOR, formoterol; GINA, Global Initiative for Asthma; ICS, inhaled corticosteroid; LABA, long-acting beta-2 agonist; LTRA, leukotriene receptor antagonist; MEOP, mepolizumab; OMAL, omalizumab; SABA, short-acting beta-2 agonist; STER, corticosteroid; TIOT, tiotropium.
[a]Intermittent asthma
[b]Persistent asthma
[c]Not approved therapy combination within the U.S. for rescue therapy
[d]Alternative: LTRA, theophylline, or cromolyn
[e]Alternative: LTRA, theophylline, or zileuton
[f]Alternative: medium-dose ICS + LTRA, theophylline, or zileuton
[g]Consider omalizumab in patients who have allergies
Adapted from National Asthma Education and Prevention Program: Expert Panel Report 3 (EPR-3): Guidelines for the Diagnosis and Management of Asthma - Summary Report 2007. *J Allergy Clin Immunol.* 2007;120(suppl 5):s94–s138; Global Initiative for Asthma. Global Strategy for Asthma Management and Prevention. Available at: https://ginasthma.org/wp-content/uploads/2020/06/GINA-2020-report_20_06_04-1-wms.pdf. Accessed April 26, 2020; National Heart Lung and Blood Institute. Asthma Care Quick Reference: Diagnosing and Managing Asthma. Available at: https://www.nhlbi.nih.gov/files/docs/guidelines/asthma_qrg.pdf. Accessed April 26, 2020; Hiday R, Abbott KD. *Asthma.* Vol 1. ACSAP2019.

- Step up if needed—assess symptom control and modifiable risk factors, comorbidities, inhaler technique and adherence, and patient preference
- Step down if possible—if asthma well controlled for at least 3 months

Remember:
- A low-dose ICS plus formoterol (a long-acting beta-2 agonist [LABA]) may be used as needed for acute asthma symptoms (maximum of 72 mcg/day of formoterol).
- Systemic oral corticosteroids are also used during exacerbations, for severe asthma, and to reduce the burden of disease.
- ICSs are first-line maintenance therapy for all patients with persistent asthma to reduce inflammation due to increased eosinophil count.
  - Inhaled LABAs are used in combination with ICSs for worsening asthma severity
    - NEVER use as monotherapy in asthma as LABAs do not address inflammation, only bronchodilation

Table 12-4 summarizes the pharmacologic therapies for the treatment of asthma. The primary strategies to control symptoms include[4]

- Adherence to controller and maintenance treatment
- Proper inhaler technique
- Reduction of environmental triggers

Chronic obstructive pulmonary disease

Chronic obstructive pulmonary disease (COPD) is an irreversible lung obstruction disease with progressive deterioration of lung function, increasing respiratory symptoms, and increased airflow limitations.[7] Symptoms may include dyspnea, cough, wheezing, and sputum production.

- Tobacco smoking is the main risk factor (others include air pollution, genetic factors, noxious exposure, age, asthma, chronic bronchitis, and infections)
- Diagnosis consists of differential and patient history and is confirmed through spirometry—post-bronchodilator FEV1/forced vital capacity <70%[7]

The Global Institute for Chronic Obstructive Lung Disease classification is presented in Figure 12-1.[7]

Remember:
- Influenza and pneumococcal vaccination lowers the risk of hospitalization and respiratory infections (see Ch. 6 for more information).[7,8]
- Pharmacologic therapy is reviewed in Table 12-5
  - Rescue short-acting bronchodilators should be prescribed to all patients for immediate symptom relief
  - Long-acting bronchodilators are preferred for maintenance therapy
    - Monotherapy—LABA or LAMA
    - Combination therapy—LABA+LAMA, LABA+ICS, or LABA+LAMA+ICS
  - In the most severe cases of COPD, roflumilast may be used; azithromycin is used with patients who formerly smoked for infection control and anti-inflammatory properties[7,8]
  - Oral corticosteroid or macrolide may be added to COPD action plan to reduce hospitalization and length of stay

Tobacco cessation

Tobacco use is a significant public health concern that can lead to cancer, heart disease, stroke, COPD, pregnancy complications, as well as complicate and exacerbate chronic health conditions.[9] Tobacco products include cigarettes, cigars, electronic cigarettes (vaping), hookah, and smokeless tobacco (i.e., snus or dip).[10]

Tobacco cessation is advised at every encounter with patients who smoke and those exposed to second-hand smoke. Nicotine dependence can create challenges for tobacco cessation and requires ongoing support. The treatment dose for nicotine dependence

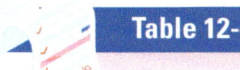

Table 12-4 Pharmacologic Treatments for Asthma[5]

TREATMENT	DRUG AGENT	DOSING			NOTES
Short-acting beta-2 agonists	Albuterol (ProAir HFA, Ventolin HFA, Proventil HFA)	1–2 inhalations Q4-6 h PRN			**SE:** Tremor, palpitations, cough, hyperglycemia **Remember:** Caution with CVD, glaucoma, diabetes, hyperthyroid, seizures
	Levalbuterol (Xopenex HFA)	1–2 inhalations Q4-6 h PRN			
Long-acting beta-2 agonists	Formoterol	1 capsule every 12 hours			**SE:** Nervousness, tremor, tachycardia, hypokalemia, cough **Remember:** NEVER use as monotherapy
	Salmeterol (Serevent)	1 inhalation BID			**BBW:** Increased risk of asthma-induced deaths ■ NEVER use as monotherapy
Long-acting muscarinic antagonists	Tiotropium (Spiriva Respimat)	2 inhalations daily			**SE:** Dry mouth, cough, urinary symptoms
		LOW DOSE	**MEDIUM DOSE**	**HIGH DOSE**	
Inhaled corticosteroids	Beclomethasone MDI (Qvar)	80–240 µg 1–4 inhalations BID	>240–480 µg	>480 µg	**CI:** Primary treatment of acute episodes of asthma **Remember:** Always rinse mouth after each use to prevent thrush. **MDI:** Slow and deep inhalation, spacer can be used, shake well **DPI:** Quick and forceful inhalation, spacer cannot be used, do not shake
	Budesonide DPI (Pulmicort Flexhaler)	180–540 µg 1–4 inhalations BID	>600–1080 µg	>1080 µg	
	Ciclesonide MDI (Alvesco)	160–320 µg 1–2 inhalations BID	>320–640 µg	>640 µg	
	Flunisolide MDI (Areobid)	320 µg 1 inhalation BID	320–640 µg	>640 µg	
	Fluticasone MDI (Flovent)	88–264 µg 2 inhalations BID	>264–440 µg	>440 µg	
	Fluticasone DPI (ArmonAir RespiClick, Arnuity Ellipta, Flovent Diskus)	100–300 µg 1–2 inhalations daily or BID	>300–500 µg	>500 µg	
	Mometasone MDI (Asmanex HFA)	200 µg 1–2 inhalations BID	400 µg	>400 µg	
	Mometasone DPI (Asmanex Twisthaler)	110–220 µg 1–2 inhalations daily	>220–440 µg	>440 µg	

Table 12-4 Pharmacologic Treatments for Asthma[5] (*Continued*)

TREATMENT	DRUG AGENT	DOSING	NOTES
		COMBINATION INHALERS	
ICS/LABA	Budesonide/ Formoterol MDI (Symbicort)	2 puffs BID	**Remember:** Rinse mouth after using to prevent fungal infections
	Fluticasone/ Salmeterol DPI (Advair Diskus, AirDuo RespiClick)	1 puff BID	
	Fluticasone/ Salmeterol MDI (Advair HFA)	2 puffs BID	
	Fluticasone/ Vilanterol DPI (Breo Ellipta)	1 puff daily	
	Mometasone/ Formoterol MDI (Dulera)	2 puffs BID	
Leukotriene receptor antagonist	Montelukast (Singulair)	▪ 10 mg QHS (adults) ▪ 4 mg and 5 mg QHS (pediatrics)	**SE:** Headache, dizziness, abdominal pain, increased LFTs **Remember:** ▪ BBW for neuropsychiatric events ▪ Only recommended for allergic asthma
Monoclonal antibody	Benralizumab (Fasenra)	30 mg SubQ every 4 wk for 3 doses, then every 8 wk	**BBW:** Anaphylaxis (administer in a health care setting) **Remember:** ▪ Used for severe allergic asthma ▪ Eosinophils predict therapeutic response
	Dupilumab (Dupixent)	300 mg SubQ every other wk	
	Mepolizumab (Nucala)	100 mg SubQ every 4 wk	
	Omalizumab (Xolair)	150–375 mg SubQ every 2–4 wk based on IgE count and weight	
	Reslizumab (Cinqair)	3 mg/kg IV every 4 wk	

Abbreviations used: BBW, black box warning; BID, twice daily; CI, contraindications; CVD, cardiovascular disease; DPI, dry-powdered inhaler; ICS, inhaled corticosteroid; IgE, immunoglobulin E; LABA, long-acting beta-2 agonist; LAMA, long-acting muscarinic antagonist; HFA, hydrofluoroalkane; LFT, liver function tests; LTRA, leukotriene receptor antagonist; MDI, metered-dose inhaler; PRN, as needed; Q, every; QHS, bedtime; SABA, short-acting beta-2 agonist; SE, side effects; SubQ, subcutaneously; µg, micrograms.

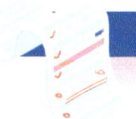

Grade	Severity	FEV1 (% predicted)
Gold 1	Mild	≥80%
Gold 2	Moderate	50%-79%
Gold 3	Severe	30%-49%
Gold 4	Very severe	<30%

	Group C	Group D
≥2 moderate exacerbations or ≥1 leading to hospitalization	LAMA	LAMA + LABA or LABA + ICS
0 or 1 moderate exacerbations not leading to hospitalization	**Group A** SABA or SAMA PRN LABA or LAMA	**Group B** LAMA or LABA
	mMRC 0-1 CAT <10	mMRC ≥2 CAT ≥10

Symptoms

Abbreviations used: CAT, COPD assessment test; FEV1, forced expiratory volume in 1 second; GOLD, Global Institute for Chronic Obstructive Lung Disease; ICS, inhaled corticosteroid; LABA, long-acting beta-2 agonist; LAMA, long-acting muscarinic antagonist; mMRC, Modified British Medical Research Council Questionnaire; PRN, as needed; SABA, short-acting beta-2 agonist; SAMA, short-acting muscarinic antagonist. Adapted from Global Initiative for Chronic Obstructive Lung Disease. Global Strategy for the Diagnosis, Management, and Prevention of Chronic Obstructive Pulmonary Disease. Available at: https://goldcopd.org/wp-content/uploads/2019/11/GOLD-2020-REPORT-ver1.0wms.pdf. Accessed April 25, 2020.

is determined by the number of cigarettes a day and the time-to-first cigarette that a patient smokes after waking up.[9]

The goal of therapy is to minimize nicotine withdrawal effects (e.g., anxiety, irritability, impatience, malaise, strong tobacco craving, and mental health issues) until the patient is free from tobacco use.[11] Additional courses of treatment may be required over time to remain tobacco free. The combination of counseling (e.g., behavioral and social support) and pharmacotherapy is the most effective treatment for tobacco cessation.[9] Currently approved treatments are outlined in Table 12-6. Patients with cardiovascular disease are recommended to use varenicline as first-line treatment.[9]

Remember:[10,12]

- Nicotine replacement therapy (NRT) combinations (i.e., patch plus short acting gum or lozenge) have shown to increase quit rates
- NRT dosing may need to be extended based on cravings or length of time the patient has been smoking to avoid treatment failure or relapse
- NRT duration—12 weeks and then requires reassessment for ongoing support
- Patients must be advised not to smoke while using NRT
  - Patients may begin NRT therapy while still smoking

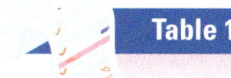

Table 12-5 Treatment Options for Chronic Obstructive Pulmonary Disease[7]

TREATMENT	DRUG AGENT	DOSING	NOTES
Short-acting muscarinic antagonists	Ipratropium MDI (Atrovent HFA)	2 inhalations QID	**SE:** Dry mouth, cough, urinary symptoms, bitter taste
Long-acting muscarinic antagonists	Aclidinium DPI (Tudorza Pressair)	1 inhalation BID	**SE:** Dry mouth, cough, urinary symptoms
	Glycopyrrolate DPI (Seebri Neohaler, Lonhala Magnair)	▪ 1 capsule via Neohaler BID ▪ 1 inhalation BID	**Remember:** Neohaler and HandiHaler come with a
	Tiotropium DPI, Respimat (Spiriva)	1 capsule via HandiHaler daily Respimat: 2.5 mcg daily	capsule, do not swallow the capsule
	Umeclidinium DPI (Incruse Ellipta)	1 inhalation daily	
Long-acting beta-2-agonists	Indacaterol DPI (Arapta Neohaler)	1 capsule via Neohaler daily	**SE:** Nervousness, tremor, tachycardia, hypokalemia, cough
	Formoterol DPI (Foradil Aerolizer)	1 capsule via Aerolizer BID	
	Olodaterol Respimat (Striverdi)	2 inhalations daily	
	Salmeterol DPI (Serevent)	1 inhalation BID	**Remember:** Toxicity is dose-related
	Arformoterol (Brovana)	Nebulizer solution 15 mcg BID	
	Formoterol (Perforomist, Foradil Aerolizer)	▪ Nebulizer solution 20 mcg BID ▪ 1 capsule every 12 h	
	COMBINATION INHALERS		
ICS/LABA	Budesonide/Formoterol MDI (Symbicort)	1 inhalation BID	
	Fluticasone/Salmeterol DPI, MDI (Advair, Wixela Inhub)	1 inhalation BID	
	Fluticasone/Vilanterol DPI (Breo Ellipta)	1 inhalation daily	
LAMA/LABA	Glycopyrrolate/Formoterol MDI (Bevespi Aerosphere)	2 inhalations BID	
	Glycopyrrolate/Indacaterol DPI (Utibron Neohaler)	1 capsule for inhalation BID	
	Tiotropium/Olodaterol Respimat (Stiolto)	2 inhalations daily	
	Umeclidinium/Vilanterol DPI (Anoro Ellipta)	1 inhalation daily	
LAMA/LABA/ICS	Umeclidinium/Vilanterol/Fluticasone DPI (Trelegy Ellipta)	1 inhalation daily	
SAMA/SABA	Ipratropium/Albuterol Respimat (Combivent)	1 inhalation Q4–6 h PRN	
Phosphodiesterase-4 inhibitors	Roflumilast (Daliresp)	500 mcg daily	**CI:** Liver impairment **SE:** Diarrhea, weight loss, insomnia, psychiatric events

Abbreviations used: BID, twice daily; CI, contraindicated; DPI, dry-powdered inhaler; ICS, inhaled corticosteroid; LABA, long-acting beta-2-agonist; LAMA, long-acting muscarinic antagonist; MDI, metered-dose inhaler; PRN, as needed; SABA, short-acting beta-2 agonist; SAMA, short-acting muscarinic antagonist; SE, side effects; Q, every; QID, 4 times a day.

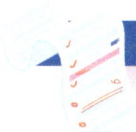

Table 12-6 Tobacco Cessation Treatment Options[10,12]

DRUG AGENT	DOSING	ADMINISTRATION	NOTES

Nicotine gum	• Starting dose:
	  ○ 4 mg if >25 cigs/d
	  ○ 2 mg if <25 cigs/d
	• After 6 wk: taper to lower dose for 2–6 wk
		• Chew until mouth tingles, then "park" gum inside cheek until tingle fades
		• Use 1 piece every 1–2 h (maximum: 24 pieces/d)
			SE: Mouth irritation, jaw soreness, heartburn, nausea
			Remember:
			• May use with patch
			• No food/drink 15 m prior to use

Nicotine inhaler*	• 10 mg/cartridge • 80 puffs in 1 cartridge	• Puff into mouth until cravings subside • Use 1 cartridge every 1–2 h (maximum: 16/d)	**SE:** Mouth and throat irritation, coughing **Remember:** • May use with patch • Not recommended with asthma or COPD • Mimics hand-to-mouth motion of smoking cigs

Nicotine lozenges	• Starting dose:
	  ○ 4 mg if 1st cig in ≤30 min of waking up
	  ○ 2 mg if 1st cig in >30 min of waking up
	• After 6 wk: taper to 1 piece daily for 3 wk, then 1 piece every 4–8 h for 3 wk
		• Place between gum and cheek, let it melt slowly
		• Use 1 piece every 1–2 h (maximum: 20 pieces/d)
			SE: Mouth irritation, hiccups, heartburn, nausea
			Remember:
			• May use with patch
			• No food/drink 15 min prior to use

Nicotine nasal spray*	• 0.5 mL per spray • Each bottle has 200 sprays	• Use 1 spray in each nostril • Use spray every 1–2 h (maximum: 80 sprays/d)	**SE:** Nasal irritation, sneezing, coughing **Remember:** • May use with patch • Use for ≥3 mo

Nicotine patch	• Starting dose:
	  ○ 21 mg for ≥ 10 cigs/d
	  ○ 14 mg for <10 cigs/d
	  ○ Low dose: 7 mg
	• After 6 wk: taper to lower dose for 2–6 wk
		• Apply a new patch each morning (remove old patch)
		• Rotate application site
		• May start patch before or on quit date
			SE: Skin irritation, trouble sleeping, vivid dreams
			Remember:
			• Can use in combination with other NRT
			• Use for ≥3 mo

Bupropion SR	Days 1–3: 150 mg/d Days 4+: 150 mg BID	Start 1–2 wk before quit date	**SE:** Insomnia, agitation, dry mouth, headache **Remember:** • Use for 3–6 mo • May increase risk of seizure in some patients
Varenicline	Days 1–3: 0.5 mg/d Days 4–7: 0.5 mg BID Days 8+: 1 mg BID	Start 1 wk before quit date	**SE:** Nausea, insomnia, vivid dreams **Remember:** • Use for 3 mo • Relieves withdrawal and competitively inhibits nicotine on nicotine receptors

Abbreviations used: BID, twice daily; cigs, cigarettes; COPD, chronic obstructive pulmonary disease; NRT, nicotine replacement therapy; SE, side effects; SR, sustained-release.

*Rarely used in clinical practice.

Adapted from Barua RS, Rigotti NA, Benowitz NL, et al. 2018 ACC Expert Consensus Decision Pathway on Tobacco Cessation Treatment: A Report of the American College of Cardiology Task Force on Clinical Expert Consensus Documents. *J Am Coll Cardiol*. 2018;72(25):3332–3365.

ADDITIONAL RESOURCES

National Asthma Education and Prevention Program. Expert panel report 3 (EPR-3): guidelines for the diagnosis and management of asthma - summary report 2007. *J Allergy Clin Immunol.* 2007;120(suppl 5):s94–s138. doi:10.1016/j.jaci.2007.09.043. Published correction appears in *J Allergy Clin Immunol.* 2007; 121(6):1330.

Global Initiative for Asthma. Pocket Guide for Asthma Management and Prevention. GINA. https://ginasthma.org/wp-content/uploads/2020/06/GINA-2020-report_20_06_04-1-wms.pdf.

Global Initiative for Chronic Obstructive Lung Disease. Pocket Guide to COPD Diagnosis, Management, and Prevention. https://goldcopd.org/wp-content/uploads/2019/11/GOLD-2020-REPORT-ver1.0wms.pdf.

American Association for Respiratory Care. Clinician's Guide to Treating Tobacco Dependence. In: American Association of Respiratory Care. Clinician's Guide to Treating Tobacco Dependence. AARC. https://www.aarc.org/wp-content/uploads/2014/11/tobacco-guide.pdf 2014:1–53

REFERENCES

1. Klinger JR, Elliott CG, Levine DJ, et al. Therapy for Pulmonary Arterial Hypertension in Adults: Update of the CHEST Guideline and Expert Panel Report. *Chest.* 2019;155(3):565–586.

2. Moote R, Attridge RL, Levine DJ. Pulmonary Arterial Hypertension. In: DiPiro JT, Yee GC, Posey LM, Haines ST, Nolin TD, Ellingrod V, eds. *Pharmacotherapy: A Pathophysiologic Approach, 11e.* New York, NY: McGraw-Hill Education; 2020.

3. Blake KV, Lang JE. Asthma. In: DiPiro JT, Yee GC, Posey LM, Haines ST, Nolin TD, Ellingrod V, eds. *Pharmacotherapy: A Pathophysiologic Approach, 11e.* New York, NY: McGraw-Hill Education; 2020.

4. National Asthma Education and Prevention Program. Expert Panel Report 3 (EPR-3): Guidelines for the Diagnosis and Management of Asthma-Summary Report 2007. *J Allergy Clin Immunol.* 2007;120 (5 Suppl):S94–138.

5. Global Initiative for Asthma. Pocket Guide for Asthma Management and Prevention. GINA. https://ginasthma.org/wp-content/uploads/2020/06/GINA-2020-report_20_06_04-1-wms.pdf. Published 2020. Accessed 26 April, 2020.

6. National Heart Lung and Blood Institute. Asthma Care Quick Reference. https://www.nhlbi.nih.gov/files/docs/guidelines/asthma_qrg.pdf. Published 2012. Accessed 26 April, 2020.

7. Global Initiative for Chronic Obstructive Lung Disease. Pocket Guide to COPD Diagnosis, Management, and Prevention. https://goldcopd.org/wp-content/uploads/2019/11/GOLD-2020-REPORT-ver1.0wms.pdf. Published 2020. Accessed 25 April, 2020.

8. Bourdet SV, Williams DM. Chronic Obstructive Pulmonary Disease. In: DiPiro JT, Yee GC, Posey LM, Haines ST, Nolin TD, Ellingrod V, eds. *Pharmacotherapy: A Pathophysiologic Approach, 11e.* New York, NY: McGraw-Hill Education; 2020.

9. Barua RS, Rigotti NA, Benowitz NL, et al. 2018 ACC Expert Consensus Decision Pathway on Tobacco Cessation Treatment: A Report of the American College of Cardiology Task Force on Clinical Expert Consensus Documents. *J Am Coll Cardiol.* 2018; 72(25):3332–3365.

10. American Association for Respiratory Care. Clinician's Guide to Treating Tobacco Dependence. In: American Association of Respiratory Care. Clinician's Guide to Treating Tobacco Dependence. AARC. https://www.aarc.org/wp-content/uploads/2014/11/tobacco-guide.pdf 2014:1–53.

11. Li RM, Dupree L, Doering P. Substance-Related Disorders II: Alcohol, Nicotine, and Caffeine. In: DiPiro JT, Yee GC, Posey LM, Haines ST, Nolin TD, Ellingrod V, eds. *Pharmacotherapy: A Pathophysiologic Approach, 11e.* New York, NY: McGraw-Hill Education; 2020.

12. Clinical Practice Guideline Treating Tobacco Use and Dependence 2008 Update Panel, Liaisons, and Staff. A clinical practice guideline for treating tobacco use and dependence: 2008 update. A U.S. Public Health Service report. *Am J Prev Med.* 2008 Aug;35(2):158-76. doi: 10.1016/j.amepre.2008.04.009. PMID: 18617085.

13. National Asthma Education and Prevention Program: Expert Panel Report 3 (EPR-3): Guidelines for the Diagnosis and Management of Asthma-Summary Report 2007. *J Allergy Clin Immunol.* 2007;120(5 Suppl):S94–138.

14. Hiday R, Abbott KD. *Asthma.* Vol 1. ACSAP2019.

CHAPTER 13

Endocrinology

With medical writing support provided by Banner Medical LLC Writer: Miriam Opara

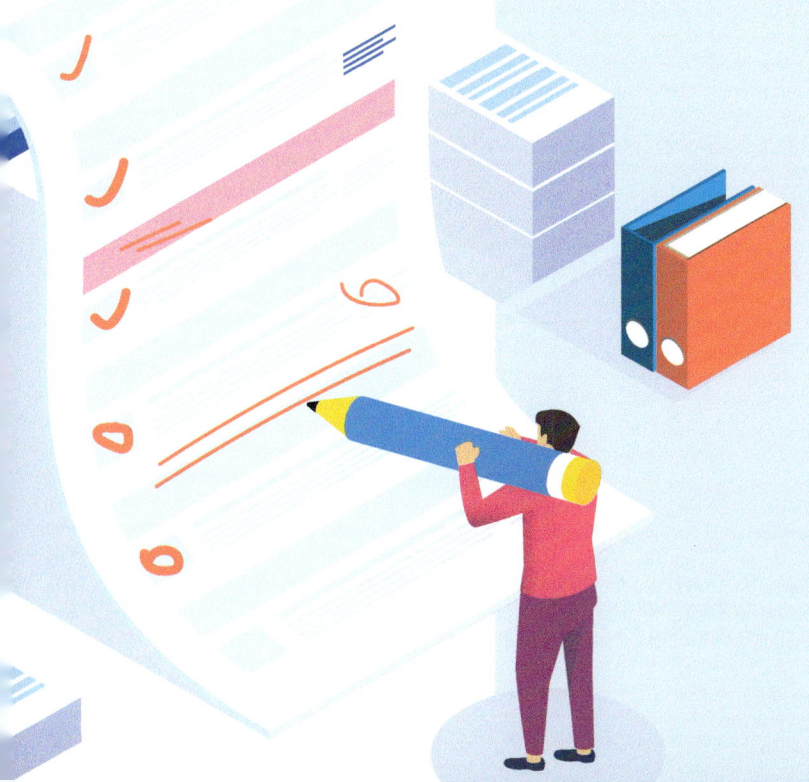

Diabetes mellitus

Diabetes mellitus (DM) is a metabolic disorder characterized by chronic hyperglycemia.[1,2]

The majority of individuals are classified with type 1 or type 2 DM.

Remember: risk for DM → impaired fasting glucose
- Fasting plasma glucose 100–125 mg/dL
- 75-g oral glucose tolerance test: 2-hour glucose 140–199 mg/dL
- A1C 5.7%–6.4%

The hallmark symptoms of diabetes are **polydipsia**, **polyuria**, and **polyphagia**. Diagnosis of DM (no hyperglycemia)—minimum of 2 abnormal blood glucose (BG) levels (see Table 13-1)[3]

- High risk requires intensive lifestyle modifications as first-line treatment[4]
  - Minimum of 7% weight loss (or 1–2 lb per week), moderate physical activity for a minimum of 150 minutes/week (e.g., brisk walking), emphasis on eating patterns, and quality of food (e.g., whole grains, fruits, vegetables)[4]

Current glycemic goals recommended by the American Diabetes Association (ADA) and the American Association of Clinical Endocrinologists (AACE) include:[4,5]

- Glycated hemoglobin (A1C): <7% (≤6.5% AACE)
  - Measured minimum of 2 times per year (stable); more frequently if uncontrolled
- Preprandial glucose: 80–130 mg/dL
- Postprandial glucose: <180 mg/dL (1–2 hours after eating)
- Risk of hypoglycemia (BG <54 mg/dL); prescribe glucagon in case of an emergency[4]

The **primary goals of care** include maintaining glycemic control, preventing complications, and optimizing quality of life.[4]

Remember the following:
- Verify currency of pneumococcal, hepatitis B series, and annual influenza vaccines
- Advise tobacco cessation (including e-cigarettes)
- Advise dental and ophthalmic exams every 6 and 12 months (respectively)
- Assess cardiovascular (CV) risk factors/complications for all patients (e.g., hypertension, hyperlipidemia); not all patients require aspirin therapy (assess CV risk)

Each patient's treatment plan should be individualized and consider factors such as CV risk/comorbidities, risk of adverse events, affordability, and patient preferences and mechanism of action (see Tables 13-2 and 13-3).

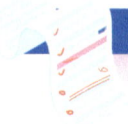

Table 13-1 2020 American Diabetes Association Prediabetes and Type 2 Diabetes Mellitus Glycemic Criteria for Screening and Diagnosis*[3]

Glycemic test	Prediabetes	Diabetes
A1C	5.7%–6.4%	≥6.5%
FPG	100–125 mg/dL	≥126 mg/dL
OGTT	140–199 mg/dL	≥200 mg/dL
RPG	—	≥200 mg/dL

Abbreviations used: A1C, glycated hemoglobin; FPG, fasting plasma glucose; OGTT, oral glucose tolerance test; RPG, random plasma glucose.
*2 abnormal blood glucose levels required (either from the same sample or from 2 separate samples).
Adapted from American Diabetes Association. Standards of Medical Care in Diabetes - 2020 Abridged for Primary Care Providers. *Clin Diabetes.* 2020;38(1):10–38.

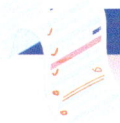

Table 13-2 Primary Mechanism of Action for Diabetes Drugs[6,7]

DECREASES GASTRIC EMPTYING	INCREASES GLUCOSE UPTAKE	INCREASES & REPLACES INSULIN RELEASE	DECREASES HEPATIC GLUCOSE OUTPUT	DECREASES GLUCAGON & INCREASES INSULIN SECRETION	INCREASES GLUCOSE EXCRETION
GLP1RA	Metformin	Insulin	Metformin	DPP4i	SGLT2i
Pramlintide	TZDs	Meglitinides		GLP1RA	
		SUs		Pramlintide	

Abbreviations used: DPP4i, dipeptidyl-peptidase 4 inhibitor; GLP1RA, glucagon-like peptide 1 receptor agonists; SGLT2i, sodium-glucose co-transporter-2 inhibitor; SU, sulfonylureas; TZD, thiazolidinedione.

Insulin therapy should mimic normal physiology (see Table 13-4).[6–8]

- Basal insulin → fasting blood glucose
- Bolus insulin → mealtime and acute elevations

First-line treatment—lifestyle modifications + metformin[4]

- Excluding any contraindications for treatment with metformin
- Lifestyle modifications should include weight management and physical activity

High risk or have established atherosclerotic cardiovascular disease (ASCVD), chronic kidney disease (CKD), or heart failure (HF)[4]

ASCVD predominates
Preferred treatment → GLP1RA with a proven CVD benefit*
OR
SGLT2i with proven CVD benefit* (if eGFR adequate)
If A1C > target, choose alternative or additional agents demonstrating CV safety

Add SGLT2i	with proven CVD benefit* if on GLP1RA
DPP4i	if not on GLP1RA
Basal insulin	Degludec or U100 glargine have CVD safety

Abbreviations used: A1C, glycated hemoglobin; CVD, cardiovascular disease; DPP4i, dipeptidyl peptidase 4 inhibitor; eGFR, estimated glomerular filtration rate; GLP1RA, glucagon-like peptide 1 receptor agonist; SGLT2i, sodium glucose co-transporter 2.
*CVD benefit = FDA labeled indication for decreasing CVD events.

HF or CKD predominates
Preferred treatment → SGLT2i
With evidence of reducing HF and/or CKD progression in CVOTs if eGFR adequate
OR
Add GLP1RA with proven CVD benefit*
If A1C > target, choose agents demonstrating CV safety (no TZD in HF)

Add GLP1RA	with proven CVD benefit* if on SGLT2i
DPP4i	in HF (if no GLP1RA not [saxagliptin])
Basal insulin	Degludec or U100 glargine have CVD safety

Abbreviations used: A1C, glycated hemoglobin; ASCV, atherosclerotic cardiovascular disease; CKD, chronic kidney disease; CVD, cardiovascular disease; CVOT, cardiovascular outcome trial; DPP4i, dipeptidyl peptidase 4 inhibitor; eGFR, estimated glomerular filtration rate; GLP1RA, glucagon-like peptide 1 receptor agonist; SGLT2i, sodium glucose co-transporter 2.
*CVD benefit = FDA labeled indication for decreasing CVD events.

If no risk/established ASCVD, CKD, or HF and above target A1C after 3 months, consider therapy based on a compelling need to minimize hypoglycemia, minimize weight gain, or affordability[4]

Minimize hypoglycemia

DPP4i	GLP1RA	SGLT2i	TZD

Minimize weight gain or promote weight loss
GLP1RA + efficacy for weight loss* OR SGLT2i

Cost is a major issue

SU**	TZD

Abbreviations used: DPP4i, dipeptidyl peptidase 4 inhibitor; GLP1RA, glucagon-like peptide 1 receptor agonist; SGLT2i, sodium glucose co-transporter 2; SU, sulfonylurea; TZD, thiazolidinedione.
*semaglutide > liraglutide > dulaglutide > exenatide > lixisenatide
**Later-generation SU preferred with < risk of hypoglycemia.

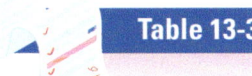

Table 13-3 Type 2 Diabetes Medications[6–8]

Drug class	Drug agent	Dose	Notes

Amylin analog	Pramlintide	T1DM:
		   Maximum of 60 mcg TID
		T2DM:
		   Maximum of 120 mcg TID
			BBW: Severe hypoglycemia with insulin
			SE: N/V, hypoglycemia, HA, weight loss
			Remember:
			 ■ Reduce mealtime insulin by 50% when starting
			 ■ Administer prior to each major meal
			 ■ Decrease A1C 0.5%–1%

Biguanide	Metformin	IR: 500 mg BID ER: 500–1000 mg/d	**BBW:** Lactic acidosis, alcohol consumption **CI:** eGFR <30 mL/min/1.73 m² **Remember:** ■ Monitor: renal function, B_{12} ■ Decrease A1C 1%–2%
Dipeptidyl peptidase 4 inhibitor	Alogliptin	25 mg/d CrCl 30–59: 12.5 mg/d CrCl <30: 6.25 mg/d	**SE:** Nasopharyngitis, URTIs, UTIs, peripheral edema, rash **Remember:** ■ Saxagliptin and alogliptin: risk of HF ■ Risk of acute pancreatitis, severe arthralgia, allergic reactions ■ Take DDP4i in the morning ■ Saxagliptin and Linagliptin are 3A4 and P-gp substrates ■ Decrease A1C 0.5%–0.8%
	Linagliptin	5 mg/d	
	Sitagliptin	100 mg/d CrCl 30–49: 50 mg/d CrCl <30: 25 mg/d	
	Saxagliptin	2.5–5 mg/d eGFR <45: 2.5 mg/d	
Glucagon-like-peptide 1 receptor agonist	Dulaglutide	1.5 mg SQ once weekly	**BBW:** Risk of thyroid C-cell carcinoma **SE:** Dulaglutide: CV effects: tachycardia, AV block **Remember:** ■ Can increase INR ■ Risk of pancreatitis ■ Semaglutide: increase complications with diabetic retinopathy ■ Exenatide and Lixisenatide: give dose within 60 min of meals ■ Exenatide/Lixisenatide/Liraglutide: pen needles not provided
	Exenatide	10 mcg BID ESRD/CrCl <30: Not recommended	
	Exenatide ER	2 mg SQ once weekly ESRD/CrCl <30: Not recommended	
	Liraglutide	1.2 mg SQ daily	
	Lixisenatide	20 mcg/d eGFR <15: Not recommended	
	Semaglutide	0.5 mg SQ once weekly	

Table 13-3 Type 2 Diabetes Medications[6–8] (*Continued*)

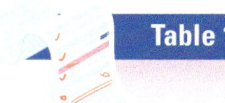

Drug class	Drug agent	Dose	Notes
			▪ Liraglutide approved to reduce risk of CV events ▪ Do not store pen with needle attached ▪ Decrease A1C 0.5%–1.5%
Meglitinides	Repaglinide Nateglinide	0.5–2 mg TID AC Maximum: 16 mg/d 60–120 mg TID AC	**CI:** T1DM, DKA, repaglinide with gemfibrozil **SE:** Weight gain, hypoglycemia **Remember:** ▪ Take 15–30 min before meals ▪ Decrease A1C 0.5%–1.5%
Sodium glucose co-transporter-2 inhibitor	Canagliflozin Dapagliflozin Empagliflozin Ertugliflozin	Maximum: 300 mg/d eGFR 45–59: 100 mg/d Maximum: 10 mg/d Maximum: 25 mg/d Maximum: 15 mg/d	**CI:** eGFR <30 mL/min/1.73 m^2, ESRD, dialysis **Remember:** ▪ Take SGLT2i in the morning ▪ Risk of ketoacidosis, genital mycotic infections, fractures, dehydration ▪ Decrease A1C 0.7%–1% ▪ Canagliflozin: Hyperkalemia, monitor meds that ↑ K ▪ Dapagliflozin: Risk of bladder cancer ▪ Empagliflozin: Reduce risk of CV mortality in T2DM and ASCVD
Sulfonylurea	Glimepiride Glipizide Glyburide Micronized glyburide	Maximum: 8 mg/d Maximum IR: 40 mg/d Maximum XR: 20 mg/d Glyburide maximum: 20 mg/d Micronized maximum: 12 mg/d	**CI:** T1DM, DKA, sulfa allergy **SE:** Weight gain, hypoglycemia **Remember:** ▪ Take with first meal of the day ▪ Reduce SU dose with TZD, GLP1 agonist, DPP4i or SGLT2i ▪ SU are 2C9 substrates ▪ Decrease A1C 1%–2%

(*continued on next page*)

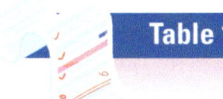

Table 13-3 Type 2 Diabetes Medications[6-8] *(Continued)*

DRUG CLASS	DRUG AGENT	DOSE	NOTES
Thiazolidinedione	Pioglitazone	HF: 15 mg/d Maximum: 45 mg/d	**BBW:** Can cause/exacerbate HF; rosiglitazone increased risk of MI
	Rosiglitazone	Maximum: 8 mg/d	**SE:** Peripheral edema, weight gain, myalgia Pioglitazone: ↑ HDL, ↓ TGs, ↓ TC **Remember:** ■ Risk of fractures ■ TZDs are major substrates of 2C8 ■ Pioglitazone increased risk of urinary bladder tumors ■ Decrease A1C 0.5%–1.4%

Abbreviations used: A1C, glycated hemoglobin; AC, before meals; ASCV, atherosclerotic cardiovascular disease; AV, atrial valve; BBW, black box warning; BID, twice daily; CI, contraindicated; CrCl, creatinine clearance; CV, cardiovascular; DDP4i, dipeptidyl-peptidase 4 inhibitor; DKA, diabetic ketoacidosis; eGFR, estimated glomerular filtration rate; ER, extended release; ESRD, end-stage renal disease; GLP1, glucagon-like-peptide 1; HA, headache; HDL, high-density lipoprotein; HF, heart failure; INR, international normalized ratio; IR, immediate release; K, potassium; MI, myocardial infarction; N/V, nausea, vomiting; SE, side effects; SGLT2i, sodium glucose co-transporter-2 inhibitor; SQ, subcutaneous; SU, sulfonylurea; TC, total cholesterol; TG, triglycerides; TID, 3 times a day; TZD, thiazolidinedione; T1DM, type 1 diabetes mellitus; T2DM, type 2 diabetes mellitus; UTI, urinary tract infection; URTI, upper respiratory tract infection, XR, extended release.

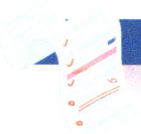

Table 13-4 Insulin Therapy for Diabetes Mellitus [6-8]

INSULIN TYPE	INSULIN NAME	ONSET & DURATION	NOTES
Rapid-acting insulin prandial or mealtime	Insulin aspart	Onset: 10–30 min Duration: 3–5 h	**CI:** Acute hypoglycemia, hypersensitivity
	Insulin glulisine	Onset: 10–30 min Duration: 3–5 h	**SE:** Weight gain, peripheral edema, lipodystrophy
	Insulin lispro	Onset: 15 min Duration: 2–3 h	**Remember:** Give up to 15 min before meals or immediately after meals
	Insulin human inhalation powder	Onset: 15 min Duration: 2–3 h	**BBW:** Acute bronchospasm in patients with asthma or COPD **Remember:** ■ Not recommended for patients who smoke ■ Replace inhaler every 15 d

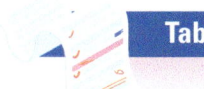

Table 13-4 Insulin Therapy for Diabetes Mellitus [6–8] (*Continued*)

INSULIN TYPE	INSULIN NAME	ONSET & DURATION	NOTES
Short-acting insulin prandial or mealtime	Regular insulin	Onset: 15–30 min Duration: 4–12 h	■ Give 30 min before meals ■ Available without prescription
	Concentrated regular insulin	Onset: 15–30 min Duration: 13–24 h	■ 5x as concentrated as regular insulin ■ Must be prescribed a U-500 insulin syringe to avoid dosing errors ■ Do NOT mix with other insulins ■ Do NOT administer IV, IM, or via insulin pump
Intermediate-acting insulin basal insulin	NPH insulin	Onset: 1–2 h Duration: 14–24 h	■ Available without prescription ■ Appears cloudy ■ Can mix with rapid/short-acting insulin ■ Draw up rapid/short-acting insulin first: **clear** before **cloudy**
	70% NPH, 30% regular	Onset: 30 min Duration: 18–24 h	All mixed insulins are named as the percentage of each component with basal first
Long-acting insulin basal insulin	Degludec	Onset: 1 h Duration: ≥24 h	**SE:** Weight gain, peripheral edema, lipodystrophy **Remember:** ■ Do NOT mix with other insulins ■ Given at same time each day
	Detemir	Onset: 2–4 h Duration: 6–23 h	**SE:** weight gain, peripheral edema, lipodystrophy
	Glargine	Onset: 3–4 h Duration: ≥24 h	**Remember:** ■ Do NOT mix with other insulins ■ Given at same time each day

Abbreviations used: BBW, black box warning; CI, contraindicated; COPD, chronic obstructive pulmonary disease; CrCl, creatinine clearance; DKA, diabetic ketoacidosis; IM, intramuscular; IV, intravenous; NPH, neutral protamine Hagedorn; SE, side effects.

Diabetic ketoacidosis is caused by insulin deficiency and excess glucagon/impaired peripheral ketone utilization.[9] Treatment includes fluid replacement, correcting of hyperglycemia and acidosis (via insulin), and correction of electrolyte imbalances.

Diabetic kidney disease (nephropathy) is caused by increased albumin excretion and low estimated glomerular filtration rate. Diabetic nephropathy can cause end-stage renal disease.[9] Treatment consists of reducing/slowing progression of nephropathy (via glucose control) and correction of acute kidney injury.

Diabetic retinopathy complications include glaucoma, cataracts, and other disorders of the eye. Screening for diabetic retinopathy is essential to prevent vision loss.

Diabetic peripheral neuropathy—no specific treatments for the underlying nerve damage. Pharmacologic agents (e.g., gabapentin/pregabalin, duloxetine, capsaicin) are recommended for pain control. Neuropathic pain manifests as burning, tingling, and numbing sensations in extremities.

Peripheral artery disease causes decreased walking speed, leg fatigue, and decreased pedal pressure. Treatment includes management of blood pressure, blood glucose, lipids, tobacco cessation, and daily foot inspections.

Hyperthyroidism

Hyperthyroidism (thyrotoxicosis) is caused by high levels of thyroid hormone in the tissues, leading to hypermetabolic state (see Figure 13-1).[10,11]

Remember the following:

- Grave's disease is the most common cause of hyperthyroidism.[10]

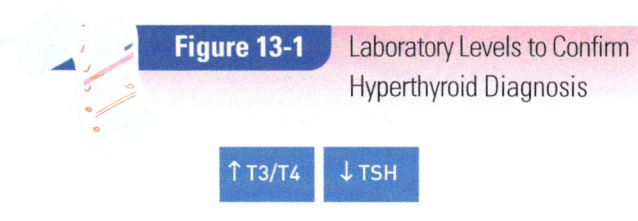

Figure 13-1 Laboratory Levels to Confirm Hyperthyroid Diagnosis

↑ T3/T4   ↓ TSH

Abbreviations used: TSH, thyroid-stimulating hormone; T3, triiodothyronine; T4, thyroxine.

- The clinical presentation is variable (asymptomatic to thyroid storm).[10]
  - Heat intolerance, palpitations, sweating, hyperdefecation, anxiety, eye lag, diaphoresis, weight loss, tremors, tachycardia, agitation, and psychosis
- Long-standing untreated hyperthyroidism can result in atrial fibrillation or heart failure.
- Adrenergic symptoms are treated with beta-blockers, regardless of the etiology of hyperthyroidism.[10]

There are three primary treatment options for hyperthyroidism:

1. Thyroidectomy is preferred in patients with contraindications to radioactive iodine (RAI) ablation or thioamides.[10]
2. RAI ablation is the most common treatment of Graves' disease.[10]
   a. Thioamides should be discontinued a minimum of 5 days before RAI ablation and restarted 3–5 days after ablation.[10]
3. Antithyroid medications (see Table 13-5)

Hypothyroidism

Hypothyroidism is a thyroid hormone deficiency of triiodothyronine (T3) and thyroxine (T4) and increase in thyroid-stimulating hormone (TSH).[13,14]

- Hashimoto's disease is the most common cause of primary hypothyroidism (autoimmune thyroiditis).[14]
- If the thyroid gland fails to produce T4 and T3, the pituitary is stimulated to increase TSH via a negative feedback loop (see Figure 13-2).[14]

Hypothyroidism has a heterogeneous presentation:[13]

- Symptomatology: fatigue, constipation, hair thinning, lethargy, voice changes, cold intolerance, dry skin, weight gain, depression, puffy face, or slowed heart rate

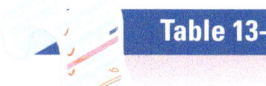
Drug agent	Drug class	Mechanism of action	Dose	Notes
Methimazole	Thioamide	■ Inhibit TH synthesis ■ PTU also inhibits peripheral conversion of T4 to T3	5–40 mg orally as single dose or divided	■ Methimazole is first-line therapy (except in pregnancy) ■ Do not d/c abruptly ■ Monitor INR closely
Propylthiouracil	Thioamide		150–300 mg orally at 8-h intervals	
Saturated solution of potassium iodide	Iodide	Temporarily inhibit hormone release and TH synthesis	1–5 drops** orally 3 times daily in water or juice	■ Rapidly decrease TH secretion (thyroid storm) ■ Not used long term
Strong iodine solution	Iodide		3–5 drops* orally 3 times daily	

Abbreviations used: d/c, discontinue; INR, international normalized ratio; PTU, propylthiouracil; TH, thyroid hormones; T3, triiodothyronine; T4, thyroxine.
*delivers 6.3 mg iodine per drop.
**delivers 38 mg iodine per drop of saturated solution.

■ Clinical suspicion → lab measurement (screening ≥60 years of age); see Figure 13-3

The goals of treatment include maintaining TSH levels within the normal range, reducing symptoms, and preventing long-term complications.[14] Treatment with thyroid hormone replacement therapy with **synthetic thyroxine** (i.e., levothyroxine) is the preferred treatment for primary hypothyroidism.[14]

■ Initial dose is dependent on patient's age, presence of co-existing CVD, and etiology of hypothyroidism (see Table 13-6).[14]
■ When indicated, initiate on the full dose of levothyroxine (1.6 mcg/kg/day).
  ● **Remember:** Use lower dose in elderly people (usually 12.5–25 mcg/day).
■ Repeat TSH value after 4–6 weeks, then every 6–12 months once stable.
■ If target values are not met, differential diagnosis should be revisited.

Myxedema coma is a rare, potentially fatal complication of hypothyroidism and a medical emergency.[14] It

Figure 13-2 Hypothyroidism Negative Feedback Loop[14]

Negative Feedback Inhibition

Hypothalamus — TRH → Pituitary — TSH → Thyroid → T3 / T4 — Periphery

Abbreviations used: TRH, thyroid releasing hormone; TSH, thyroid-stimulating hormone; T3, triiodothyronine; T4, thyroxine.

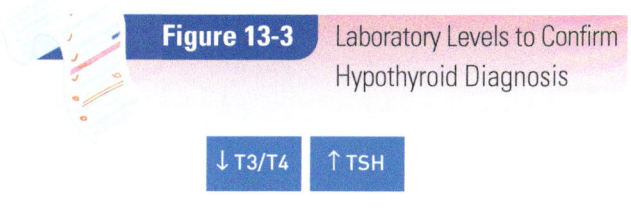

Figure 13-3 Laboratory Levels to Confirm Hypothyroid Diagnosis

↓ T3/T4   ↑ TSH

Abbreviations used: TSH, thyroid-stimulating hormone; T3, triiodothyronine; T4, thyroxine.

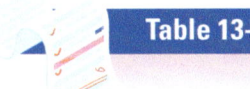

Table 13-6 Comparison of Hypothyroidism Drug Treatments[14]

Drug agent	Mechanism of action	Dose	Notes
Levothyroxine	Synthetic T4	Full dose: 1.6 mcg/kg/d	■ Dose ↓ in CAD and older patients ■ PO tablets are taken on empty stomach 60 min before breakfast or 3 h after last meal at bedtime ■ IV:PO ratio is 0.75:1
Liothyronine	T3	Maintenance: 25–75 mcg/d	■ Titrate in 12.5–25 mcg increments ■ Shorter half-life = fluctuations in T3 levels
Thyroid, Desiccated USP	T3/T4	CAD: 15 mg/d Maintenance: 60–120 mg/d	■ Titrate in 15-mg increments ■ Porcine-derived ■ Less-predictable potency and stability

Abbreviations used: CAD, coronary artery disease; IV, intravenous; PO, by mouth; T3, triiodothyronine; T4, thyroxine.

typically occurs in patients who have had untreated hypothyroidism for a long time or their hypothyroidism decompensates. Myxedema coma is characterized by poor circulation, hypothermia, and hypometabolism. First-line treatment usually consists of intravenous levothyroxine.[14]

Cushing's syndrome

Cushing's syndrome is caused by excess cortisol or overused glucocorticoids.[15] The pathogenesis of Cushing's syndrome is outlined in Figure 13-4.[15]

The symptomatology of Cushing's syndrome is very broad because of the pleiotropic actions of cortisol

(e.g., acne, amenorrhea, depression, hirsutism, obesity, osteopenia, diabetes).[15]

The goal of treatment is to lower cortisol concentrations to a normal level, and treat any associated comorbidities.[16]

■ Iatrogenic—minimize glucocorticoid exposure with acute or chronic steroid treatment as outlined in Table 13-7[17]
■ Endogenous—minimize cortisol production
  • The preferred treatment is surgical resection of the source of the hypercortisolism[15]
  • Pharmacologic agents used in the treatment of Cushing's syndrome are outlined in Table 13-8[15,18]

Figure 13-4 Pathogenesis of Cushing's Syndrome[15]

Negative Feedback Inhibition

Hypothalamus →(CRH)→ Pituitary →(ACTH)→ Adrenal Glands → Cortisol

Abbreviations used: CRH, corticotropin-releasing hormone; ACTH, adrenocorticotropic hormone.

Addison's disease

Addison's disease is an autoimmune condition known as primary adrenal insufficiency; the pathogenesis is outlined in Figure 13-5.[20]

Adrenal insufficiency causes increased adrenocorticotropic hormone and decreased cortisol levels. Signs and symptoms include fatigue, weakness, anorexia, hyperpigmentation, nausea, and hypotension.[20]

Table 13-7　Ways to Minimize Glucocorticoid Exposure in Acute and Chronic Use[17]

ACUTE USE OF GLUCOCORTICOIDS	CHRONIC USE OF GLUCOCORTICOIDS
■ High loading dose followed by tapering of therapy (e.g., steroid "dose packs") ■ Targeted compartmental dosage forms (e.g., ICS or joint injections)	■ Lowest possible dose for the shortest period of time ■ Alternate-day vs. daily therapy ■ Once daily vs. split doses ■ Agents with low systemic absorption

Abbreviations used: ICS, inhaled corticosteroids.

Treatment includes lifelong replacement therapy with glucocorticoids and mineralocorticoids.[21]

- Cortisol: replaced by any steroid (e.g., prednisone, hydrocortisone)
- Aldosterone: replaced by fludrocortisone

Remember: systemic steroids can cause the adrenal gland to stop producing cortisol due to feedback inhibition; discontinuation of long-term steroids should be tapered.

Multiple sclerosis

Multiple sclerosis is an autoimmune disease that attacks the myelin sheath, causing tissue injury. Inflammation, demyelination, and axonal degeneration are the major pathologic mechanisms (characterized by periods of active disease and intervals of remission).[22] The location of inflammatory lesions dictates symptomatology:

- Early symptoms: fatigue, weakness, tingling, and blurred vision[22]

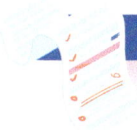

Table 13-8　Pharmacologic Agents Used in Management of Cushing's Syndrome[18,19]

DRUG AGENT	DRUG CLASS	MECHANISM OF ACTION	NOTES
Cabergoline	Dopamine D2R agonist	Inhibits D2R in corticotrope tumors	Hypotension, depression, headache, nausea
Etomidate Ketoconazole Metyrapone	Adrenal steroid inhibitors	Inhibits steroidogenesis	■ Doses required for cortisol suppression are often toxic ■ Ketoconazole CYP 3A4 inhibitor
Miotane	Adrenolytic		■ Limited by GI and neurologic side effects ■ Requires cortisol monitoring
Osilodrostat	11-beta-hydroxylase inhibitor		■ ↑ testosterone in women ■ Monitor for adrenal insufficiency
Mifepristone	Anti-progestational	GCR antagonist	■ CI in pregnancy ■ Monitor for adrenal insufficiency
Pasireotide	Somatostatin analog	↓ ACTH = ↓ cortisol	■ Indicated in adults unable to undergo surgery; or was not curative

Abbreviations used: ACTH, adrenocorticotropic hormone; CI, contraindicated; D2R, dopamine 2 receptor; GCR, glucocorticoid receptor; GI, gastrointestinal.

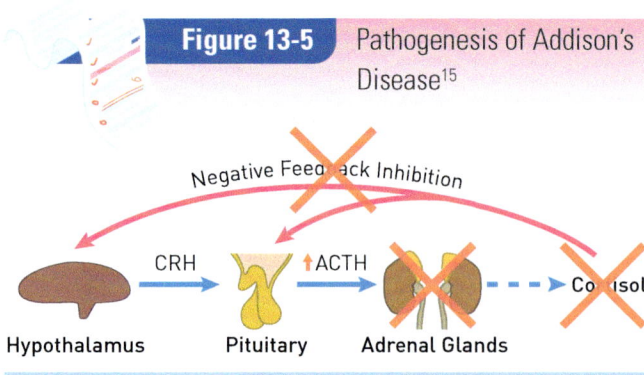

Figure 13-5 Pathogenesis of Addison's Disease[15]

Abbreviations used: CRH, corticotropin-releasing hormone; ACTH, adrenocorticotropic hormone.

- With disease progression: decreased cognitive function, muscle spasms, incontinence, difficulty walking, and visual disturbances[22]

The primary goal of therapy is to reduce exacerbations, relapses, or clinical attacks and to prevent disease progression.[23] Disease-modifying therapies are the primary treatment options for slowing the progression (see Table 13-9).

Systemic lupus erythematosus

Systemic lupus erythematosus (SLE) is a multisystem autoimmune disease affecting musculoskeletal, skin, renal, neuropsychiatric, cardiovascular, pulmonary, hematologic, and reproductive systems (characterized by flare-ups and periods of remission).[24,25] Nonspecific symptomatology makes diagnosis challenging:[24,25]

- Fatigue, weight loss, fever, arthralgia, myalgia, and **malar rash** (butterfly rash)
- High clinical suspicion—present with symptoms in ≥2 organ systems

Treatment depends on symptomatology and organ system involvement (see Table 13-10).[24]

- Hydroxychloroquine (Plaquenil)—gold standard; reduces flare-ups/other symptoms[24]
- Immunosuppressants and cytotoxic drugs—symptom control in SLE[24]
- Belimumab—control ongoing disease activity or frequent flare-ups[24]

- Consult Ch. 17, 18, and 20 for more in-depth drug therapy information
- Nonpharmacologic therapy: beneficial for symptom control and increased quality of life
  - Sun protection, vaccinations, exercise, smoking cessation, and body mass index control[24]

Sjögren's disease

Sjögren's disease is a chronic inflammatory autoimmune disorder.

- Goals for treatment: symptom palliation, prevention of complications, and optimization of immunosuppressive therapy[26]
  - Oral symptoms: topical fluoride or non-fluoride re-mineralizing agent, sugar-free lozenges or gum (xylitol), pilocarpine, chlorhexidine rinse
  - Ocular symptoms: topical azithromycin, steroids, artificial tears, cyclosporine
  - Musculoskeletal pain: azathioprine, corticosteroids, hydroxychloroquine, leflunomide, methotrexate, sulfasalazine
  - Fatigue: Dehydroepiandrosterone, exercise, hydroxychloroquine, tumor necrosis factor alpha inhibitors

Psoriasis

Psoriasis is a chronic autoimmune inflammatory disease. It is recognized as a skin disease, but it has multisystem inflammatory effects. Symptoms include raised, scaly, red plaques (patches) with silvery buildup on the skin.[27]

Mild-to-moderate psoriasis can be adequately controlled with topical medications or phototherapy. Moderate-to-severe psoriasis may require combinations with biologic agents or systemic medications.[27] Topical and systemic treatments are outlined in Table 13-11.

Psoriasis comorbidities are important to manage including cardiovascular disease, metabolic syndrome, mental health, obesity, inflammatory bowel disease, malignancy, sleep apnea, chronic obstructive pulmonary disease, and hepatic disease.[27]

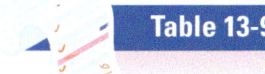

Table 13-9 Disease-Modifying Therapy for Multiple Sclerosis[23]

Drug agent	Dose	Route	Notes
Interferon-beta-1a	30 mcg once weekly	IM	▪ HA, flu-like symptoms, injection site pain, depression
Interferon-beta-1a	22 mcg or 44 mcg 3 times/wk	SQ	▪ Monitor LFTs, CBC, thyroid every 6 mo
Interferon beta-1b	0.25 mg every other d	SQ	
Pegylated Interferon beta-1a	125 mcg every 14 d	SQ	
Glatiramer Acetate	20 mg every other d or 40 mg 3 times/wk	SQ	▪ Injection site reaction, flushing, SOB, rash, chest pain ▪ Preferred in pregnancy
Cladribine	Weight-based treatment course once a y for 2 y	PO	URTI, HA, low WBC
Dimethyl fumarate	120 mg BID for 1 wk then 240 mg BID	PO	Flushing, GI symptoms
Dimethyl fumarate	231 mg BID for 1 wk then 462 mg BID	PO	
Fingolimod	0.5 mg daily	PO	▪ HA, flu, diarrhea, abdominal pain ▪ Monitor LFTs, CBC, macular edema, bradycardia
Siponimod	Titrate each day over 4–5 d to 1 mg or 2 mg daily	PO	▪ HA, increased BP ▪ Monitor LFTs, CBC
Teriflunomide	7 mg or 14 mg daily	PO	▪ HA, hair thinning, N/D ▪ Monitor LFTs
Alemtuzumab	12 mg daily for 5 d, then 12 mg daily for 3 d 1 y later	IV	▪ **BBW:** Autoimmune condition, infusion reaction, malignancy ▪ REMS program ▪ Monitor thyroid, infections
Natalizumab	300 mg once every 28 d	IV	▪ **BBW:** PML ▪ REMS program
Ocrelizumab	600 mg every 6 mo	IV	Infusion site reaction, increased risk of infection and malignancy

Abbreviations used: BBW, black box warning; BP, blood pressure; CBC, complete blood count; GI, gastrointestinal; HA, headache; IM, intramuscular; IV, intravenous; LFT, liver function test; N/D, nausea, diarrhea; PML, progressive multifocal leukoencephalopathy; PO, by mouth; REMS, risk evaluation and mitigation strategies; SOB, shortness of breath; SQ, subcutaneous; URTI, upper respiratory tract infection; UTI, urinary tract infection; WBC, white blood cells.

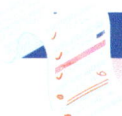

Table 13-10 Symptom Control for Lupus[24,25]

Symptoms	Treatment	Notes
Arthralgia	Glucocorticoids, hydroxychloroquine, methotrexate, NSAIDs	Goal is low chronic steroid exposure
Cutaneous lupus	Topical glucocorticoids, hydroxychloroquine	Use sunscreen and avoid sun exposure
Hematologic	Azathioprine, mycophenolate, rituximab	Monitor infection
Renal	Azathioprine, cyclophosphamide, glucocorticoids, mycophenolate	Monitor SCr, urinalysis
Cardiovascular	Antihypertensive agents, cholesterol-lowering agents	See Ch. 10; treat risk factors aggressively
Neuropsychiatric	Anticonvulsants, antidepressants, antipsychotics, glucocorticoids	Control exacerbating factors
Pulmonary	Azathioprine, cyclophosphamide, glucocorticoids, mycophenolate, rituximab	Monitor lung function

Abbreviations used: NSAIDs, nonsteroidal anti-inflammatory drugs; SCr, serum creatinine.
Adapted from Fanouriakis A, Kostopoulou M, Alunno A, et al. 2019 update of the EULAR recommendations for the management of systemic lupus erythematosus. *Ann Rheum Dis*. 2019;78(6):736–745. Lam NC, Ghetu MV, Bieniek ML. Systemic lupus erythematosus: primary care approach to diagnosis and management. *Am Fam Physician*. 2016;94(4):284–294.

Table 13-11 Topical and Systemic Treatment Options for Psoriasis[27–30]

Drug agent	Drug class	Notes
Topical steroids	Anti-inflammatory	Reduce swelling and redness of plaques
Calcipotriene Calcitriol	Vitamin D₃	Slow cell growth, removes scales, reduce itching and inflammation
Tazarotene	Vitamin A	Slow skin cell growth
Anthralin	Chrysarobin	▪ From bark of the Araroba tree ▪ Reduce rapid growth of skin cells
Methotrexate	Antimetabolite	Monitor folic acid, LFTs, GI effects
Apremilast	Phosphodiesterase 4 inhibitor	Monitor renal function, depression, suicidal ideations
Cyclosporine	Calcineurin inhibitor	Monitor BP, renal function, BUN, LFTs
Acitretin	Retinoid	Monitor LFTs, CBC
Adalimumab Certolizumab Etanercept Infliximab	TNF-alfa inhibitor	▪ For moderate to severe psoriasis ▪ Monitor: CBC, CMP, TB test, hepatitis screening, infections ▪ All therapies may be switched with a different biologic agent if clinically needed
Brodalumab Ixekizumab Secukinumab	IL-17 inhibitor	
Guselkumab Tildrakizumab	IL-23 inhibitor	
Ustekinumab	IL-12/IL-23 inhibitor	

Abbreviations used: BP, blood pressure; BUN, blood urea nitrogen; CBC, complete blood count; CMP, complete metabolic panel; GI, gastrointestinal; IL, interleukin; LFT, liver function test; TB, tuberculosis; TNF, tumor necrosis factor.

ADDITIONAL RESOURCES

American Diabetes Association. Standards of medical care in diabetes - 2020 abridged for primary care providers. *Clin Diabetes.* 2020;38(1):10–38.

American Diabetes Association. Abridged for primary care providers. *Clin Diabetes.* 2020;38(1):10–38.

National Multiple Sclerosis Society. Disease-modifying therapies for MS. Available at: https://www.nationalmssociety.org/NationalMSSociety/media/MSNationalFiles/Brochures/Brochure-The-MS-Disease-Modifying-Medications.pdf.

Menter A, Gelfand JM, Connor C, et al. Joint American Academy of Dermatology-National Psoriasis Foundation guidelines of care for the management of psoriasis with systemic nonbiologic therapies. *J Am Acad Dermatol.* 2020.

REFERENCES

1. Trujillo J, Haines S. Diabetes mellitus. In: DiPiro JT, Yee GC, Posey LM, Haines ST, Nolin TD, Ellingrod V, eds. *Pharmacotherapy: A Pathophysiologic Approach.* 11th ed. New York, NY: McGraw-Hill; 2020.

2. Wu Y, Ding Y, Tanaka Y, Zhang W. Risk factors contributing to type 2 diabetes and recent advances in the treatment and prevention. *Int J Med Sci.* 2014;11(11):1185–1200.

3. American Diabetes Association. Standards of medical care in diabetes - 2020 abridged for primary care providers. *Clin Diabetes.* 2020;38(1):10–38.

4. Riddle MC, Bakris G, Blonde L, et al. Standards of medical care in diabetes - 2020. *Diabetes Care.* 2020;43.

5. Garber AJ, Handelsman Y, Grunberger G, et al. Consensus statement by the American Association of Clinical Endocrinologists and American College of Endocrinology on the comprehensive type 2 diabetes management algorithm - 2020 executive summary. *Endocr Pract.* 2020;26(1):107–139.

6. American Diabetes Association. Abridged for primary care providers. *Clin Diabetes.* 2020;38(1):10–38.

7. Garber AJ, Handelsman Y, Grunberger G, et al. Consensus statement by the American Association of Clinical Endocrinologists and American College Of Endocrinology on the comprehensive type 2 diabetes management algorithm - 2020. *Endocr Pract.* 2020; 26(1):107–139.

8. American Diabetes Association. 9. pharmacologic approaches to glycemic treatment. *Diabetes Care.* 2020;43(suppl 1):s98–s110.

9. American Diabetes Association. 11. microvascular complications and foot care. *Diabetes Care.* 2020;43(suppl 1):s135–s151.

10. Kravets I. Hyperthyroidism: diagnosis and treatment. *Am Fam Physician.* 2016;93(5):363–370.

11. LiVolsi VA, Baloch ZW. The pathology of hyperthyroidism. *Front Endocrinol (Lausanne).* 2018;9:737.

12. Calissendorff J, Falhammar H. Lugol's solution and other iodide preparations: perspectives and research directions in Graves' disease. *Endocrine.* 2017;58(3):467–473.

13. Chaker L, Bianco AC, Jonklaas J, Peeters RP. Hypothyroidism. *Lancet.* 2017;390(10101):1550–1562.

14. Chiovato L, Magri F, Carlé A. Hypothyroidism in context: Where we've been and where we're going. *Adv Ther.* 2019;36(suppl 2): s47–s58.

15. Raff H, Sharma ST, Nieman LK. Physiological basis for the etiology, diagnosis, and treatment of adrenal disorders: Cushing's syndrome, adrenal insufficiency, and congenital adrenal hyperplasia. *Compr Physiol.* 2014;4(2):739–769.

16. Nieman LK. Recent updates on the diagnosis and management of cushing's syndrome. *Endocrinol Metab (Seoul).* 2018; 33(2):139–146.

17. Nicolaides NC, Pavlaki AN, Maria Alexandra MA, Chrousos GP. Glucocorticoid therapy and adrenal suppression. In: Feingold KR, Anawalt B, Boyce A, et al., eds. *Endotext.* South Dartmouth, MA: MDText.com, Inc.; 2000.

18. Nieman LK. Update in the medical therapy of Cushing's disease. *Curr Opin Endocrinol Diabetes Obes.* 2013;20(4):330–334.

19. Cuevas-Ramos D, Lim DST, Fleseriu M. Update on medical treatment for Cushing's disease. *Clin Diabetes Endocrinol.* 2016; 1:16.

20. Bornstein SR, Allolio B, Arlt W, et al. Diagnosis and treatment of primary adrenal insufficiency: an Endocrine Society clinical practice guideline. *J Clin Endocrinol Metab.* 2016;101(2):364–389.

21. Michels A, Michels N. Addison disease: early detection and treatment principles. *Am Fam Physician.* 2014;89(7):563–568.

22. Thompson AJ, Baranzini SE, Geurts J, Hemmer B, Ciccarelli O. Multiple sclerosis. *Lancet.* 2018;391(10130):1622–1636.

23. National Multiple Sclerosis Society. Disease-modifying therapies for MS. Available at: https://www.nationalmssociety.org/NationalMSSociety/media/MSNationalFiles/Brochures/Brochure-The-MS-Disease-Modifying-Medications.pdf.

24. Fanouriakis A, Kostopoulou M, Alunno A, et al. 2019 update of the EULAR recommendations for the management of systemic lupus erythematosus. *Ann Rheum Dis.* 2019;78(6):736–745.

25. Lam NC, Ghetu MV, Bieniek ML. Systemic lupus erythematosus: primary care approach to diagnosis and management. *Am Fam Physician.* 2016;94(4):284–294.

26. Vivino FB, Carsons SE, Foulks G, et al. New treatment guidelines for Sjögren's disease. *Rheum Dis Clin North Am.* 2016;42(3): 531–551.

27. Menter A, Strober BE, Kaplan DH, et al. Joint AAD-NPF guidelines of care for the management and treatment of psoriasis with biologics. *J Am Acad Dermatol.* 2019;80(4):1029–1072.

28. Menter A, Gelfand JM, Connor C, et al. Joint American Academy of Dermatology-National Psoriasis Foundation guidelines of care for the management of psoriasis with systemic nonbiologic therapies. *J Am Acad Dermatol.* 2020.

29. National Psoriasis Foundation. Prescription non-steroidal topical treatments. Available at: https://www.psoriasis.org/about-psoriasis/treatments/topicals/non-steroid. Accessed April 29, 2020.

30. National Psoriasis Foundation. Prescription topical steroid treatments. Available at: https://www.psoriasis.org/about-psoriasis/treatments/topicals/steroids. Accessed April 29, 2020.

CHAPTER 14

Male and Female Health

With medical writing support provided by
Banner Medical LLC Writer: Miriam Opara

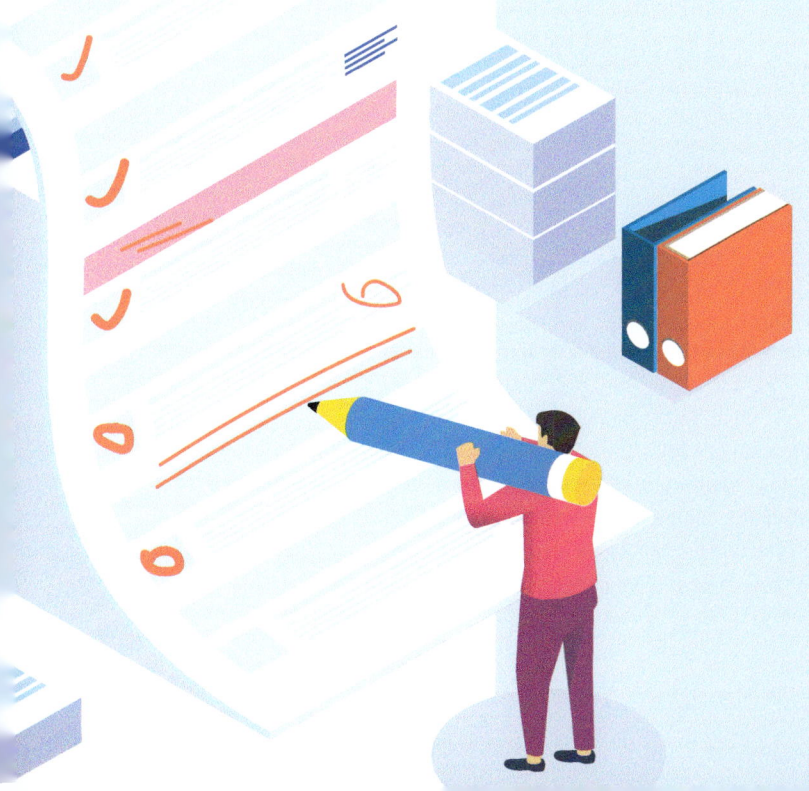

Fertility and Contraception

A typical menstrual cycle is 23–35 days with an average of 28 days (see Table 14-1).[1]

Remember, infertility agents mimic endogenous hormones.[2–4]

- Clomiphene increases LH/FSH; causes ovulation
- Ganirelix prevents premature LH surge during fertility treatments
- Gonadotropins act as LH, FSH, or hCG; cause follicle stimulation/ovulation
- hCG or leuprolide commonly used to trigger ovulation
- Due to the growth of multiple follicles/release of eggs, multiple births are more common among women who undergo fertility treatments

Remember the following regarding contraception:[1,5,6]

- Combined oral contraceptives (COCs)—mono-, bi-, tri-, or quad-phasic
  - Wait minimum 3 weeks post-delivery—deep vein thrombosis risk; 4–6 weeks ↑ risk factors
  - Same-day start—take active pill first day of menses (no backup method [BUM] needed)
  - Sunday start—take active pill first Sunday after menses begins (use BUM for 7 days)

- COC warning signs: **ACHES**
  - **A**bdominal pain—may be a sign of liver problems
  - **C**hest pain, shortness of breath, coughing up blood—may be a sign of blood clot in lungs
  - **H**eadache—may be a sign of stroke or blood clot
  - **E**ye problems (blurred vision, flashing lights, blindness)—may be a sign of stroke, blood clots, optic neuritis
  - **S**evere leg pain with or without swelling—may be a sign of deep vein thrombosis
- Transdermal patch increases adherence (may be less effective with weight >198 lbs [90kg])
  - Increased incidence of blood clots caused by higher systemic estrogen exposure
  - For missed dose >24 hours in first 3 weeks, apply new patch and use BUM for 7 days
- Vaginal ring has **lowest estrogen exposure** among combined hormonal products
  - If ring is removed or expelled on week 1 or 2 for >3 hours, reinsert and use BUM for 7 days
  - If ring is removed or expelled on week 3, insert **new** ring and use BUM for 7 days
- Progestin-only products are preferred during **breastfeeding**; oral progestin less efficacious than COCs
  - Timing of administration matters—If missed dose >3 hours, use BUM for 48 hours

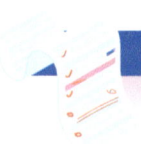

Table 14-1 The Menstrual Cycle[1]

CYCLE DAY	DESCRIPTION
1	Begins with day 1 of menses; can last for 4–8 d; hormone levels are low (start of follicular phase)
1–5	Follicles develop on the ovaries (each follicle contains 1 egg)
5–8	One follicle continues to develop and will begin to release estrogen; by day 8 menses usually stops; lining of uterus thickens and grows
9–13	Estrogen levels peak; ↑ luteinizing hormone (surge ~36 hr before ovulation)
14	Ovulation occurs (end of follicular phase, start of luteal phase)
15–24	Fallopian tubes assist egg on journey to the uterus; progesterone released to further ↑ uterine lining thickness; fertilization may occur if sperm is present; pregnancy occurs if embryo implants into uterine wall
24–28	Unfertilized egg breaks apart; around day 24 estrogen and progesterone levels drop (not pregnant); uterine lining and egg are shed with day 1 of menses (end of luteal phase, start of follicular phase)

- Injectable depot medroxyprogesterone acetate causes weight gain, menstrual irregularity, bone loss, and it may take longer to conceive after discontinuation; safe to use during pregnancy
- Intrauterine devices (IUD)—**most effective reversible contraception**; contraindicated in pregnancy, active pelvic infection, and significantly distorted uterine anatomy
- IUD warning signs: **PAINS**
  - **P**eriod late
  - **A**bdominal pain or pain during intercourse
  - **I**nfection or abnormal odorous discharge
  - **N**ot feeling well—fever or chills
  - **S**trings missing or one shorter than the other
- Subdermal progestin-releasing implant—can try to conceive within 1 week of removal; menstrual irregularity; decreased efficacy possible (>130% ideal body weight)
- Emergency contraception—within 72 hours (Plan B 1-step) or 120 hours (5 days, Ella) after unprotected sex; copper IUD within 5 days of unprotected sex
  - Reduced efficacy:
    - Plan B with body mass index >26 (can use Ella or IUD)
    - Ella with body mass index >35 (can use IUD)

The efficacy of various contraception methods and their failure rate is outlined in Figure 14-1.

Postmenopausal hormone therapy

Treatment of menopausal symptoms should be initiated based on the presence of vasomotor symptoms and vulvovaginal symptoms, weighing risks versus benefits. Benefits outweigh the risks in women who are symptomatic and healthy within 10 years of menopause ≤60 years.

- **Intact uterus**—estrogen + progesterone; decreased risk of cancer/endometrial hyperplasia
- **Hysterectomy**—monotherapy with unopposed estrogen ok

- **Transdermal**—preferred in women with venous thromboembolism risk, hypertension, hypertriglyceridemia, obesity, diabetes, and gallbladder disease
- **Vulvovaginal** symptoms only—use low-dose vaginal estrogen or ospemifene and/or lubricants
- **Nonhormonal options**—SNRI, SSRI, gabapentin, clonidine

Remember:
- **CI:** history/active breast cancer, deep vein thrombosis, or pulmonary embolism, and arterial thromboembolic disease (not all-inclusive)
- CYP 3A4 inducers decrease effects of estrogen and inhibitors increase effects of estrogen

Osteoporosis

Osteoporosis causes low bone mineral density, which causes decreased bone tissue, increased bone fragility, and risk of bone fracture (most commonly hip, spine, and wrist).[7]

- **Osteopenia:** T-score −1 to −2.5 standard deviations below the young adult mean
- **Osteoporosis:** T-score below −2.5 standard deviations below the young adult mean

A dual-energy x-ray absorptiometry (DXA) scan is used to diagnose osteoporosis. Treatment initiation is recommended by the National Osteoporosis Foundation[8] in postmenopausal women and men ≥50 years presenting with the following:

- History of hip or vertebral fracture
- T-score ≤ −2.5 (femoral neck, total hip, or lumbar spine) by DXA
- T-score −1 to −2.5 (femoral neck or lumbar spine) by DXA
  - PLUS 10-year hip fracture probability ≥3% or 10-year any major fracture probability ≥20% (using FRAX at https://www.sheffield.ac.uk/FRAX/)

Pharmacologic therapy includes calcium and vitamin D supplementation, bisphosphonates, selective

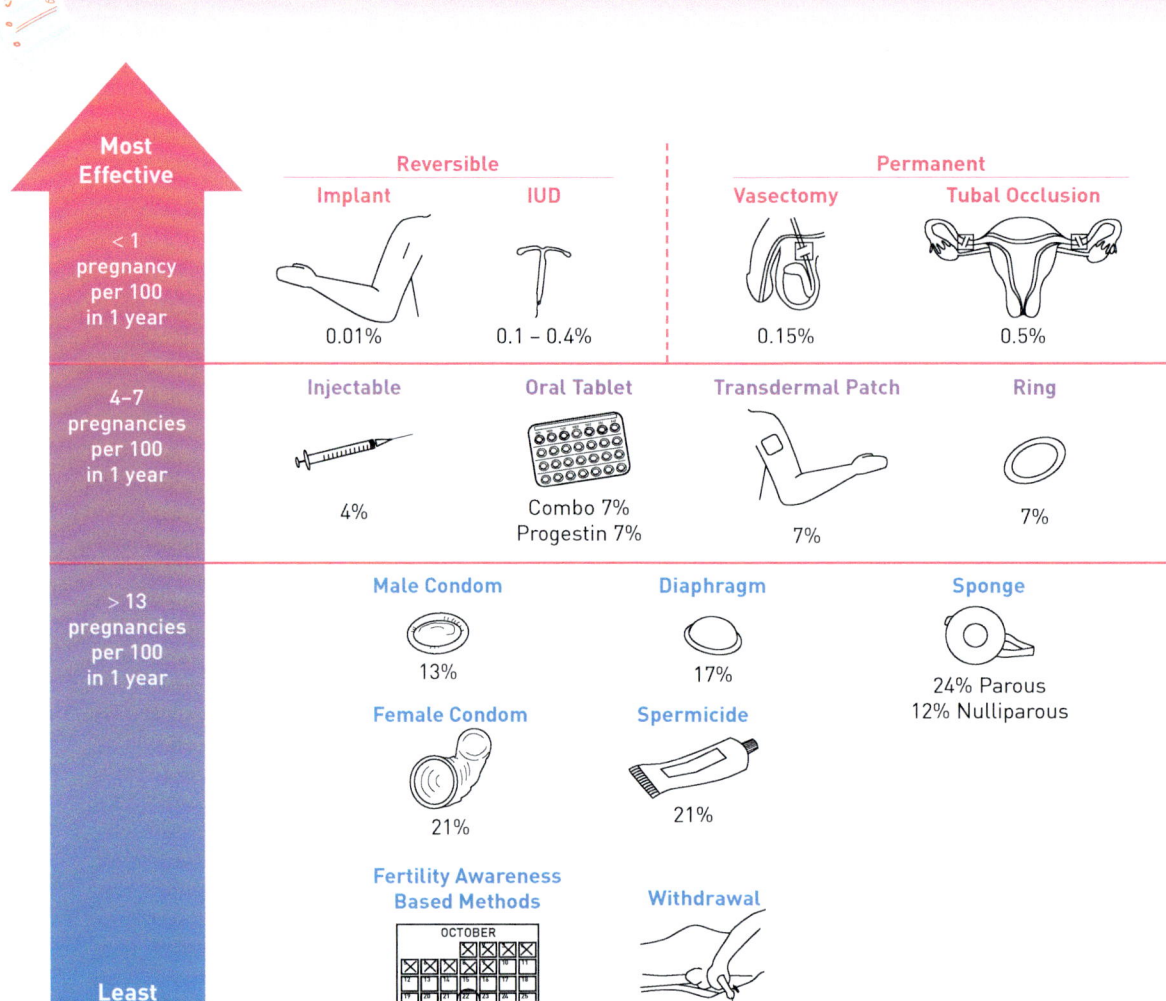

estrogen receptor modulators (SERMs), parathyroid hormone analogs, calcitonin, RANKL inhibitor, and sclerostin inhibitor. **Remember** the following:

- Maximum of 500 mg of calcium per dose because of limited GI tract absorption
- Take calcium carbonate with food to maximize absorption; calcium citrate can be taken with or without food
- Adequate calcium and vitamin D supplementation:
  - Calcium 1000 mg → females ≤50 years; men ≤70 years

- Calcium 1200 mg → females ≥51 years; men ≥71 years
- Vitamin D 800 IU/day → goal: vitamin D level 30 ng/mL in adults
- Calcium decreases bioavailability of fluoroquinolones, tetracyclines, and levothyroxine
- Must stay upright after oral bisphosphonate administration for minimum of 30 minutes; contraindicated in CrCL <30–35 mL/min
- SERMs are used for shortest period of time at the lowest dose
  - Side effects: hot flashes, increased risk of venous thromboembolism

- Hypocalcemia needs to be resolved before starting denosumab, bisphosphates, and romosozumab
- Romosozumab—increases the risk of myocardial infarction, stroke, and cardiovascular death
- Teriparatide and alaboparatide contraindicated—high risk of osteosarcoma

Male hypogonadism

Male hypogonadism is a result of decreased functional activity of the gonads.[9] The gonads (testes) produce hormones (testosterone) and gametes (sperm). Testosterone has an essential role in male sexual, cognitive, and body development. Male hypogonadism causes deficiency in serum testosterone <300 ng/dL.

Symptoms include the following:

- Anemia
- Muscle wasting
- Reduced bone mass
- Erectile dysfunction
- Reduced energy and stamina and
- Depressed mood

Testosterone replacement therapy (see Table 14-2) is the primary treatment strategy (only in men with clinical symptoms and confirmed low testosterone). **Remember** FDA warning for cardiovascular risk.[9]

Erectile dysfunction

Erectile dysfunction (ED) is persistent failure to achieve a penile erection for sexual intercourse for ≥3 months.[10] ED can result from reduced blood flow to the penis in patients with hypertension, atherosclerosis, and diabetes. Medications may also cause or contribute to ED (see Table 14-3).[10,11]

Treatment for ED begins by ruling out secondary causes (e.g., medication) with the goal of improving the quantity and quality of penile erections. First-line pharmacologic therapy is phosphodiesterase type-5 (PDE-5) inhibitors (sildenafil, tadalafil, avanafil, and vardenafil).[10,11]

- Mechanism of action: blocks PDE-5 from degrading cGMP so that the smooth muscle

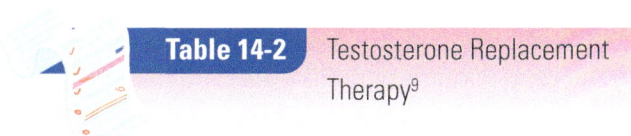

Table 14-2 Testosterone Replacement Therapy[9]

FORMULATION	NOTES
Topical gels & solutions Buccal tablets Transdermal patch Implantable pellets Intramuscular injections Oral tablets	<ul><li>Gels/solutions: apply at the same time every morning</li><li>Patch: use only one patch, remove, and apply a new patch each night</li><li>Oral agents have increased risk of hepatotoxicity<ul><li>Except undecanoate; bypasses first-pass metabolism</li></ul></li><li>Wash hands thoroughly after application; avoid secondary exposure to women and children</li><li>**Side effects:** gynecomastia, increased appetite, increased risk of clotting</li></ul>

relaxation occurs and allows blood flow into the penis
- **Remember** the following:
  - Absolute contraindication with nitrates causes increased risk of severe hypotension
  - May cause vision changes
  - Dose adjust when combined with alpha-1 blockers and antihypertensives
  - Requires stimulation for efficacy
  - Erections lasting >4 hours/painful (priapism)—MUST seek medical help

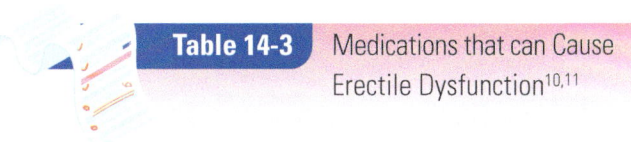

Table 14-3 Medications that can Cause Erectile Dysfunction[10,11]

MEDICATION	
Alcohol	Beta-blockers
Anticholinergics	BPH medications
Antidepressants	Diuretics
Antipsychotics	Opioids

Abbreviation used: BPH, benign prostatic hyperplasia.

Benign prostatic hyperplasia

Benign prostatic hyperplasia is an overgrowth of prostate stromal/epithelial cells that causes constriction of the bladder neck and obstruction of urinary outflow.[12] The bladder contracts with small amounts of urine causing frequent urination, slow urinary stream, urgency, and straining to urinate. Eventually, the bladder weakens and loses the ability to empty itself.[12] Diagnosis requires a physical exam, including a urinalysis and serum prostate-specific antigen. Treatment depends on the severity of symptoms and is outlined in Table 14-4.[12,13]

Overactive bladder

Overactive bladder (OAB) is characterized by the presence of bothersome urinary symptoms defined by symptoms of [14,15]

- Urgency: sudden and compelling desire to urinate
- Frequency: up to 7 micturitions a day
- Nocturia: interruption of sleep because of the need to void
- Urgency incontinence: involuntary leakage of urine

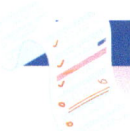

Table 14-4 Benign Prostatic Hyperplasia Treatment Options Based on Severity[12,13]

DRUG AGENT	MOA	NOTES
MILD SYMPTOMS		
Watchful waiting	Behavioral modifications	Reassessment every 6–12 mo
MODERATE SYMPTOMS		
Alpha antagonists		
Doxazosin Terazosin	Nonselective alpha-1 blocker	Improves AUA symptom score, ↑ urinary flow rate, and ↓ PVR volume Nonselective agents: require titration and BP monitoring
Alfuzosin Silodosin Tamsulosin	Selective alpha-1A blocker	**SE:** dizziness, fatigue, headache, fluid retention, orthostatic hypotension, floppy iris syndrome (> with selective agents)
5 Alpha-reductase inhibitors		
Dutasteride Finasteride	Inhibits 5-alpha reductase enzyme, which blocks the conversion of testosterone to dihydrotestosterone	Helps to reduce prostate size **SE:** decreased libido, gynecomastia **CI:** women of child-bearing age/children Monitor: prostate-specific antigen
Phosphodiesterase type 5 inhibitors		
Tadalafil	Increased muscle relaxation in LUT	Improves LUTS and erectile dysfunction, can be used in combination with other BPH agents **SE:** Headache, flushing, dizziness, hypotension
SEVERE SYMPTOMS		
Surgery or prostatectomy	Symptom improvement	Risk of complications

Abbreviations used: AUA, American Urological Association; BPH, benign prostatic hyperplasia; CI, contraindicated; LUTS, lower urinary tract symptoms; MOA, mechanism of action; PVR, post-void residual; SE, side effects.

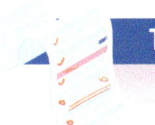

DRUG AGENT	**MECHANISM OF ACTION**	**NOTES**
Antimuscarinics		
Darifenacin*	Blocks acetylcholine from binding and	**SE:** dizziness, drowsiness, dry mouth, constipation, dry eyes
Fesoterodine	limits the contractions of detrusor	Do not use in narrow-angle glaucoma, caution in impaired gastric
Oxybutynin	muscles	emptying and history of urinary retention
Solifenacin*		
Tolterodine		
Trospium		
Beta-3 agonist		
Mirabegron	Relaxes the detrusor muscle and increases	**SE:** hypertension, headache, constipation, dizziness
	bladder capacity	

Table 14-5 Treatment Options for Overactive Bladder Disease[14,15]

Abbreviation used: SE, side effects.
*M3 selective agent.

OAB urgency is caused by an overactive detrusor muscle. There are five classifications of urinary incontinence:[14,15]

1. Stress urinary incontinence: involuntary loss of small volume of urine induced by exercise, coughing, sneezing, lifting
2. Urge urinary incontinence: cannot hold urine long enough to reach the toilet; large amounts of leakage
3. Overflow incontinence: constant dribbling of urine, frequent urination of small amounts
4. Mixed incontinence: combination of urgency and stress urinary incontinence
5. Functional incontinence: not caused by bladder or urethra abnormalities; usually occurs in dementia, cognitive, or mobility deficiencies

Remember the following:[14,15]
- The risk factors for OAB include age (>40 years), diabetes, obesity, prior vaginal delivery, hysterectomy, and pelvic injury

- Goal of treatment: to manage urgency incontinence (see Table 14-5)
- Behavioral therapy (bladder training, pelvic floor muscle training) is first-line treatment
- Antimuscarinics (i.e., anticholinergics) and Beta-3 agonists are second-line therapies for urge urinary incontinence
- Extended-release antimuscarinics are preferred over immediate release; causes less dry mouth

Desmopressin is the treatment of choice for nocturia. Desmopressin is an antidiuretic hormone analog that temporarily decreases urine production. It is contraindicated in patients with severe hyponatremia, polydipsia, and use with loop diuretics.[15]

ADDITIONAL RESOURCES

Curtis KM, Tepper NK, Jatlaoui TC, et al. U.S. medical eligibility criteria for contraceptive use, 2016. *MMWR Recomm Rep.* 2016;65(3):1–103

Camacho PM, Petak SM, Binkley N, et al. American Association of Clinical Endocrinologists/American College of Endocrinology clinical practice guidelines for the diagnosis and treatment of postmenopausal osteoporosis-2020 update. *Endocr Pract.* 2020;26(suppl 1):1–46.

Bhasin S, Brito JP, Cunningham GR, et al. Testosterone therapy in men with hypogonadism: an Endocrine Society clinical practice guideline. *J Clin Endocrinol Metab.* 2018;103(5):1715–1744.

Burnett AL, Nehra A, Breau RH, et al. Erectile dysfunction: AUA guideline. *J Urol.* 2018;200(3):633–641.

Lightner DJ, Gomelsky A, Souter L, Vasavada SP. Diagnosis and treatment of overactive bladder (non-neurogenic) in adults: AUA/SUFU guideline amendment 2019. *J Urol.* 2019;202(3): 558–563.

REFERENCES

1. Office of Women's Health. Your menstrual cycle. U.S. Department of Health & Human Services. Available at: https://www.womenshealth.gov/menstrual-cycle/your-menstrual-cycle. Updated July 12, 2017. Accessed May 26, 2020.

2. Lindsay TJ, Vitrikas KR. Evaluation and treatment of infertility. *Am Fam Phys.* 2015;91:308–314.

3. Cunningham J. Infertility: A primer for primary care providers. *Jaapa.* 2017;30(9):19–25.

4. Gunn DD, Bates GW. Evidence-based approach to unexplained infertility: a systematic review. *Fertil Steril.* 2016;105(6):1566–1574. e1561.

5. Curtis KM, Tepper NK, Jatlaoui TC, et al. U.S. medical eligibility criteria for contraceptive use, 2016. *MMWR Recomm Rep.* 2016;65(3):1–103.

6. Therapeutic Research Center. The art of selecting and prescribing hormonal contraception (Course 160246). Pharmacist's Letter. 2016. Available at: https://pharmacist.therapeuticresearch.com/Content/Segments/PRL/2016/Sep/The-Art-of-Selecting-Prescribing-Hormonal-Contraception-10112. Accessed May 26, 2020.

7. Theraupeutic Research Center. Managing osteoporosis: screening, treatment, and more. Pharmacist's Letter. Available at: https://pharmacist.therapeuticresearch.com/Content/Segments/PRL/2012/Jul/Managing-Osteoporosis-Screening-Treatment-and-More-4529. June 2019.

8. Cosman F, de Beur SJ, LeBoff MS, et al. Clinician's guide to prevention and treatment of osteoporosis. *Osteoporos Int.* 2014; 25(10):2359–2381.

9. Bhasin S, Brito JP, Cunningham GR, et al. Testosterone therapy in men with hypogonadism: an Endocrine Society clinical practice guideline. *J Clin Endocrinol Metab.* 2018;103(5): 1715–1744.

10. Lee M, Sharifi R. Erectile dysfunction. In: DiPiro JT, Yee GC, Posey LM, Haines ST, Nolin TD, Ellingrod V, eds. *Pharmacotherapy: A Pathophysiologic Approach.* 11th ed. New York, NY: McGraw-Hill; 2020.

11. Burnett AL, Nehra A, Breau RH, et al. Erectile dysfunction: AUA guideline. *J Urol.* 2018;200(3):633–641.

12. Lee M, Sharifi R. Benign prostatic hyperplasia. In: DiPiro JT, Yee GC, Posey LM, Haines ST, Nolin TD, Ellingrod V, eds. *Pharmacotherapy: A Pathophysiologic Approach.* 11th ed. New York, NY: McGraw-Hill; 2020.

13. American Urological Association. Management of benign prostatic hyperplasia. In: American Urological Association Guidelines, 2010. Available at: https://www.auanet.org/guidelines/benign-prostatic-hyperplasia-(bph)-guideline/benign-prostatic-hyperplasia-(2010-reviewed-and-validity-confirmed-2014).

14. Lightner DJ, Gomelsky A, Souter L, Vasavada SP. Diagnosis and treatment of overactive bladder (non-neurogenic) in adults: AUA/SUFU guideline amendment 2019. *J Urol.* 2019;202(3): 558–563.

15. Rovner ES, Wyman J, Lam S. Urinary incontinence. In: DiPiro JT, Yee GC, Posey LM, Haines ST, Nolin TD, Ellingrod V, eds. *Pharmacotherapy: A Pathophysiologic Approach.* 11th ed. New York, NY: McGraw-Hill; 2020.

CHAPTER 15

Gastroenterology

With medical writing support provided by
Banner Medical LLC Writer: Miriam Opara

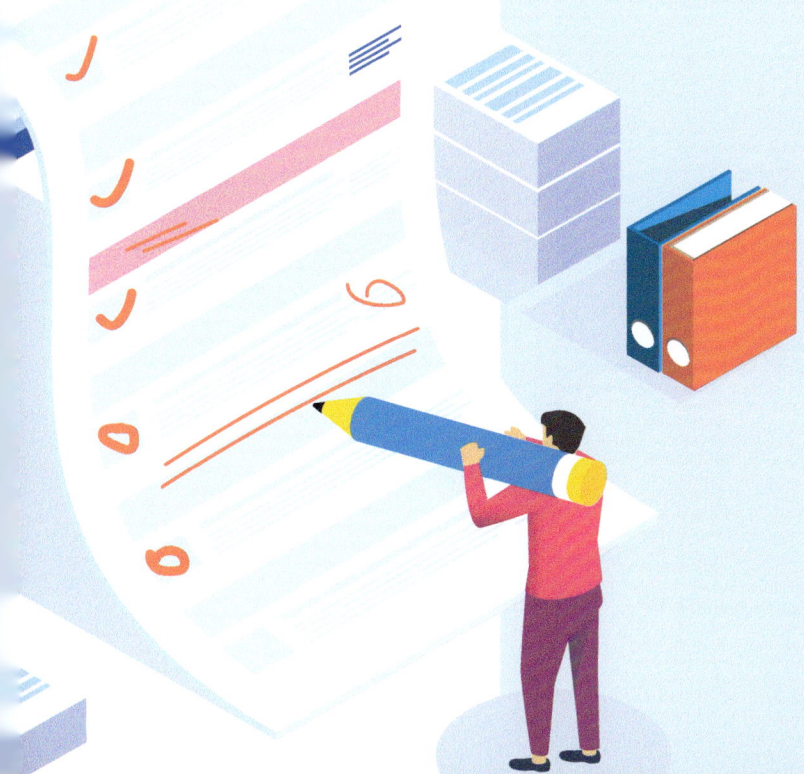

Gastrointestinal reflux disease and peptic ulcer disease

Gastrointestinal reflux disease (GERD) occurs when refluxed acidic stomach contents flow back into the esophagus or oral cavity resulting from decreased lower esophageal sphincter pressure.[1] Symptoms may include heartburn, dysphagia, reflux chest pain, and regurgitation. There are various drugs and foods that exacerbate GERD (see Table 15-1).[1]

The goal of therapy is to alleviate symptoms and prevent complications. Treatment includes lifestyle changes, over the counter antacids, histamine-2 receptor antagonists (H2RA), or proton-pump inhibitors (PPIs) for 2 weeks.[2] If symptoms do not improve, the patient should seek medical advice. The recommended initial treatment is a PPI at the lowest effective dose (see Figure 15-1).[2]

The onset and duration of action varies among antacids, H2RAs, and PPIs (see Table 15-2).

Antacids neutralize gastric acid, which increases gastric pH (see Table 15-3).[1] H2RAs reversibly inhibit histamine-2 receptors on the gastric parietal cells, which decreases gastric acid secretion (see Table 15-3). PPIs irreversibly bind to the gastric H/K-ATPase pump in the parietal cells and block gastric acid secretion (see Table 15-3).[1,2]

Peptic ulcer disease is defined by the etiology of the ulcer: *Heliobacter pylori*, nonsteroidal anti-inflammatory drug–induced, and stress-related damage (see Table 15-4).[3] Symptoms typically include dyspepsia, gastric pain, and burning sensation (exacerbated by eating).[3]

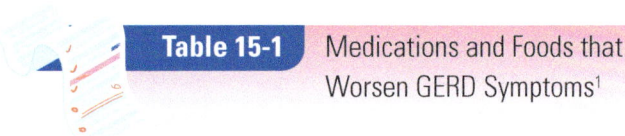

Table 15-1 Medications and Foods that Worsen GERD Symptoms[1]

DRUG AGENT	FOOD
Aspirin	Alcohol
Bisphosphonates	Chocolate
Estrogen	Coffee, tea
Iron supplements	Fatty meals
Nicotine replacement therapy	Garlic
NSAIDs	Onions
Steroids	Orange juice
Tetracycline	Spicy foods

Abbreviation used: NSAIDs, nonsteroidal anti-inflammatory drug.

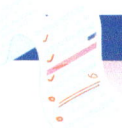

Figure 15-1 GERD Treatment Approach[1,2]

Lifestyle modifications
- Weight loss
- Elevate the head of the bed
- Avoid eating within 2-3 h of bedtime

Initial drug treatment
- PPI once daily for 8 w
- Partial response—may consider dose/frequency adjustment
- Nonresponders—require further evaluation

Maintenance therapy
- Consider when symptoms continue after PPI discontinuation or complications occur*
- PPI at the lowest effective dose
- Alternative: H2RA

Abbreviations used: H2RA, histamine-2 receptor antagonist; PPI, proton-pump inhibitor.
*complications include erosive esophagitis and Barret's esophagus.

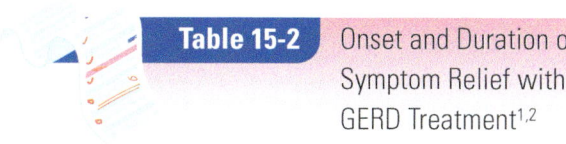

Table 15-2 Onset and Duration of Symptom Relief with GERD Treatment[1,2]

Drug agent	Onset	Duration
Antacids	<5 m	20–30 m
H2RA	30–40 m	4–10 h
H2RA + antacid	<5 m	8–10 h
PPI	2–3 h	12–24 h

Abbreviations used: H2RA, histamine-2 receptor antagonist; PPI, proton-pump inhibitor.

Inflammatory bowel disease

Inflammatory bowel disease is a condition that includes ulcerative colitis (inflammation in the colon) and Crohn's disease (inflammation throughout the intestines).[5,6] Symptoms include abdominal pain, frequent bowel movements, fistulas, weight loss, and chronic diarrhea.[5]

The **goal of therapy** is to treat acute exacerbations and maintain remission. Steroids (e.g., prednisone, budesonide, hydrocortisone) are often used to treat acute exacerbations and should be tapered over 8–12 weeks once remission is achieved.[6,7] Maintenance of remission depends on the severity of the disease (see Tables 15-5 and 15-6).[6,7]

Constipation and diarrhea

Constipation is difficult or infrequent passage of stool including straining on defecation, sensations of incomplete evacuations, and hard or lumpy stool.[8]

- Chronic constipation—symptoms ≥3 months[8]
- Drug-induced constipation is commonly associated with opioids, anticholinergics, calcium channel blockers (e.g., verapamil), bile acid sequestrants (e.g., colesevelam), and antacids (e.g., calcium carbonate, aluminum hydroxide).[9]

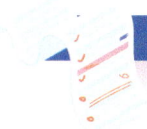

Table 15-3 GERD Treatment Options[1,2]

Treatment	Generic name	Brand name
Antacids	Aluminum hydroxide + magnesium carbonate	Gaviscon
	Aluminum hydroxide + magnesium hydroxide	Mylanta Ultimate Strength
	Aluminum hydroxide + magnesium hydroxide + simethicone	Maalox and Mylanta
	Aspirin + citric acid + sodium bicarbonate	Alka-Seltzer
	Calcium carbonate	Tums
	Calcium carbonate + magnesium hydroxide	Rolaids
	Magnesium hydroxide	Milk of Magnesia
Histamine-2 receptor antagonists	Cimetidine	Tagamet
	Famotidine	Pepcid
	Nizatidine*	Tazac
	Ranitidine	Zantac
Proton-pump inhibitors	Dexlansoprazole*	Dexilant
	Esomeprazole	Nexium
	Lansoprazole	Prevacid
	Omeprazole	Prilosec
	Omeprazole + sodium bicarbonate	Zegerid
	Pantoprazole*	Protonix
	Rabeprazole*	Aciphex

*Rx only

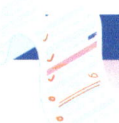

Table 15-4 | Peptic Ulcer Disease[3,4]

CHARACTERISTIC	H.PYLORI-INDUCED	NSAID-INDUCED	STRESS-INDUCED
Condition	Chronic	Chronic	Acute
Site of damage	Duodenum > stomach	Stomach > duodenum	Stomach > duodenum
Symptoms	Gastric pain	Asymptomatic	Asymptomatic
Ulcer depth	Superficial	Deep	Superficial
GI bleeding	Less severe	More severe	More severe
Treatment	Typically involves a combination of ≥2 antimicrobials* + PPI	◾ Misoprostol ◾ PPI ◾ Sucralfate	◾ Antacids ◾ H2RA ◾ PPI ◾ Sucralfate

Abbreviations used: H2RA, histamine-2 receptor antagonist; NSAID, nonsteroidal anti-inflammatory drug; PPI, proton-pump inhibitor.
*Antimicrobial selection is dependent on *H. pylori* sensitivity, previous antibiotic exposure, and patient allergies. Agents selected may include amoxicillin, bismuth subsalicylate, clarithromycin, a fluroquinolone, metronidazole (or another nitroimidazole antibiotic), and tetracycline.

◾ Treatment for constipation includes lifestyle management, increased fiber intake, and laxative agents based on the etiology of the constipation (see Figure 15-2 and Table 15-7).[8,9]

Diarrhea is increased loose bowel movements[9] caused by drugs (e.g., antibiotics, colchicine, metoclopramide), food poisoning, viral infections, or bacterial infection (most commonly *E. coli*).

◾ Nonpharmacologic therapy: oral rehydration therapy; BRAT diet (bananas, rice, applesauce, and toast)
◾ Pharmacologic therapy—if pain is uncontrolled (see Table 15-8)[9]

Motion sickness

Motion sickness is typically caused by travel, seasickness, or airsickness. Symptoms include nausea, dizziness, and fatigue.[10] Prophylactic treatment is most effective 30 minutes to 2 hours before traveling to reduce the severity or duration of symptoms, usually with anticholinergics or antihistamines as first-line therapy.

Anticholinergics:

◾ Scopolamine patch (Tranderm Scop): 1 patch is applied 4 hours before travel; new patch applied every 3 days as needed. The patch is applied behind the ear; wash hands after applying the patch
  • Side effects: sedation (do not drive, avoid alcohol), dry mouth, dizziness, dry eyes, sensitivity to bright light

Antihistamines:

◾ Use first generation (nonsedating antihistamines are not effective)
  • Cyclizine (Marezine)
  • Dimenhydrinate (Dramamine)
  • Diphenhydramine (Benadryl)
  • Meclizine (Antivert, Bonine)
  • Promethazine (Phenergan)
◾ Side effects: sedation, dry eyes, blurry vision, dry mouth

Nausea associated with motion sickness can be treated with ondansetron (Zofran), promethazine (Phenergan), prochlorperazine (Compazine), and metoclopramide (Reglan).[10]

Table 15-5	Ulcerative Colitis Induction and Remission Therapy[5,7]

INDUCTION AND MAINTENANCE FOR MODERATE TO SEVERE UC

Anti-TNF agents	**Integrin receptor antagonist**
▪ Adalimumab (Humira)	▪ Vedolizumab (Entyvio)
▪ Golimumab (Simponi)	
▪ Infliximab (Remicade)	
Janus kinase inhibitor	**IL-12/23 Inhibitor (AGA)**
▪ Tofacitinib (Xeljanz)	▪ Ustekinumab (Stelara)

INDUCTION OF REMISSION FOR UC

Mildly active	**Mildly active left-sided colitis**
▪ Rectal 5-ASA	▪ 5-ASA enemas
	▪ Rectal 5-ASA + Oral 5-ASA
Fail 5-ASA therapy or moderately active	**Moderate to severely active**
▪ Oral budesonide	▪ Adalimumab (Humira)
	▪ Golimumab (Simponi)
	▪ Infliximab (Remicade) ± thiopurine
	▪ Tofacitinib (Xeljanz)
	▪ Vedolizumab (Entyvio)
	▪ Methotrexate
Moderate to severe, biologics naïve	**Moderate to severe, prior infliximab use**
▪ Infliximab (Remicade)	▪ Ustekinumab (Stelara)
▪ Vedolizumab (Entyvio)	▪ Tofacitinib (Xeljanz)

MAINTENANCE OF REMISSION FOR UC

Distal disease	**Moderate to severe**
▪ Sulfasalazine, balsalazide, olsalazine, mesalamine (oral + topical)	▪ Tofacitinib (Xeljanz)
	▪ Methotrexate
	▪ Combinations:
	● Anti-TNF agents, vedolizumab, ustekinumab + thiopurines or methotrexate

Abbreviations used: UC, ulcerative colitis; 5-AGA, American Gastroenterological Association; ASA, mesalamine; TNF, tumor necrosis factor.
Adapted from Feuerstein JD, Isaacs KL, Schneider Y, et al. AGA Clinical Practice Guidelines on the Management of Moderate to Severe Ulcerative Colitis. *Gastroenterology*. 2020;158(5):1450–1461.

Nausea and Vomiting

Multiple disease processes, conditions, and certain medications are associated with nausea and vomiting (e.g., pregnancy, antineoplastic agents, postoperative).[11] The most common causes of nausea and vomiting include[11]

- Irritation of the chemoreceptor trigger zone (e.g., chemotherapy, narcotics, alcohol)
- Vestibular disorders (e.g., motion sickness, Meniere's syndrome)
- Central nervous system disorders (e.g., migraines, psychogenic vomiting
- Gastrointestinal disorders (e.g., obstruction, gastroparesis, gastroenteritis)

Depending on the etiology of the nausea and vomiting, patients may initially choose to self-treat with

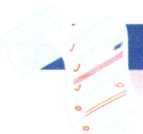

Table 15-6 Crohn's Disease Recommended Therapy[5,6]

INDUCTION OF REMISSION FOR CROHN'S DISEASE

Mild to moderate active CD
- Sulfasalazine

Moderate to severe CD
- Vedolizumab (Entyvio) ± immunomodulator
- Natalizumab (Tysarbi)

Severely active CD
- Adalimumab (Humira)
- Certolizumab (Cimzia)
- Infliximab (Remicade)

Perianal fistulas
- Infliximab
- Adalimumab
- Certolizumab
- Thiopurines
- Tacrolimus**

Mild to moderate ileal or right-sided CD
- Ileal release budesonide

Moderate to severe CD: who fail steroids, thiopurines, methotrexate, or anti-TNF agents (or no prior exposure to anti-TNF agents)
- Ustekinumab (Stelara)

Fulminant CD
- IV corticosteroids
- Infliximab (Remicade)

Steroid sparing therapy
Thiopurine
- Azathioprine (Imuran)

Anti-TNF agents
- Adalimumab (Humira)
- Certolizumab (Cimzia)
- Infliximab (Remicade)

Methotrexate

MAINTENANCE OF REMISSION

- Thiopurine* ± Anti-TNF therapy
- Methotrexate ± Anti-TNF therapy

Refractory azathioprine/mercaptopurine
- Anti-TNF agents (infliximab, adalimumab, certolizumab pegol)

Use the following if agent was used for induction:
- Natalizumab (Tysarbi)
- Vedolizumab (Entyvio)
- Ustekinumab (Stelara)

Failed steroids, thiopurines, methotrexate, or anti-TNF inhibitors, or anti-TNF inhibitor naïve
- Ustekinumab (Stelara)

Abbreviations used: CD, Crohn's disease; TNF, tumor necrosis factor.
*thiopurine methyltransferase testing should be considered before initial use.
**short-term for perianal and cutaneous fistulas.
Adapted from Lichtenstein GR, Loftus EV, Isaacs KL, Regueiro MD, Gerson LB, Sands BE. ACG Clinical Guideline: Management of Crohn's Disease in Adults. *Am J Gastroenterology.* 2018;113(4):481–517.

Figure 15-2 Treatment Algorithm for Constipation[8,9]

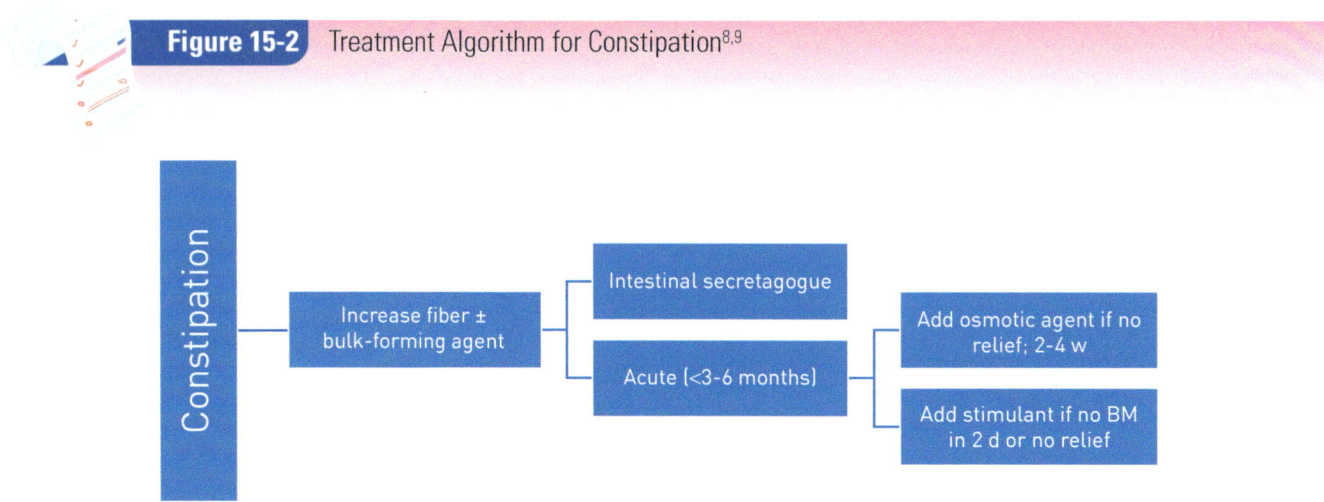

Abbreviations used: BM, bowel movement.

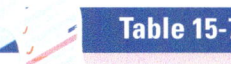

Table 15-7 Pharmacologic Agents for Constipation[8,9]

DRUG AGENT	DRUG CLASS & NAME	NOTES
Bulk-forming agents	Calcium polycarbophil (Fiber-Lax, FiberCon) Methylcellulose (Citrucel) Psyllium (Metamucil)	Creates a gel-like matrix in the stool Causes softening of feces in 1–3 d
Osmotic agents	Glycerin (Fleet, Pedia-Lax) Lactulose (Enulose, Kristalose) Magnesium hydroxide (Milk of Magnesia) PEG 3350 (Miralax) Sorbitol	Draws fluid into the bowel lumen through osmosis Causes watery evacuation in 1–6 h Causes softening of feces in 1–3 d
Stimulant agents	Bisacodyl (Dulcolax) Sennosides (Senna, Sennokot)	Directly stimulates colonic neurons Causes soft stool in 6–12 h
Emollients (stool softeners)	Docusate (Colace, DocQLace, Dulcolax stool softener)	Reduces surface tension of stool Causes softening of feces in 1–3 d
Intestinal secretagogue agents	Linaclotide (Linzess)	Guanylate cyclase C agonist Increases the speed of GI transit
	Lubiprostone (Amitiza)	Activates chloride channels ↑ fluid in the gut and peristalsis
	Plecanatide (Trulance)	Guanylate cyclase C agonist Increases the speed of GI transit
Opioid antagonists	Methylnaltrexone (Relistor) Naloxegol (Movantik) Naldemedine (Symproic)	Peripherally acting mu-opioid receptor antagonists to ↓ constipation
Other agents	Prucalopride (Motegrity)	Selective 5-HT$_4$ receptor agonist

Abbreviations used: 5-HT$_4$, 5-hydroxytryptamine-4; PEG, polyethylene glycol.

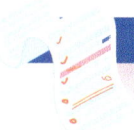

Table 15-8 Antidiarrheal Medications[9]

GENERIC NAME	BRAND NAME	MECHANISM OF ACTION
Bismuth subsalicylate	Pepto-Bismol	Antisecretory and antimicrobial effects
Dicyclomine	Bentyl	Antispasmodic
Diphenoxylate + atropine	Lomotil	Antimotility agents that slow intestinal motility
Loperamide	Imodium	

nonprescription medications or nondrug modalities (see Table 15-9).[11] If symptoms worsen, or are the result of a serious medical issue (e.g., cancer), the use of prescription agents becomes more common (see Table 15-9).[11]

Remember:

- Use of antihistamines with anticholinergic properties should be avoided in elderly adults and those with benign prostatic hyperplasia, narrow-angle glaucoma, and asthma.
- Cannabinoids are used for breakthrough chemotherapy-induced nausea and vomiting (CINV). Droperidol has limited use for CINV (risk of extrapyramidal symptoms and QTc prolongation); used as a rescue antiemetic only for postoperative nausea and vomiting (PONV).

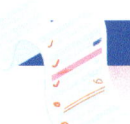

Table 15-9 Nonprescription and Prescription Agents for Treatment of Nausea and Vomiting*[11]

NONDRUG & NONPRESCRIPTION	PRESCRIPTION
Lifestyle changes	Antihistamines
• Avoidance of spicy or fried foods	• Hydroxyzine (Vistaril, Atarax)
• Restricting oral intake	• Scopolamine (Transderm Scop)
• Smaller meals	• Trimethobenzamide (Tigan)
Behavioral interventions	Benzodiazepine
• Acupuncture	• Lorazepam (Ativan)
• Biofeedback	Butyrophenones
• Chewing gum	• Haloperidol (Haldol)
• Cognitive distraction	• Droperidol (Inapsine)
• Guided imagery	Cannabinoids
• Hypnosis	• Dronabinol (Marinol)
• Relaxation	• Nabilone (Cesamet)
• Systematic desensitization	
• Transcutaneous electrical stimulation	
• Yoga	
BRAT diet	5-HT$_3$ receptor antagonists
• Bananas, rice, applesauce, toast	• Dolasetron (Anzemet)
	• Granisetron (Sancuso; Sustol)
	• Ondansetron (Zofran)
	• Palonosetron (Aloxi)
Herbal supplements	Miscellaneous
• Ginger	• Metoclopramide (Reglan)
• Lemongrass	• Olanzapine (Zyprexa)
Nonprescription drug agents	Phenothiazines
• Antacids	• Chlorpromazine (Thorazine)
• Antihistamines[+]	• Prochlorperazine (Compazine)
• Bismuth subsalicylate	• Promethazine (Phenergan)
• Doxylamine succinate	Substance P/Neurokinin-1 receptor antagonist
• H2RAs	• Aprepitant (Emend)
• Phosphorylated carbohydrate solution (Emetrol)	• Fosaprepitant (Emend)
• Pyridoxine	• Netupitant/palonosetron (Akynzeo)
	• Rolapitant (Varubi)

Abbreviation used: 5HT$_3$, 5-Hydroxytryptamine-3.
*Treatment should be based on the etiology of the nausea and vomiting and follow known guidelines when applicable.
[+]Antihistaminic-anticholinergic drugs such as dimenhydrinate, diphenhydramine, and meclizine.

- Corticosteroids and 5-Hydroxytryptamine-3 receptor antagonists can be used as monotherapy or in combination for prophylaxis of CINV or PONV.
- Haloperidol should not be used first-line for uncomplicated nausea and vomiting because of the risk of extrapyramidal symptoms and QTc prolongation; may consider for breakthrough CINV or palliative care.
- 5-HT3 receptor antagonists are equivalent when used in equipotent doses/schedules for CINV. Selection should be based on route of administration, side effect potential, and cost. No IV dolasetron for CINV because of risk of QTc prolongation.
- Lorazepam is used for anticipatory nausea and vomiting associated with CINV.
- Avoid olanzapine in elderly adults and concomitant use with benzodiazepines.

ADDITIONAL RESOURCES

DeVault KR, Castell DO, Gastroenterology ACo. Updated guidelines for the diagnosis and treatment of gastroesophageal reflux disease. *Am J Gastroenterol.* 2005;100(1):190–200.

Lichtenstein GR, Loftus EV, Isaacs KL, Regueiro MD, Gerson LB, Sands BE. ACG Clinical Guideline: Management of Crohn's Disease in Adults. *American Journal of Gastroenterology.* 2018; 113(4):481–517.

Feuerstein JD, Isaacs KL, Schneider Y, et al. AGA Clinical Practice Guidelines on the Management of Moderate to Severe Ulcerative Colitis. *Gastroenterology.* 2020;158(5):1450–1461.

Brainard A, Gresham C. Prevention and treatment of motion sickness. *Am Fam Physician.* 2014;90(1):41–46.

REFERENCES

1. May D, Thiman M, Rao SSC. Gastroesophageal reflux disease. In: DiPiro JT, Yee GC, Posey LM, Haines ST, Nolin TD, Ellingrod V, eds. *Pharmacotherapy: A Pathophysiologic Approach.* 11th ed. New York, NY: McGraw-Hill; 2020.

2. DeVault KR, Castell DO, Gastroenterology ACo. Updated guidelines for the diagnosis and treatment of gastroesophageal reflux disease. *Am J Gastroenterol.* 2005;100(1):190–200.

3. Love BL, Mohorn PL. Peptic ulcer disease and related disorders. In: DiPiro JT, Yee GC, Posey LM, Haines ST, Nolin TD, Ellingrod V, eds. *Pharmacotherapy: A Pathophysiologic Approach.* 11th ed. New York, NY: McGraw-Hill; 2020.

4. Chey WD, Leontiadis GI, Howden CW, Moss SF. ACG clinical guideline: treatment of helicobacter pylori infection. *Am J Gastroenterology.* 2017;112(2):212–239.

5. Hemstreet BA. Inflammatory bowel disease. In: DiPiro JT, Yee GC, Posey LM, Haines ST, Nolin TD, Ellingrod V, eds. *Pharmacotherapy: A Pathophysiologic Approach.* 11th ed. New York, NY: McGraw-Hill; 2020.

6. Lichtenstein GR, Loftus EV, Isaacs KL, Regueiro MD, Gerson LB, Sands BE. ACG clinical guideline: Management of Crohn's disease in adults. *Am J Gastroenterology.* 2018;113(4): 481–517.

7. Feuerstein JD, Isaacs KL, Schneider Y, et al. AGA clinical practice guidelines on the management of moderate to severe ulcerative colitis. *Gastroenterology.* 2020;158(5):1450–1461.

8. Bharucha AE, Pemberton JH, Locke GR. American Gastroenterological Association technical review on constipation. *Gastroenterology.* 2013;144(1):218–238.

9. Fabel PH, Shealy KM. Diarrhea, constipation, and irritable bowel syndrome. In: DiPiro JT, Yee GC, Posey LM, Haines ST, Nolin TD, Ellingrod V, eds. *Pharmacotherapy: A Pathophysiologic Approach.* 11th ed. New York, NY: McGraw-Hill; 2020.

10. Brainard A, Gresham C. Prevention and treatment of motion sickness. *Am Fam Physician.* 2014;90(1):41–46.

11. Gravatt LAH, Donohoe KL, Gatesman ML. Nausea and Vomiting. In: DiPiro JT, Yee GC, Posey LM, Haines ST, Nolin TD, Ellingrod V, eds. *Pharmacotherapy: A Pathophysiologic Approach.* 11th ed. New York, NY: McGraw-Hill; 2020.

CHAPTER 16

Psychiatry and Neurology

With medical writing support provided by
Banner Medical LLC Writer: Miriam Opara

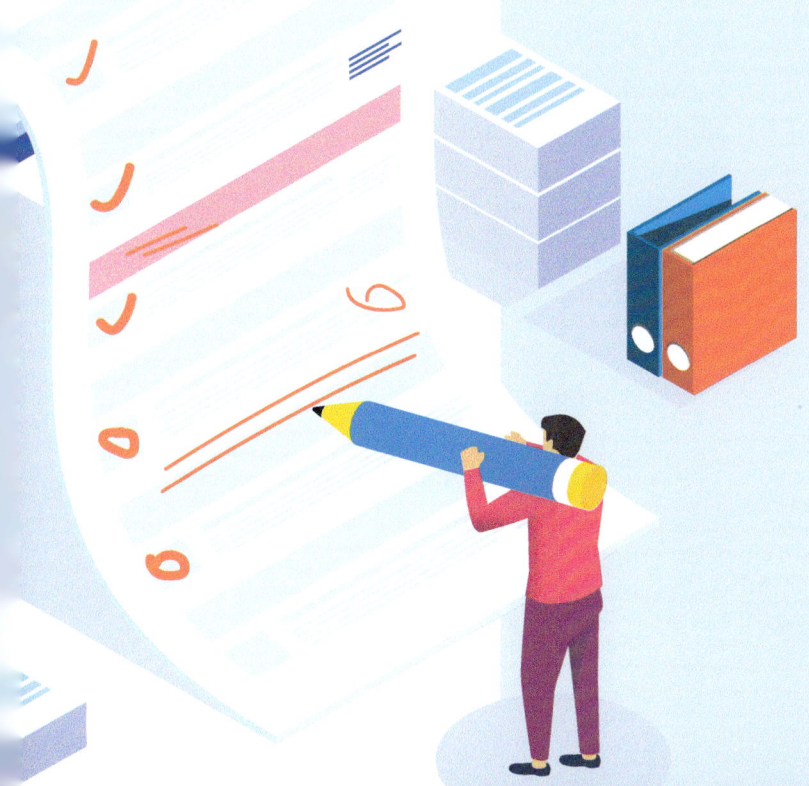

Attention deficit hyperactivity disorder

Attention deficit hyperactivity disorder (ADHD) is a neurodevelopmental disorder involving genetic and environmental risk factors, marked by a pattern of inattention and/or hyperactivity and impulsivity that can have a negative impact on social, academic, and/or occupational functioning.[1,2]

- Symptoms (see Table 16-1) are usually present before age 12
- **Remember: 6–6–2 → ≥6** symptoms (age ≥17) for **≥6** months in **≥2** settings (e.g., home, school)

Treatment combines behavioral therapy and pharmacologic treatment (see Table 16-2). Risk versus benefits must be considered when initiating pharmacologic treatment in children.[2]

Remember the following:

- Give stimulants with or after breakfast to help minimize weight loss
  - Stimulant side effects: Increased BP possible, increased abuse potential,

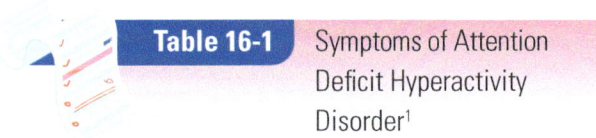

Table 16-1	Symptoms of Attention Deficit Hyperactivity Disorder[1]

Inattention
- Avoids tasks requiring continuous attention
- Forgets daily activities
- Has difficulty organizing tasks
- Loses things
- Has trouble listening
- Does not follow through on instructions
- Distracts easily

Hyperactivity and impulsivity
- Fidgets with hands or feet
- Leaves seat unexpectedly
- Runs and climbs at inappropriate times
- Has difficulty playing quietly
- Blurts out answers
- Often interrupts others
- Has difficulty taking turns
- Talks excessively

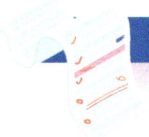

Table 16-2	Treatment Options for Attention Deficit Hyperactivity Disorder[2]

CALM

Clonidine (Catapres)

Atomoxetine (Strattera)

Lisdexamfetamine (Vyvanse)

Methylphenidate (Ritalin, Concerta, Daytrana)

GRAD

Guanfacine (Intuniv)

R

Amphetamine/Dextroamphetamine (Adderall)

Dexmethylphenidate (Focalin)

dilated pupils, loss of appetite, insomnia
- Atomoxetine: Increased risk of suicidal ideation in children and adolescents
- Extended-release doses should be titrated up every 7 days
- Patch: Apply 2 hours before desired effect and remove after 9 hours
- Alpha 2 agonists can lower BP
- Watch for drug interactions with CYP450 inducers, CYP450 inhibitors, and CYP2D6 substrates

Schizophrenia

Schizophrenia is a psychiatric disorder that causes altered brain structure/chemistry, primarily dopamine.[3,4] Patients may suffer from a profound disruption in perception, cognition, and emotion. Symptoms may include[3,4]

- Acute psychotic behavior, such as hallucinations, delusions, and ideas of influence
- Disconnected thought processes, inability to hold logical conversations (alogia), or contradictory thoughts (ambivalence)
- Patients may display flat affect, or affect may be inappropriate or labile

- Uncooperative, hostile, verbal, or physical aggression (resulting from misperception of reality)
- Residual symptoms (differentiating feature) may include anxiety; suspiciousness; and lack of volition, motivation, insight, and judgment

DSM-5 criteria classify schizophrenia symptoms into positive (e.g., hallucinations, delusions, confused thoughts, movement disorders, difficulty concentrating) and negative symptoms (e.g., lack of pleasure, alogia, flat affect, lack of follow-through). A third category, cognitive dysfunction (verbal fluency, working memory, attention, verbal learning and memory, executive functioning), is also a central feature.

Treatment includes medications that target neurotransmitter receptors (see Table 16-3).

Long-acting injectable (LAI) antipsychotics are administered by injection in various weekly or monthly intervals. LAIs are an option for patients with adherence struggles or who respond well to oral antipsychotic medications, but experience increased

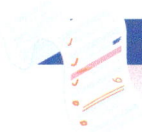

Table 16-3 Antipsychotics for Treatment of Schizophrenia[3,4]

FIRST-GENERATION ANTIPSYCHOTICS

Low potency	**Side effects**
Chlorpromazine (Thorazine)	▪ Increased risk of death in elderly patients with dementia-related psychosis
Thioridazine (Mellaril)	▪ Sedation
Mid potency	▪ EPS (see Table 16-4)
Loxapine (Loxitane)	▪ Cardiac and metabolic effects
Perphenazine (Trilafon)	▪ Seizures
Thiothixene (Navane)	▪ QT prolongation
Trifluoperazine (Stelazine)	▪ Anticholinergic effects
High potency	
Fluphenazine (Prolixin)	
Haloperidol (Haldol)	

SECOND-GENERATION ANTIPSYCHOTICS[3,4]

AABCC . . . I . . . L . . . OPQR . . . Z	**Side effects**
Asenapine (Saphris)	▪ Metabolic SE
Aripiprazole (Abilify)	● Highest risk: clozapine, olanzapine, quetiapine
Brexpiprazole (Rexulti)	● Lowest risk: aripiprazole, ziprasidone
Cariprazine (Vraylar)	▪ EPS (see Table 16-4)
Clozapine (Clozaril)	● Highest risk: quetiapine
Iloperidone (Fanapt)	▪ Hematological effects
Lurasidone (Latuda)	● Highest risk: clozapine (REMS program requiring regular ANC monitoring)
Olanzapine (Zyprexa)	▪ QT Prolongation
Paliperidone (Invega)	● Highest risk: ziprasidone
Quetiapine (Seroquel)	▪ Hyperprolactinemia
Risperidone (Risperdal)	● Highest risk: risperidone, paliperidone
Ziprasidone (Geodon)	▪ Seizure
	● Highest risk: clozapine

Abbreviations used: ANC, absolute neutrophil count; EPS, extrapyramidal side effects; REMS, risk evaluation and mitigation strategies; SE, side effects.

side effects and/or poor absorption. The following are available LAI antipsychotics:

- First generation
  - Haloperidol
  - Fluphenazine
- Second generation
  - Aripiprazole
  - Olanzapine
  - Paliperidone
  - Risperidone

Extrapyramidal side effects are listed in Table 16-4.

Bipolar disorder

Bipolar disorder is a mood disorder that causes fluctuations between elevated and depressed symptoms.[5] Bipolar is classified as bipolar I or bipolar II:[5]

- **Bipolar I:** Mania ± depression; psychosis possible
  - Mania is a state of abnormally elevated or irritable mood ≥1 week (e.g., inflated self-esteem, less sleep, talkative, easily distracted, and increased risky behavior)
- **Bipolar II:** Depression ± hypomania

The **goal of therapy** is to stabilize the patient's mood without inducing a depressive or manic episode.[6] Combination therapy with psychotherapy and mood

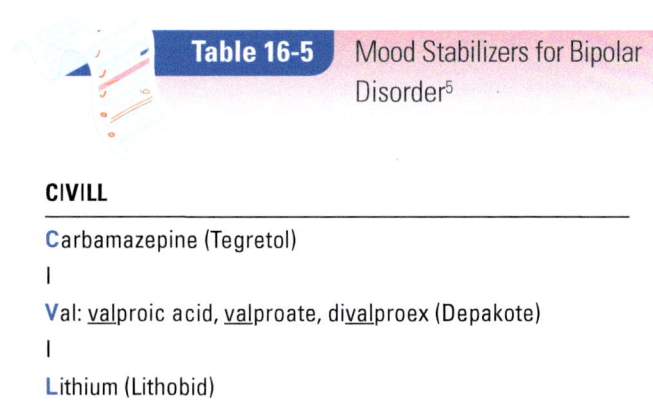

Table 16-5 Mood Stabilizers for Bipolar Disorder[5]

CIVILL

Carbamazepine (Tegretol)

I

Val: <u>val</u>proic acid, <u>val</u>proate, di<u>val</u>proex (Depakote)

I

Lithium (Lithobid)

Lamotrigine (Lamictal)

stabilizers (see Table 16-5) provides the best efficacy for most patients with bipolar disorder.[6]

Lithium (see Table 16-6) is effective for both manic and depressive components.

- Use caution with thyroid disorders, sodium depletion, and concomitant diuretics
- Side effects: GI (diarrhea); CNS, renal (polydipsia, polyuria); hypothyroidism; cardiac effects; weight gain; teratogenicity

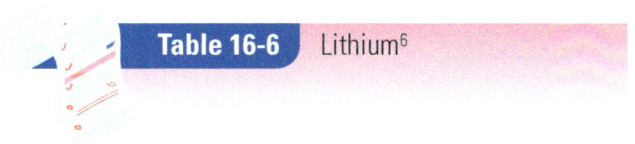

Table 16-6 Lithium[6]

TROUGH GOAL RANGE: 0.6–1.2 mEq/L

Lithium levels increase with
- Decreased sodium (ACEi, ARBs, thiazide)
- NSAIDs

Lithium levels decrease with
- Increased sodium
- Caffeine and theophylline

Increased risk of neurotoxicity if the following are taken with lithium:
- Verapamil
- Diltiazem
- Phenytoin
- Carbamazepine

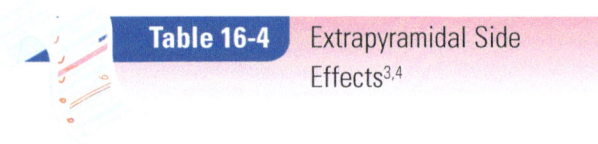

Table 16-4 Extrapyramidal Side Effects[3,4]

ADAPT

Akathisia: motor restlessness

Dystonia: muscle spasms

A

Parkinsonism: bradykinesia, rigidity

Tardive dyskinesia: involuntary movements (treated with deutetrabenazine or valbenazine)

Abbreviations used: ACEi, angiotensin-converting enzyme inhibitor; ARB, angiotensin receptor blocker; NSAIDs, nonsteroidal anti-inflammatory drugs.

Second-generation antipsychotics (e.g., quetiapine and lurasidone) are used with or without mood stabilizers for the treatment of patients with bipolar disorder.[5]

Depression

Major depressive disorder can include feelings of hopelessness, worthlessness, guilt, loss of pleasure, constant worry, lack of energy, changes in weight and/or sleep patterns, and/or suicidal thoughts.[7] Depression is thought to be caused by decreased brain levels of serotonin (5-HT), dopamine, and norepinephrine.[8]

- Treatment: Psychotherapy + pharmacologic agents outlined in Table 16-7

- Selective serotonin reuptake inhibitors (SSRIs) are generally the preferred initial treatment options followed by serotonin-norepinephrine reuptake inhibitors (SNRIs)[7]

"Atypical" antidepressants may be considered for the following:

- Brexanolone—post-partum depression
- Bupropion—comorbid smoking and ADHD
- Esketamine—treatment-resistant depression or acute suicidality
- Mirtazapine—weight gain and sleep
- Trazodone—insomnia

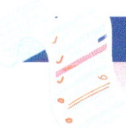

| **Table 16-7** | Antidepressants for Treatment of Depression[8] |

SSRIs: EFFECTIVVE Serotonin Prescriptions	SNRIs: VALIDD
Escitalopram (Lexapro)	Venlafaxine (Effexor)
Fluoxetine (Prozac)	A
Fluvoxamine (Luvox)*	Levomilnacipran (Fetzima)
E	I
Citalopram (Celexa)	Duloxetine (Cymbalta)
T	Desvenlafaxine (Pristiq)
I	
Vilazodone (Viibryd)	
Vortioxetine (Trintellix)	
E	
Sertraline (Zoloft)	
Paroxetine (Paxil)	
TCAs: ADDING	**Side effects: LASSO**
Amitriptyline (Elavil)	Loss or impairment of memory
Desipramine (Norpramin)	Anticholinergic
Doxepin (Silenor)	Sedation
Imipramine (Tofranil)	Suicidal risk
Nortriptyline (Pamelor)	Orthostatic hypotension
G	
MAOIs: TIPS[8]	
Tranylcypromine (Parnate)	
Isocarboxazid (Marplan)	
Phenelzine (Nardil)	
Selegiline (Eldepryl)	

Abbreviations used: MAOIs, monoamine oxidase inhibitors; SNRIs, serotonin-norepinephrine reuptake inhibitors; SSRIs, selective serotonin reuptake inhibitors; TCAs, tricyclic antidepressants.
*specifically indicated for obsessive compulsive disorder.

Second-generation antipsychotics may be used to augment antidepressant therapy or for treatment-resistant depression (at lower doses than schizophrenia)

Remember the following:[8]
- Black Box Warning: Suicidal thinking/ideation for all antidepressants
- Efficacy lag time: Can take 4–6 weeks to start feeling a benefit in mood (maximum 12 weeks for full benefit)
- Monoamine oxidase inhibitors: Avoid tyramine-containing foods (red wine, aged cheese, marmite)
- Risk of fatal overdose with tricyclic antidepressants (TCAs); TCAs/SNRIs also used in neuropathic pain and migraine
- Do not stop abruptly, titrate dose down in most cases to avoid discontinuation syndrome
- Pregnancy concerns—discontinuation can cause depression relapse; antidepressants can cause low birth weight, poor maternal weight gain, and suicidality
  - If continuing antidepressants during pregnancy, choose low–fetal risk medication
- Watch for QT prolongation (greatest risk with citalopram), increased BP with SNRIs, serotonin syndrome when multiple serotoninergic agents are combined, and decreased libido

Anxiety

Anxiety disorders are categorized as generalized anxiety disorder (GAD), panic disorder, agoraphobia, social anxiety disorder (SAD), and separation anxiety disorder. The goal of treatment is to reduce the severity and duration of anxiety symptoms (see Table 16-8) and improve overall functioning.[9]

Anxiety disorders require an acute treatment phase, maintenance phase, and a discontinuation phase. Psychotherapy plus pharmacologic therapy has produced the best overall results.[9]

First-line pharmacologic therapy options:

- GAD—duloxetine, escitalopram, paroxetine, sertraline, venlafaxine

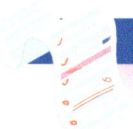

Table 16-8 Generalized Anxiety Disorder Symptoms[9]

Psychological symptoms
- Excessive anxiety
- Uncontrolled worrying
- Feeling on edge
- Difficulty concentrating

Physical symptoms
- Restlessness
- Fatigue
- Irritability
- Sleep disturbance

- Panic disorder—SSRIs, venlafaxine
- SAD—escitalopram, fluvoxamine, paroxetine, sertraline, venlafaxine

The antianxiety response of antidepressants can take 6–8 weeks or longer. Careful titration is important because some patients experience increased anxiety symptoms (jitteriness) initially and require lower doses.

Second-line pharmacological therapy options include buspirone, hydroxyzine, gabapentin/pregabalin, clomipramine (OCD), prazosin (PTSD), and benzodiazepines (see Tables 16-9 and 16-10).[9]

Remember the following:
- Benzodiazepine side effects: falls/fractures, CNS depression, depressed mood, cognitive impairment, accidental overdose, addiction/dependency

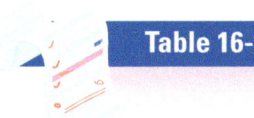

Table 16-9 Four Effects of Benzodiazepines[10]

MAAS

Muscle relaxant
Anxiolytic
Anticonvulsant
Sedative

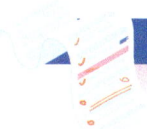

Table 16-10	Benzodiazepine Onset and Duration of Action[10]

ONSET OF ACTION		
RAPID: ~15 MIN (PEAK ONSET IN HOURS)	**INTERMEDIATE: 15–30 MIN (PEAK ONSET IN HOURS)**	**SLOW: 30–60 MIN (PEAK ONSET IN HOURS)**
Midazolam (0.5–1)	Alprazolam (0.7–1.6)	Temazepam (0.75–1.5)
Diazepam (1)	Triazolam (0.75–2)	Oxazepam (2–3)
	Lorazepam (1–1.5)	
	Clonazepam (1–4)	
	Chlordiazepoxide (2–4)	
DURATION OF ACTION		
SHORT-ACTING TriM	**INTERMEDIATE-ACTING ALTO**	**LONG-ACTING CDC**
Triazolam (Halcion)	**A**lprazolam (Xanax)	**C**lonazepam (Klonipin)
Midazolam (Versed)	**L**orazepam (Ativan)	**D**iazepam (Valium)
	Temazepam (Restoril)	**C**hlordiazepoxide (Librium)
	Oxazepam (Serax)	

- **LOT** (**L**orazepam, **O**xazepam, **T**emazepam)—preferred in older patients and hepatic dysfunction; less likely to accumulate due to conjugation metabolism
- Avoid use in pregnancy (especially 1st trimester) because of fetal risk of cleft palate
- Chlordiazepoxide preferred for alcohol withdrawal treatment
  - Careful consideration required due to abuse potential and risk of accumulation of hepatic metabolites
- Never abruptly discontinue; risk of withdrawal seizures and death
- Benzodiazepines are recommended for short-term use → 2–4–week duration

Alzheimer's disease

Alzheimer's disease (AD) features neuron degeneration in executive functioning brain areas, amyloid plaques and neurofibrillary tangles accumulation, destruction of cholinergic pathways, and insidious dementia. AD initially begins with complaints of vague memory loss and forgetfulness.[11] Cognitive decline is gradual, with loss of daily function in advanced stages. Symptoms of AD are described as cognitive, neuropsychiatric, and behavioral (see Table 16-11).[11]

There is no treatment to reverse or halt progression; the primary goal of treatment is to preserve patient function and slow cognitive decline.[12] Acetylcholinesterase inhibitors and N-methyl-d-aspartate (NMDA) receptor antagonists are indicated for the treatment of AD. Pharmacologic therapy is based on the severity of the disease (see Table 16-12)[12] and should be combined with non-pharmacologic strategies and monitoring for cognitive decline.[11] Behavioral disturbances can be treated based on severity; antipsychotics should be avoided in AD.[11]

Remember:
- Cholinesterase inhibitor side effects: dizziness, falls, syncope, bradycardia, insomnia, vivid dreams, daytime drowsiness
- NMDA receptor antagonist side effects: confusion, hallucinations, dizziness, falls, constipation

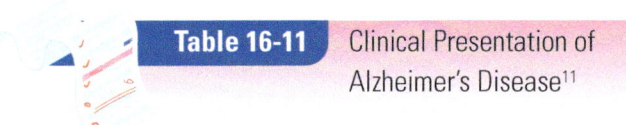

Table 16-11 Clinical Presentation of Alzheimer's Disease[11]

Cognitive
- Memory loss (recall)
- Aphasia
- Difficulty identifying objects
- Disorientation
- Impaired executive function

Neuropsychiatric
- Depression
- Hallucinations/delusions
- Apathy
- Irritability

Behavioral
- Inability to care for self
- Verbal or physical aggression
- Wandering
- Motor hyperactivity
- Sexual promiscuity

Parkinson Disease

Parkinson Disease (PD) → chronic, progressive neurologic disorder → ↓ motor function, bradykinesia, tremor at rest, rigidity, postural instability, and gait difficulties.[13, 14]

- Results from degeneration of the substantia nigra in the brain → ↓ dopaminergic cells

Primary treatment for PD is dopamine replacement (Table 16-13)[13, 14] → initial agent selected varies based on provider, patient preference, and severity of symptoms. Levodopa is considered for patients > 65 years and dopamine agonists are typically used in younger patients.[13, 14]

- Levodopa (L-dopa) → prodrug of dopamine + carbidopa (prevents peripheral metabolism of L-dopa before it can cross the blood-brain barrier). Long term L-dopa therapy eventually leads to motor complications.
  - "OFF" time refers to periods of poor movement (i.e., poor symptom control when drug is not efficacious)
    - ↑ off-time is a complication of long-term L-dopa therapy
  - "ON" time refers to periods of good movement (i.e., good symptom control when drug is efficacious)
  - Dyskinesia may occur during on-time while taking L-dopa[13, 14]
    - Abnormal movements that can occur at peak drug concentration

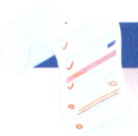

Table 16-12 Pharmacological Therapy for Alzheimer's Disease[12]

Drugs: "MERGED"	Mechanism of action	Severity of disease
Memantine (Namenda)	NMDA receptor antagonist	Moderate-to-severe
E	—	—
Rivastigmine (Exelon)	Cholinesterase inhibitor	Mild-to-moderate Transdermal: severe
Galantamine (Razadyne)	Cholinesterase inhibitor	Mild-to-moderate
E	—	—
Donepezil (Aricept)	Cholinesterase inhibitor	Mild-to-severe

Abbreviations used: NMDA, N-methyl-D-aspartate.

Table 16-13 Parkinson Disease Treatment Options[13, 14]

DRUG AGENT	NOTES
CARBIDOPA/LEVODOPA (SINEMET)	
Carbidopa/Levodopa	Carbidopa does not cross BBB, reduces the peripheral conversion of L-dopa to dopamine
DOPAMINE AGONISTS	
Pramipexole (Mirapex)	Stimulate dopamine receptors
Ropinirole (Requip)	Preferred therapy for younger patients
Rotigotine (Neurpro)	Can induce dyskinesia, psychosis
COMT INHIBITORS	
Entacapone (Comtan)	↑ the duration of action of L-dopa by preventing peripheral conversion of L-dopa
ANTICHOLINERGICS	
Benztropine (Cogentin)	↓ cholinergic activity
Trihexyphenidyl (Artane)	Useful for tremors but no dopamine activity
MOA-B INHIBITORS	
Rasagiline (Azilect)	Blocks the breakdown of dopamine
Safinamide (Xadago)	Caution when used in combination with other serotonergic agents
Selegiline (Eldepryl, Zelapar)	
OTHERS	
Amantadine (Gocovri, Osmolex)	Treats dyskinesia resulting from levodopa-based therapy
Istradfylline (Nourianz)	↑ the duration of action of L-dopa
Pimavanserin (Nuplazid)	Treats Parkinson Disease psychosis

Abbreviations used: BBB, blood-brain barrier; L-dopa, levodopa.

Dyskinesia, motor fluctuations, and wearing off of L-dopa therapy → adjunctive therapy to optimize L-dopa (e.g., COMT inhibitors, istradefylline)

Seizure Disorders

Epilepsy is a chronic neurologic condition → hyperexcitable, hypersynchronized neurons repetitively fire action potentials→ ≥ 2 involuntary/unprovoked seizures (or 1 with probability of recurrence).[15]

- Seizures are classified as focal, generalized, or unknown onset[15]

Seizure types can be described based on symptomatology:[15]

- Motor symptoms → sustained jerking movements (chronic), limp or weak muscles (atonic), muscle twitching (myoclonus), and rigid or tense muscles (tonic)
- Non-motor symptoms → changes in sensation, emotions, thinking, cognition, awareness

Acute Seizure Management

Duration of most seizures < 2 minutes and do not require medical intervention. Status epilepticus is a seizure lasting > 5 minutes.[16] Treatment is completed in three phases:[16]

1. Stabilization: check airway, start EEG, oxygen, fluids
2. Initial treatment: IV/IM benzodiazepine (lorazepam or midazolam)

3. Second treatment: IV fosphenytoin
   a. Second line: valproic acid or phenobarbital
   b. Third line: levetiracetam or lacozamide

Chronic seizure management

Antiseizure drugs (ASDs) are first-line therapy for epilepsy to decrease seizure frequency (see Table 16-14).[15, 17, 18] Titrating initial dose is important along with monitoring for adverse effects. All ASDs have increased risk of suicidal behavior/ideation and CNS side effects. Most ASDs have good bioavailability (except gabapentin and vigabatrin).

Remember:[15]

Phenytoin levels must be monitored and dose changes must be made appropriately. Phenytoin follow Michaelis-Menten pharmacokinetics. Phenytoin is highly protein-bound and only unbound, free phenytoin is active. Monitoring concentration levels will determine the dosing strategy.

Target concentration → Total: 10–20 mcg/mL

$$Phenytoin\ Dose\ Correction = \frac{Total\ phenytoin\ measured}{(0.2 \times albumin) + 0.1}$$

Valproic acid is also extensively bound to albumin. However, free valproate levels are not commonly monitored.

- Target concentration → Total: 50–100 mcg/mL
- Concentrations >100 mcg/mL are associated with thrombocytopenia

Sleep disorders

Insomnia is the most common sleep disorder[19], characterized by difficulty falling/staying asleep and reduced quality of sleep.

- Sleep hygiene is first-line therapy for insomnia
- Natural products commonly used for sleep include melatonin and valerian

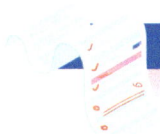

Table 16-14	Antiseizure Drugs[15,17]	

DRUG AGENT	INDICATIONS	NOTES
FIRST GENERATION		
Carbamazepine (Tegretol)	Monotherapy Adjunctive: focal-onset, TC, and mixed seizure (except absence seizure)	■ Inhibitor of CYP2C19 ■ Inducer of CYP3A4 (autoinducer) **BBW:** Increased risk of SJS/TEN with HLA-B*1502 allele **SE:** CNS effects, dizziness, drowsiness
Clonazepam (Klonopin)	Monotherapy Adjunctive: LGS, myoclonic, absence	**SE:** sedation, irritability, aggression, nightmares, hallucinations
Ethosuximide (Zarontin)	Monotherapy Adjunctive: absence in patients ≥ 3 years old	Drug of choice for absence seizures **SE:** N/V, weight loss
Phenobarbital	Used for focal-onset and generalized seizures	**SE:** drowsiness, confusion, paroxysmal effects, vertigo
Phenytoin (Dilantin) Fosphenytoin (Cerebyx)	Monotherapy Adjunctive: focal-onset, TC	■ Strong enzyme inducer ■ Increased risk of SJS/TEN with HLA-B*1502 allele **SE:** slurred speech, confusion, insomnia
Primidone (Mysoline)	Monotherapy Adjunctive: focal-onset, TC	**SE:** N/V, emotional disturbances
Valproic acid (Depakene)	Monotherapy Adjunctive: focal-onset, multiple seizure types	**SE:** abdominal pain, weight gain, anorexia, blurred vision, tremor Teratogenicity

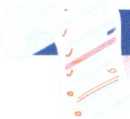

Table 16-14 Antiseizure Drugs[15,17] (*Continued*)

Drug agent	Indications	Notes
SECOND GENERATION		
Felbamate (Felbatol)	Used for severe refractory epilepsy only	**SE:** anorexia, N/V, CNS effects, insomnia, dizziness
Gabapentin (Neurontin)	Adjunctive: focal-onset	**SE:** peripheral edema, weight gain
Lamotrigine (Lamictal)	Monotherapy focal-onset (patients ≥16yo) Adjunctive: focal-onset, TC, generalized seizures of LGS (patients ≥2 yo)	Should be considered in patients ≥60 yo **BBW:** rash including SJS/TEN **SE:** tremor, rhinitis, pharyngitis
Levetiracetam (Keppra)	Adjunctive: focal-onset, myoclonic, generalized TC	**SE:** psychosis, aggression, apathy, depression, irritability
Oxcarbazepine (Trileptal)	Monotherapy Adjunctive: focal-onset	▪ Inhibitor of CYP2C19 ▪ Inducer of CYP3A4 **SE:** abnormal vision, tremor, rash (SJS/TEN)
Tiagabine (Gabitril)	Adjunctive: focal-onset	**SE:** lack of energy, irritability
Topiramate (Topamax)	Monotherapy Adjunctive: focal-onset, primary generalized TC	**SE:** slurred speech, tremor, nervousness, rash (SJS/TEN)
Zonisamide (Zonegran)	Adjunctive: focal-onset	**SE:** depression, difficulty recalling words, rash (SJS/TEN)
THIRD GENERATION		
Brivaracetam (Briviact)	Monotherapy Adjunctive: focal-onset	**SE:** aggressive behavior, anxiety, angioedema
Cannabadiol (Epidiolex)	Monotherapy Adjunctive: LGS, Dravet syndrome	**SE:** insomnia, decreased appetite, hepatotoxicity
Clobazam (Onfi)	Adjunctive: LGS	▪ Inhibitor of CYP2C9 ▪ Inducer of CYP3A4 **BBW:** increased risk of death with opioids, rash (SJS/TEN)
Eslicarbazepine (Aptiom)	Monotherapy Adjunctive: focal-onset	▪ Used for treatment resistance ▪ Inhibitor of CYP2C19 **SE:** blurred vision, tremor, rash (SJS)
Lacosamide (Vimpat)	Monotherapy Adjunctive: focal-onset	**SE:** tremor, cardiac effects
Perampanel (Fycompa)	Monotherapy: focal-onset Adjunctive: TC	First line for treatment resistance **BBW:** aggression, hostility, irritability, homicidal ideations
Pregabalin (Lyrica)	Adjunctive: focal-onset	First line for treatment resistance **SE:** blurred vision, dry mouth, edema, weight gain
Rufinamide (Banzel)	Adjunctive: LGS	**SE:** gait disturbances, rash (SJS)
Vigabatrin (Sabril)	Adjunctive: refractory focal-onset	**BBW:** peripheral vision loss **SE:** seizure exacerbation

Abbreviations used: BBW, black box warning; CNS, central nervous system; HLA, human leukocyte antigen; LGS, Lennox-Gastaut syndrome; N/V, nausea, vomiting; SE, side effects; SJS, Stevens-Johnson syndrome; TEN, toxic epidermal necrolysis; TC, tonic-clonic; yo, years old.
Adapted from Nguyen V-HV, Dergalust S, Chang E. Epilepsy. In: DiPiro JT, Yee GC, Posey LM, Haines ST, Nolin TD, Ellingrod V, eds. *Pharmacotherapy: A Pathophysiologic Approach.* 11th ed. New York, NY: McGraw-Hill; 2020.

- First-generation sedating antihistamines (e.g., diphenhydramine, doxylamine, hydroxyzine) are for short-term use only

Chronic insomnia is treated when symptoms ≥3× per week >3 months (see Table 16-15).[19]

Remember: Non-benzodiazepines—complex sleep behavior (sleep-walking, sleep-driving, engaging in activities while not fully awake), CNS depression, dizziness, daytime drowsiness

Restless leg syndrome is the urge to move lower legs during the night.[19]

- Dopamine agonists are first-line treatment (only pramipexole [Mirapex] and ropinirole [Requip]) are FDA-approved)
- Gabapentin enacarbil (Horizant) also FDA-approved

Narcolepsy is characterized by excessive daytime somnolence and can be accompanied by cataplexy, hypnagogic hallucinations, and sleep paralysis.[19]

- Excessive daytime somnolence—modafinil or armodafinil first-line, then dextroamphetamine or methylphenidate, then sodium oxybate
  - Solrimafetol is newly approved and therapy use is still being determined
- Cataplexy (sudden paralysis)—TCAs, SSRIs, SNRIs first-line

ADDITIONAL RESOURCES

Wolraich ML, Hagan JF, Allan C, et al. Clinical practice guideline for the diagnosis, evaluation, and treatment of attention-deficit/hyperactivity disorder in children and adolescents. *Pediatrics.* 2019;144(4).

American Psychiatric Association. The American Psychiatric Association practice guideline for the treatment of patients with schizophrenia. 3rd ed. 2020. Available at: https://psychiatryonline.org/doi/book/10.1176/appi.books.9780890424841.

Yatham LN, Kennedy SH, Parikh SV, et al. Canadian Network for Mood and Anxiety Treatments (CANMAT) and International Society for Bipolar Disorders (ISBD) 2018 guidelines for the management of patients with bipolar disorder. *Bipolar Disord.* 2018;20(2):97–170.

American Psychological Association Guideline Development Panel for the Treatment of Depressive Disorders. Clinical practice guideline for the treatment of depression across three age cohorts. 2019. Available at: https://www.apa.org/depression-guideline/guideline.pdf.

Anxiety and Depression Association of America. Clinical practice review for GAD. Available at: https://adaa.org/resources-professionals/practice-guidelines-gad. Updated July 2, 2015.

Kanner AM, Ashman E, Gloss D, et al. Practice guideline update summary: efficacy and tolerability of the new antiepileptic drugs I: treatment of new-onset epilepsy. Report of the Guideline Development, Dissemination, and Implementation Subcommittee of the American Academy of Neurology and the American Epilepsy Society. *Epilepsy Curr.* 2018;91(2):74–81.

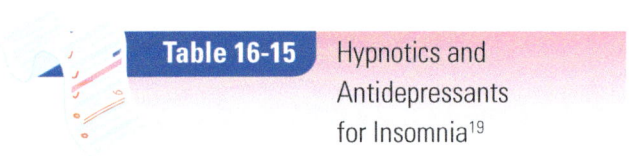

Table 16-15 Hypnotics and Antidepressants for Insomnia[19]

Drug agent	Mechanism of action
Eszopiclone (Lunesta) Zaleplon (Sonata) Zolpidem (Ambien)	Non-benzodiazepine: ↑ GABA
Flurazepam (Dalmane) Temazepam (Restoril) Triazolam (Halcion)	Benzodiazepine
Ramelteon (Rozerem)	Melatonin receptor agonist
Lemborexant (Dayvigo) Survorexant (Belsomra)	Orexin receptor antagonist
Amitriptyline (Elavil) Doxepin (Silenor) Mirtazapine (Remeron) Nortriptyline (Pamelor) Trazodone (Desyrel)	Antidepressant

Abbreviations used: GABA, gamma aminobutyric acid.

REFERENCES

1. Dopheide JA, Stutzman DL, Pliszka SR. Attention deficit/hyperactivity disorder. In: DiPiro JT, Yee GC, Posey LM, Haines ST, Nolin TD, Ellingrod V, eds. *Pharmacotherapy: A Pathophysiologic Approach.* 11th ed. New York, NY: McGraw-Hill; 2020.
2. Wolraich ML, Hagan JF, Allan C, et al. Clinical practice guideline for the diagnosis, evaluation, and treatment of attention-deficit/hyperactivity disorder in children and adolescents. *Pediatrics.* 2019;144(4).
3. American Psychiatric Association. The American Psychiatric Association practice guideline for the treatment of patients with schizophrenia. 3rd ed. 2020. Available at https://psychiatryonline.org/doi/book/10.1176/appi.books.9780890424841.
4. Crismon ML, Smith T, Buckley PF. Schizophrenia. In: DiPiro JT, Yee GC, Posey LM, Haines ST, Nolin TD, Ellingrod V, eds. *Pharmacotherapy: A Pathophysiologic Approach.* 11th ed. New York, NY: McGraw-Hill; 2020.
5. Yatham LN, Kennedy SH, Parikh SV, et al. Canadian Network for Mood and Anxiety Treatments (CANMAT) and International Society for Bipolar Disorders (ISBD) 2018 guidelines for the management of patients with bipolar disorder. *Bipolar Disord.* 2018;20(2):97–170.

6. Drayton SJ, Fields CS. Bipolar Disorder. In: DiPiro JT, Yee GC, Posey LM, Haines ST, Nolin TD, Ellingrod V, eds. *Pharmacotherapy: A Pathophysiologic Approach*. 11th ed. New York, NY: McGraw-Hill; 2020.

7. American Psychological Association Guideline Development Panel for the Treatment of Depressive Disorders. Clinical practice guideline for the treatment of depression across three age cohorts. 2019. Available at: https://www.apa.org/depression-guideline/guideline.pdf.

8. VandenBerg AM. Major Depressive Disorder. In: DiPiro JT, Yee GC, Posey LM, Haines ST, Nolin TD, Ellingrod V, eds. *Pharmacotherapy: A Pathophysiologic Approach*. 11th ed. New York, NY: McGraw-Hill; 2020.

9. Anxiety and Depression Association of America. Clinical practice review for GAD. ADAA. Available at: https://adaa.org/resources-professionals/practice-guidelines-gad. Udated July 2, 2015. Accessed May 8, 2020.

10. Melton ST, Kirkwood CK. Anxiety disorders: generalized anxiety, panic, and social anxiety disorders. In: DiPiro JT, Yee GC, Posey LM, Haines ST, Nolin TD, Ellingrod V, eds. *Pharmacotherapy: A Pathophysiologic Approach*. 11th ed. New York, NY: McGraw-Hill; 2020.

11. Peron EP, Zimmerman KM, Crouse EL, Slattum PW, Hobgood SE. Alzheimer disease. In: DiPiro JT, Yee GC, Posey LM, Haines ST, Nolin TD, Ellingrod V, eds. *Pharmacotherapy: A Pathophysiologic Approach*. 11th ed. New York, NY: McGraw-Hill; 2020.

12. Cummings JL, Isaacson RS, Schmitt FA, Velting DM. A practical algorithm for managing Alzheimer's disease: what, when, and why? *Ann Clin Transl Neurol*. 2015;2(3):307–323.

13. American Parkinson Disease Association. Parkinson's Disease Handbook. Staten Island, NY: APDA; 2019.

14. Chen JJ, Dashtipour K. Parkinson Disease. In: DiPiro JT, Yee GC, Posey LM, Haines ST, Nolin TD, Ellingrod V, eds. *Pharmacotherapy: A Pathophysiologic Approach, 11e*. McGraw-Hill Education; 2020.

15. Nguyen V-HV, Dergalust S, Chang E. Epilepsy. In: DiPiro JT, Yee GC, Posey LM, Haines ST, Nolin TD, Ellingrod V, eds. *Pharmacotherapy: A Pathophysiologic Approach*. 11th ed. New York, NY: McGraw-Hill; 2020.

16. Glauser T, Shinnar S, Gloss D, et al. Evidence-Based Guideline: Treatment of Convulsive Status Epilepticus in Children and Adults: Report of the Guideline Committee of the American *Epilepsy Society*. Epilepsy Curr. 2016 Jan-Feb 2016;16(1):48-61. doi:10.5698/1535-7597-16.1.48

17. Kanner AM, Ashman E, Gloss D, et al. Practice guideline update summary: efficacy and tolerability of the new antiepileptic drugs I: treatment of new-onset epilepsy. Report of the Guideline Development, Dissemination, and Implementation Subcommittee of the American Academy of Neurology and the American Epilepsy Society. *Epilepsy Curr*. 2018;91(2):74–81.

18. Krumholz A, Shinnar S, French J, Gronseth G, Wiebe S. Evidence-based guideline: management of an unprovoked first seizure in adults: Report of the Guideline Development Subcommittee of the American Academy of Neurology and the American Epilepsy Society. *Neurology*. 2015;85(17):1526–1527.

19. Dopp JM, Phillips BG. Sleep–wake disorders. In: DiPiro JT, Yee GC, Posey LM, Haines ST, Nolin TD, Ellingrod V, eds. *Pharmacotherapy: A Pathophysiologic Approach*. 11th ed. New York, NY: McGraw-Hill; 2020.

CHAPTER 17

Fever and Pain

With medical writing support provided by
Banner Medical LLC Writer: Miriam Opara

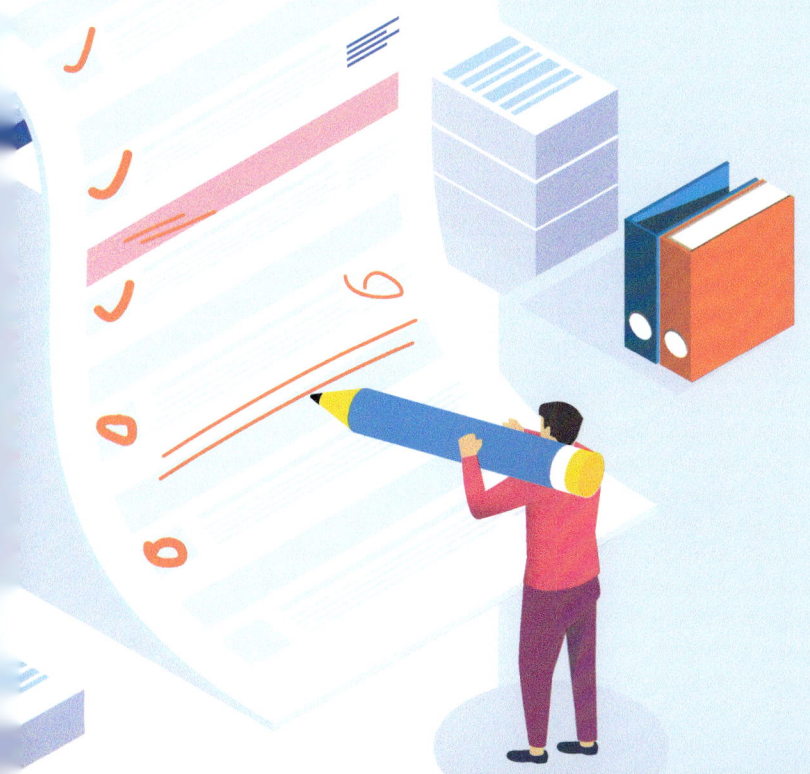

Fever

Fever is caused by microbial infections and noninfectious factors. Fever is determined based on the site of measurement (see Table 17-1).[1] Rectal measurement is the gold standard.

Treatment for fever is antipyretics (acetaminophen [APAP], nonsteroidal anti-inflammatory drug (NSAIDs), acetylsalicylic acid) that inhibit prostaglandin E2 synthesis through inhibition of the cyclooxygenase enzyme.[1]

- **APAP** dosing:
  - Children/infants: 10–15 mg/kg every 4–6 hours
  - Adults: 325–1000 mg every 4–6 hours
- **Ibuprofen** dosing:
  - Children/infants: 5–10 mg/kg every 6–8 hours (**≥6 months** of age only)
  - Adults: 200–400 mg every 4–6 hours

Pain

Pain is defined as nociceptive (somatic or visceral), neuropathic, and functional.[2] Pain is classified as acute or chronic. The severity of pain on a pain score scale from 1–10 determines treatment, as outlined in Figure 17-1.[2]

Non-opioid treatment for pain is outlined in Table 17-2.[2]

Remember: NSAIDs
- Black Box Warning: increase cardiovascular (CV) thrombotic events
- Monitor: creatinine clearance, blood pressure, hemoglobin, and hematocrit

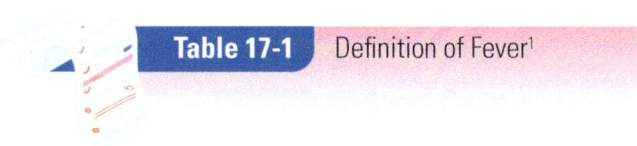

Table 17-1 Definition of Fever[1]

Measurement site	Fever (°F)
Rectal	101
Oral	100.4
Temporal	101

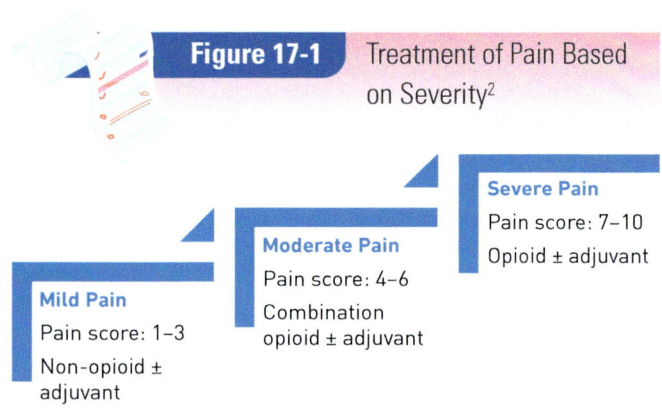

Figure 17-1 Treatment of Pain Based on Severity[2]

Severe Pain
Pain score: 7–10
Opioid ± adjuvant

Moderate Pain
Pain score: 4–6
Combination opioid ± adjuvant

Mild Pain
Pain score: 1–3
Non-opioid ± adjuvant

- Adverse effects: dyspepsia, CV events, gastrointestinal (GI) bleeding, renal impairment

Opioids are mu receptor agonists in the central nervous system (CNS), which primarily produce pain relief, but also euphoria and respiratory depression. Opioids and equianalgesic dosing are listed in Table 17-3.[3,4]

Rules of thumb:
- Transdermal fentanyl conversion—determine total daily dose of oral morphine
  - **Remember:** 2:1 (2 mg/day of oral morphine = 1 mcg/hr of fentanyl)[5]

Dosing conversions:[6]
1. Calculate total 24-hour dose requirement for each opioid being used
2. Convert each opioid to morphine milligram equivalents (MME); use ratio-conversion to calculate the dose of the new drug
3. Divide to attain appropriate interval and dose for new drug
4. Always have breakthrough pain medication available while making changes (dosing ranges from 5%–17% of the total daily baseline opioid dose)

Important considerations:
- Exercise caution with methadone; conversion factor increases at higher doses
- Fentanyl is dosed in mcg/hr vs. mg/day

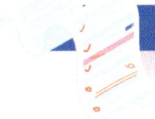

Table 17-2 Non-opioid Pain Treatment[2]

Acetaminophen	Inhibition of PG synthesis in the CNS resulting in reduced pain impulse generation
	Adults: Maximum 4000 mg/d
	Pediatrics (≤12 years): Maximum 2600 mg/day
	OVERDOSE: Antidote is N-acetylcysteine—restores intracellular glutathione
NSAIDs	Inhibition of COX, leading to blockade of PG synthesis

PAIN	**MEDS**	**KICK**
Piroxicam	Meloxicam*	Ketoprofen
A	Etodolac*	Indomethacin
Ibuprofen	Diclofenac*	Celecoxib*
Naproxen	Sulindac	Ketorolac**

Salicylate NSAIDs	**Non-acetylated salicylates**
Aspirin	Salsalate
Irreversible COX1 inhibitor	Magnesium salicylate
	Diflunisal

Abbreviations used: CNS, central nervous system; COX, cyclooxygenase; NSAIDs, nonsteroidal anti-inflammatory drugs; PG, prostaglandin.
*COX2 selective NSAIDs
**Use lowest effective dose for shortest period of time; maximum of 5 d of treatment; in the setting of acute pain, oral treatment should only be used after IV or IM administration.

- Do not use the calculated dose in MMEs for converting between opioids.
  - The lowest effective dose should be prescribed of the new opioid to avoid unintentional overdose resulting from incomplete cross-tolerance and unique pharmacokinetic profiles

Opioid side effects:[2]
Usually lessen over time (except constipation)

- CNS: sedation, mental clouding, confusion
- GI: constipation, nausea, and vomiting
- Miosis: pinpoint pupils

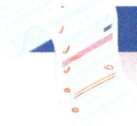

Table 17-3 Opioid Equianalgesic Doses[3,4]

	EQUIANALGESIC DOSE (MG)			
DRUG AGENT	**PARENTERAL**	**ORAL**	**ONSET (MIN)**	**HALF-LIFE (HR)**
Morphine	10	30	10–20	2
Fentanyl	0.1	—	7–15	3–4
Hydromorphone	1.5	7.5	10–20	2–3
Oxycodone	—	20	30–60	2–3
Methadone	5	10	30–60	12–190
Meperidine	75	300	10–20	3–4
Codeine	120	200	30	3

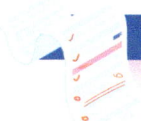

Table 17-4	Substance Abuse Terminology[2]

Dependence	Physiological state in which withdrawal symptoms occur if a drug is not given. Withdrawal symptoms: anxiety, tachycardia, shakiness, shortness of breath
Addiction	A strong compulsion to take a drug despite harm; drug-seeking behavior, including exaggerating the pain, getting prescriptions from multiple prescribers and/or forgery
Pseudo-addiction	Behaviors may suggest addiction, but in reality, behaviors are due to unrelieved pain
Tolerance	Higher opioid dose is needed to produce the same level of analgesia that a lower dose previously provided

- Respiratory depression
- Histamine release: pruritis

Opioid abuse disorder (see Table 17-4):[2]

Signs and symptoms of acute opioid overdose:

- Extreme sleepiness
- Slow or shallow breathing
- Fingernails or lips turning blue or purple
- Extremely small "pinpoint" pupils
- Bradycardia and/or hypotension

Opioid abuse treatment:[2,4]
- Naltrexone (nasal spray: 1 spray [4 mg])
- Buprenorphine +/– naloxone (Suboxone)

Adjuvant pain treatment (see Table 17-5) may be used for uncontrolled pain and when patients develop tolerance or adverse effects on opioid treatment. Adding adjuvant medication to opioid therapy improves pain management by non-opioid mechanisms of action.

Neuropathic pain is caused by a disorder of the somatosensory nervous system. Neuropathic pain often leads to a lack of sensation or numbness. Risk factors include trauma, diabetes, multiple sclerosis, vitamin deficiencies, varicella-zoster, and carpal tunnel syndrome.

First-line therapy (4–6–week trial; see Ch. 16 for more information):[1]

- Tricyclic antidepressants: amitriptyline, nortriptyline

- Serotonin-norepinephrine reuptake inhibitors (SNRIs): duloxetine, venlafaxine
- Gabapentinoids: gabapentin, pregabalin
- Topicals for focal pain: capsaicin, lidocaine

Second-line therapy (exacerbation or inadequate response; 4–6–week trial):[2]

- Tramadol
- Combinations of first-line therapies (e.g., gabapentinoid + SNRI)

Arthritis

Osteoarthritis (OA) is the most common form of arthritis that occurs in weight-bearing joints (hands, knees, hips, spine), causing pain with motion and joint

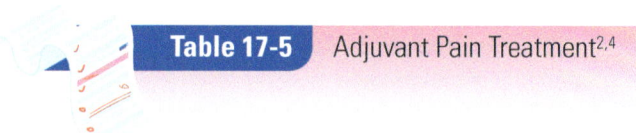

Table 17-5	Adjuvant Pain Treatment[2,4]

DRUG CLASS	DRUG AGENT
Tricyclic antidepressants	Amitriptyline
	Nortriptyline
Anticonvulsants	Gabapentin
	Pregabalin
	Carbamazepine
	Lamotrigine
Corticosteroids	Dexamethasone
	Prednisone

stiffness at rest (<30 min) that resolves with motion. Pain presentation is typically unilateral.[7] Treatment focuses on symptom control—primary goal is pain relief.[7]

- Nonpharmacologic—exercise strongly recommended for all forms of OA
  - Weight loss, Tai Chi, and cane use in knee and hip OA
- Over-the-counter—first-line therapy for pain
  - Oral NSAIDs
    - Dose is scheduled, not as needed
- Topical NSAIDs (knee OA, not hip OA)
- Intraarticular injections (not hand OA): corticosteroids, hyaluronic acid
- Acetaminophen (scheduled, not as needed)
- Topical capsaicin (not hand OA)

Rheumatoid arthritis (RA) is a chronic, progressive autoimmune disorder that primarily affects smaller joints (fingers, wrist, ankles, feet).[8,9] Bilateral, symmetrical symptoms usually develop over several weeks. Hallmark symptoms of RA include swelling and morning stiffness (>30 min).

Classic symptoms of RA: [8,9]

- Joint swelling
- Pain
- Stiffness
- Bone deformity
- Weakness
- Difficulty moving
- Edema
- Erythema

RA is classified as mild, moderate, or severe. Patients with RA should be started on a disease-modifying antirheumatic drug (DMARD) regardless of severity (see Table 17-6).[8,9]

- **Methotrexate** is the preferred initial DMARD therapy
  - Mechanism of action—irreversibly binds and inhibits dihydrofolate reductase, inhibiting folate, thymidylate synthetase, and purine
  - **Remember:** folic acid supplementation given concomitantly

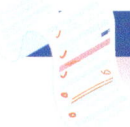

Table 17-6 Disease-Modifying Antirheumatic Drugs for Rheumatoid Arthritis Treatment[8,92]

NON-BIOLOGICAL DMARDs	
Methotrexate	ONCE Weekly dosing
Hydroxychloroquine	
Sulfasalazine	Prodrug
Leflunomide	Prodrug of teriflunomide

BIOLOGIC DMARDs	
TNF-alpha inhibitors (CEASING)	**Non-TNF-alpha inhibitors (B MATTARS)**
Certolizumab pegol	**B**aricitinib
Etanercept	M
Adalimumab	**A**batacept
S	**T**ocilizumab
Infliximab	**T**ofacitinib
N	**A**nakinra
Golimumab	**R**ituximab
	Sarilumab

Abbreviations used: DMARDs, disease-modifying antirheumatic drugs; TNF, tumor necrosis factor.

Moderate-to-severe RA despite methotrexate: combination of DMARDs is recommended

DMARD onset of action may take several weeks or months after initiation; low-dose corticosteroids may be considered for immediate pain relief. Glucocorticoids are commonly used in RA flares; use the lowest dose for the shortest time.

Remember:
- Live vaccines should NOT be given during treatment with DMARDs; avoid for 3 months after discontinuation of therapy
- Increased risk of infection with DMARD therapy
- Methotrexate and leflunomide—contraindicated during pregnancy

Gout

Gout occurs from an excess accumulation of uric acid—overproduction or underexcretion. Several conditions are associated with the accumulation of uric acid, leading to hyperuricemia:[10]

- Congestive heart failure
- Diabetic ketoacidosis
- Hypothyroidism
- Impaired kidney function
- Lactic acidosis
- Lead toxicity
- Obesity
- Pernicious anemia
- Psoriasis
- Starvation

Symptoms of gout include severe pain, warmth, swelling, and inflammation of involved joints. Asymptomatic patients may not need pharmacologic therapy, but are encouraged to implement lifestyle measures (e.g., weight loss, DASH diet, reduce alcohol intake, limit purine-rich foods) to reduce urate concentrations.[10]

- Gout attack—drug therapy for acute attack + prevention of future attacks (see Table 17-7)
  - Preventative therapy is indicated for an occurrence of two or more gout attacks per year

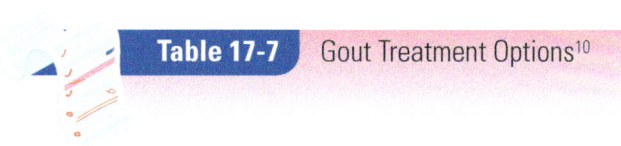

Table 17-7 Gout Treatment Options[10]

Acute attack treatment—pain and inflammation
- Colchicine (Colcrys)
- NSAIDs
- Steroids (PO, IV, IM, Intra-articular)

Chronic urate lowering treatment—prevention of future attacks

XO inhibitors are first-line—blocking XO stops the production of UA and produces a nontoxic product
- Allopurinol
- Febuxostat

Uricosurics—inhibit reabsorption of UA in the kidneys, which increases UA excretion
- Lesinurad
- Probenecid

Recombinant uricase—converts UA to allantoin, which is excreted
- Pegloticase

Abbreviations used: IM, intramuscular; IV, intravenous; NSAIDs, nonsteroidal anti-inflammatory drugs; PO, by mouth; UA, uric acid; XO, xanthine oxidase.

- The goal of therapy is to reduce uric acid level to <6 mg/dL.[10]

Colchicine considerations:[10]

- Start medication within 12–36 hours of an acute attack
- Dosing: 1.2 mg initially, followed by 0.6 mg 1 hour later
- Drug interactions:
  - CYP3A4 inhibitors: reduce colchicine dose to 0.6 mg followed by 0.3 mg 1 hour later; do not repeat dose earlier than 3 days

Migraines

Migraine is a chronic neurovascular disorder causing severe headaches/autonomic nervous system dysfunction. Migraines are classified based on the presence of aura or visual symptoms (e.g., flashes of light, blind spots, zig-zag lines).[11]

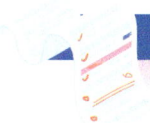

Table 17-8	ACUTE Drug Treatment for Migraines[12]

Analgesics

Acetaminophen/aspirin/caffeine

Diclofenac, ibuprofen, ketorolac, naproxen

Triptans: selective agonists for the serotonin receptor → vasoconstriction of cranial blood vessels

Dose	Take at the onset of headache; can repeat once after 2 h if no symptom relief (except Naratriptan; repeat after 4 h)
Long-acting but slow onset	Frovatriptan Naratriptan
Shorter acting but faster onset	Almotriptan Eletriptan Rizatriptan Sumatriptan Zolmitriptan

Ditans: serotonin 5-H1F receptor agonists with no vasoconstriction effect

Lasmiditan	Risk of driving impairment and CNS depression (e.g., dizziness, sedation)

Ergotamines: nonselective agonist of serotonin receptor → cerebral vasoconstriction

Dihydroergotamine	Ergotamine + caffeine

Remember: Migraines are unilateral, pulsating, and aggravated by routine physical activity. Treatment consists of abortive therapy (see Table 17-8) or prophylactic therapy.

Prophylactic treatment is considered if the patient uses acute treatment >2 days/week or >3 times per month.[11]

- Beta-blockers: propranolol, timolol, metoprolol
- Antiepileptics: divalproex, topiramate
- Antidepressants: amitriptyline, venlafaxine, duloxetine
- Calcitonin gene-related peptide inhibitors: erenumab, fremanezumab, galcanezumab
- Botulinum toxin

ADDITIONAL RESOURCES

Kolasinski SL, Neogi T, Hochberg MC, et al. 2019 American College of Rheumatology/Arthritis Foundation guideline for the management of osteoarthritis of the hand, hip, and knee. *Arthritis Care Res (Hoboken).* 2020;72(2):149–162.

Singh JA, Furst DE, Bharat A, et al. 2012 update of the 2008 American College of Rheumatology recommendations for the use of disease-modifying antirheumatic drugs and biologic agents in the treatment of rheumatoid arthritis. *Arthritis Care Res (Hoboken).* 2012;64(5):625–639.

Dowell D, Haegerich TM, Chou R. CDC guideline for prescribing opioids for chronic pain—United States, 2016. *MMWR Reconm Rep.* 2016;65:1–49.

FitzGerald JD, Dalbeth N, Mikuls T, et al. 2020 American College of Rheumatology guideline for the management of gout. *Arthritis Care Res.* 2020;72:744–760.

Gilmore B, Michael M. Treatment of acute migraine headache. *Am Fam Physician.* 2011;83(3):271–280.

REFERENCES

1. Bates D, Schultheis BC, Hanes MC, et al. A comprehensive algorithm for management of neuropathic pain. *Pain Med.* 2019; 20(suppl 1):s2–s12.

2. Herndon CM, Ray JB, Kominek CM. Pain management. In: DiPiro JT, Yee GC, Posey LM, Haines ST, Nolin TD, Ellingrod V, eds. *Pharmacotherapy: A Pathophysiologic Approach.* 11th ed. New York, NY: McGraw-Hill; 2020.

3. Centers for Disease Control and Prevention. CDC guideline for prescribing opioids for chronic pain. Available at: https://www.cdc.gov/drugoverdose/prescribing/guideline.html. Updated August 28, 2019. Accessed May 24, 2020.

4. Dowell D, Haegerich TM, Chou R. CDC guideline for prescribing opioids for chronic pain—United States, 2016. *MMWR Reconm Rep.* 2016;65:1–49.

5. American Society of Health Systems Pharmacists. Demystifying opioid conversion calculations. Available at: https://www.ashp.org/-/media/store-files/p1985-sample-chapter-5.ashx. Accessed July 27, 2020.

6. Centers for Disease Control and Prevention. Calculating total daily dose of opioids for safer dosage. Available at: https://www.cdc.gov/drugoverdose/pdf/calculating_total_daily_dose-a.pdf. Accessed September 13, 2020.

7. Kolasinski SL, Neogi T, Hochberg MC, et al. 2019 American College of Rheumatology/Arthritis Foundation guideline for the management of osteoarthritis of the hand, hip, and knee. *Arthritis Care Res.* 2020;72(2):149–162.

8. Singh JA, Saag KG, Bridges SL Jr, et al. 2015 American College of Rheumatology Guideline for the Treatment of Rheumatoid Arthritis. *Arthritis Rheumatol.* 2016 Jan;68(1):1–26. doi: 10.1002/art.39480. Epub 2015 Nov 6. PMID: 26545940

9. Gruber S, Lezcano B, Hylland S. Rheumatoid arthritis. In: DiPiro JT, Yee GC, Posey LM, Haines ST, Nolin TD, Ellingrod V, eds. *Pharmacotherapy: A Pathophysiologic Approach.* 11th ed. New York, NY: McGraw-Hill; 2020.

10. Fravel MA, Ernst ME. Gout and hyperuricemia. In: DiPiro JT, Yee GC, Posey LM, Haines ST, Nolin TD, Ellingrod V, eds. *Pharmacotherapy: A Pathophysiologic Approach.* 11th ed. New York, NY: McGraw-Hill; 2020.

11. Harrell TK, Minor DS. Headache disorders. In: DiPiro JT, Yee GC, Posey LM, Haines ST, Nolin TD, Ellingrod V, eds. *Pharmacotherapy: A Pathophysiologic Approach.* 11th ed. New York, NY: McGraw-Hill; 2020.

12. Gilmore B, Michael M. Treatment of acute migraine headache. *Am Fam Physician.* 2011;83(3):271–280.

CHAPTER 18

Oncology

With medical writing support provided by Banner Medical
LLC Writers: Jennifer Miller and Miriam Opara

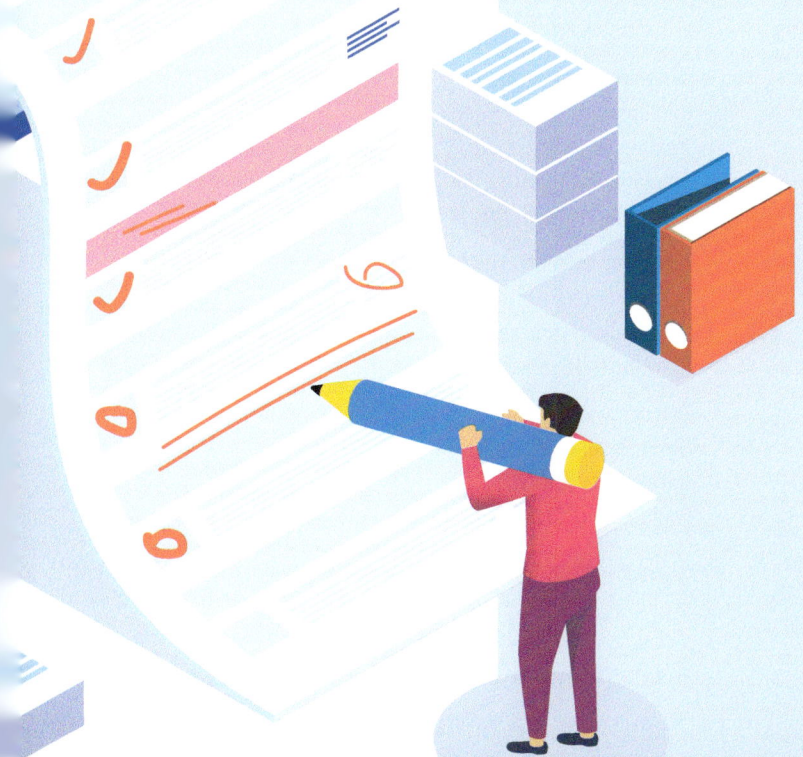

Oncology

Treatment regimens are based on the type of cancer (and stage), prognostic factors, age, and performance status of the patient. The effect on the cell cycle (specific or nonspecific) is the basis for which chemotherapy agents are classified (see Figure 18-1, and Tables 18-1 and 18-2).[1,2]

Oncology agents can also be classified as targeted therapies outlined in Table 18-3.

Breast cancer

Treatment of breast cancer is based on

- Hormone receptor status
  - Estrogen receptor + or −
  - Progesterone receptor + or −
  - Menopausal status
- Stage of cancer
  - Lymph node involvement
- Histology
  - Biomarker status
    - HER2 + or −
    - BRCA

Table 18-4 outlines neoadjuvant/adjuvant regimens and Table 18-5 outlines endocrine therapies.

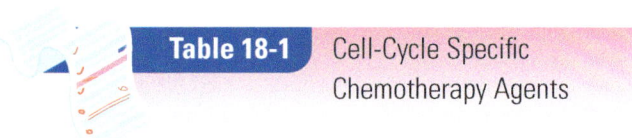

Table 18-1 Cell-Cycle Specific Chemotherapy Agents

PHASE	DRUG AGENT
Phase G1	Asparaginase
	Steroids
Phase S	Azacitidine (Vidaza)
	Decitabine (Dacogen)
	Fluorouracil (Adrucil)
	Gemcitabine (Gemzar)
	Irinotecan (Camptosar)
	Pemetrexed (Alimta)
Phase G2	Bleomycin (Blenoxane)
	Etoposide (Toposar)
Phase M	Docetaxel (Taxotere)
	Paclitaxel (Taxol)
	Vinblastine (Velban)
	Vincristine (Oncovin)
	Vinorelbine (Navelbine)

Source: Adapted from Medina P, Shord S. Cancer Treatment and Chemotherapy. In: DiPiro J, Talbert R, Yee G, Matzke G, Wells B, Posey L, eds. *Pharmacotherapy: A Pathophysiologic Approach.* 8th ed. McGraw-Hill; 2011:2191–2227; Teicher BA. Newer Cytotoxic Agents: Attacking Cancer Broadly. *Clin Cancer Res.* 2008;14(6):1610–1617.

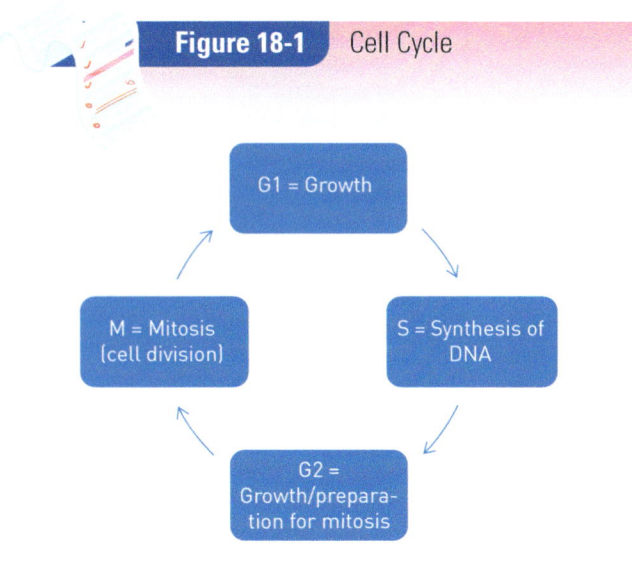

Figure 18-1 Cell Cycle

- G1 = Growth
- S = Synthesis of DNA
- G2 = Growth/preparation for mitosis
- M = Mitosis (cell division)

Source: Adapted from Medina P, Shord S. Cancer Treatment and Chemotherapy. In: DiPiro J, Talbert R, Yee G, Matzke G, Wells B, Posey L, eds. *Pharmacotherapy: A Pathophysiologic Approach.* McGraw-Hill; 2011:2191–2227.

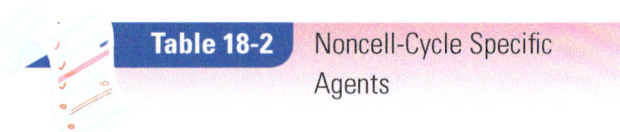

Table 18-2 Noncell-Cycle Specific Agents

Alkylating agents
Cyclophosphamide (Cytoxan)
Ifosfamide (Ifex)
Cisplatin (Platinol)
Carboplatin (Paraplatin)

Anthracycline antibiotics*
Daunorubicin (Cerubidine)
Doxorubicin (Adriamycin)
Idarubicin (Idamycin)

Others
Dacarbazine (DTIC)
Carmustine (BiCNU)
Lomustine (CCNU)

*Associated with maximum lifetime cumulative dose.

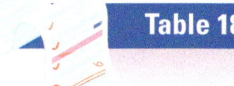

Table 18-3 — Targeted Oncology Agents

Human epidermal growth factor receptor-2 (HER2)
Ado-trastuzumab emtansine (Kadcyla)
Pertuzumab (Perjeta)
Trastuzumab (Herceptin)

Epidermal growth factor receptor (EGFR)
Cetuximab (Erbitux)
Panitumumab (Vectibix)

Cytotoxic T-lymphocyte-associated protein 4 (CTLA-4)
Ipilimumab (Yervoy)

Vascular endothelial growth factor (VEGF)
Bevacizumab (Avastin)

CD20
Obinutuzumab (Gazyva)
Ofatumumab (Arzerra)
Rituximab (Rituxan)

Programmed death receptor-1 (PD-1)
Nivolumab (Opdivo)
Pembrolizumab (Keytruda)

Programmed death-ligand 1 (PD-L1)
Avelumab (Bavencio)
Atezolizumab (Tecentriq)
Durvalumab (Imfinzi)

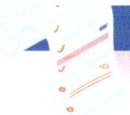

Table 18-5 — Endocrine Therapies Commonly Used in Breast Cancer Management* [3,4]

Drug class	Drug Agents
Aromatase inhibitors	Nonsteroidal
	▪ Anastrozole (Arimidex)
	▪ Letrozole (Femara)
	Steroidal
	▪ Exemestane (Aromasin)
Antiestrogens	SERM
	▪ Tamoxifen (Novaldex; Soltamox)
	▪ Toremifene (Fareston)
	SERD
	▪ Fulvestrant (Faslodex)
LHRH analogs	Goserelin (Zoladex)
	Leuprolide (Lupron)
	Triptorelin (Triptodur)

Abbreviations used: LHRH, luteinizing hormone–releasing hormone; SERD, selective estrogen receptor down regulator; SERM, selective estrogen receptor modulator.
*Endocrine therapies used if tumor is hormone-receptor-positive.
Adapted from National Comprehensive Cancer Network. NCCN Guidelines (version 3.2020): Breast Cancer. Available at: https://www.nccn.org/professionals/physician_gls/pdf/breast.pdf; Michaud LB, Barnett C, Esteva F. Breast Cancer. In: DiPiro J, Talbert R, Yee G, Matzke G, Wells B, Posey L, eds. *Pharmacotherapy: A Pathophysiologic Approach*. 8th ed. McGraw-Hill; 2011:2229–2270.

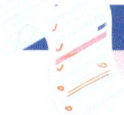

Table 18-4 — Neoadjuvant/Adjuvant Regimens Commonly Used in Breast Cancer Treatment[3]

Regimen	Drug agents
AC	Doxorubicin + Cyclophosphamide
EC	Epirubicin + Cyclophosphamide
AC → Paclitaxel	Doxorubicin + Cyclophosphamide → Paclitaxel
AC → Docetaxel	Doxorubicin + Cyclophosphamide → Docetaxel
TAC	Docetaxel + Doxorubicin + Cyclophosphamide
TC	Docetaxel + Cyclophosphamide
CMF	Cyclophosphamide + Methotrexate + 5-Fluorouracil
AC → T + Trastuzumab*	Doxorubicin + Cyclophosphamide → Paclitaxel + Trastuzumab → Trastuzumab
TCH*	Docetaxel + Carboplatin + Trastuzumab → Trastuzumab
AC → T*H	Doxorubicin + Cyclophosphamide → Docetaxel + Trastuzumab → Trastuzumab
T*CHP	Docetaxel + Carboplatin + Trastuzumab + Pertuzumab → Trastuzumab + Pertuzumab
Paclitaxel + Trastuzumab	Paclitaxel + Trastuzumab

*Trastuzumab and Pertuzumab used only if HER2+.
Adapted from National Comprehensive Cancer Network. NCCN Guidelines (version 3.2020): Breast Cancer. Available at: https://www.nccn.org/professionals/physician_gls/pdf/breast.pdf.

Prostate cancer

The main goal of prostate cancer treatment is to reduce testosterone to slow tumor development. Life expectancy plays a major role in determining tests and treatment options. Table 18-6 outlines the therapy approach for prostate cancer.

Lung cancer

Lung cancer is generally classified as either small-cell lung cancer or non-small cell lung cancer. The treatment strategies differ based on this classification and the state of disease (see Tables 18-7 and 18-8).

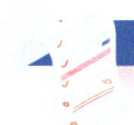

Table 18-6 Therapies Used in Prostate Cancer Management[5,6]

THERAPY	PROCEDURE/DRUG AGENT	NOTES
Nonpharmacologic	Active surveillance Orchiectomy Radiation Radical prostatectomy	■ Generally used for low-to-intermediate recurrence risk ■ Orchiectomy = surgical castration
LHRH/GnRH agonists	Goserelin (Zoladex) Histrelin (Supprelin) Leuprolide (Lupron) Triptorelin (Triptodur)	■ Used as androgen deprivation therapy ■ Used for intermediate, high, very high-risk recurrence ■ Goserelin and Histrelin available as implant ■ Triptorelin available as implant or depot ■ Leuprolide available as implant or depot ■ May cause decrease in bone mineral density ■ Associated with tumor flare and need for antiandrogen treatment with therapy initiation
GnRH antagonists	Degarelix (Firmagon)	■ Advantage over LHRH agonists: castrate levels achieved rapidly (~1 w vs. 1 m with LHRH agonists) ■ Eliminates tumor flare and need for antiandrogen treatment

Antiandrogens	Flutamide
	Bicalutamide (Casodex)
	Nilutamide (Nilandron)
		■ Indicated only in combination with androgen deprivation therapy
		■ Combinations
		  ● Flutamide and bicalutamide indicated in combination with LHRH agonist
		  ● Nilutamide indicated in combination with orchiectomy

Systemic regimens	Docetaxel + Prednisone Cabazitaxel + Prednisone Mitoxantrone Radium-223	■ Chemotherapy used in this castrate-resistant prostate cancer ■ Radium-223 used for symptomatic bone metastases ■ Mitoxantrone recommended for those with visceral metastases
Secondary hormone therapy	Abiraterone (Zytiga) + Prednisone Apalutamide (Erleada) Darolutamide (Nubeqa) Enzalutamide (Xtandi)	■ Used in metastatic hormone-refractory prostate cancer (also known as castrate resistant prostate cancer)
Immunotherapy	Sipuleucel-T (Provenge)	Option for castrate-resistant prostate cancer following progression

Abbreviations used: GnRH, gonadotropin-releasing hormone antagonists; LHRH, luteinizing hormone–releasing hormone.
Adapted from National Comprehensive Cancer Network. NCCN Guidelines (version 1.2020): Prostate Cancer. Available at: https://www.nccn.org/professionals/physician_gls/pdf/breastprostate.pdf; Norris L, Kolesar J. Prostate Cancer. In: DiPiro J, Talbert R, Yee G, Matzke G, Wells B, Posey L, eds. *Pharmacotherapy: A Pathophysiologic Approach.* 8th ed. McGraw-Hill; 2011:2319–2332.

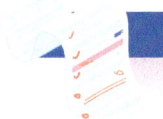

Table 18-7 Common Regimens Used in Small-Cell Lung Cancer Treatment[7,8]

STAGE	MANAGEMENT
Limited	Chemo-radiation ■ Cisplatin-Etoposide ■ Carboplatin may be substituted for Cisplatin if patient is not able to tolerate
Extensive	Carboplatin + Etoposide + Atezolizumab or Durvalumab Cisplatin + Etoposide Carboplatin + Etoposide Carboplatin + Irinotecan Cisplatin + Irinotecan
Single agents/ second-line therapy	Nivolumab ± Ipilimumab Pembrolizumab Topotecan Irinotecan Gemcitabine Docetaxel Paclitaxel Vinorelbine Temozolamide

Adapted from Frieze D, Adams V. Lung Cancer. In: DiPiro J, Talbert R, Yee G, Matzke G, Wells B, Posey L, eds. *Pharmacotherapy: A Pathophysiologic Approach.* 8th ed. McGraw-Hill; 2011:2271–2285; National Comprehensive Cancer Network. NCCN Guidelines (version 3.2020): Small Cell Lung Cancer. Available at: https://www.nccn.org/professionals/physician_gls/pdf/breastsclc.pdf.

Non-small cell lung cancer treatment overview

General points:

- Chemotherapy is not recommended in Stages IA or IIA.
- Cisplatin-based regimen is recommended for Stages IIA, IIB, and IIIA.
- Therapy should be driven by histology (see Table 18-8).

Adverse event management

Tables 18-9 and 18-10 outline adverse events and pharmacist considerations associated with chemotherapy and immunotherapy, respectively.[3,10–14]

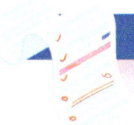

Table 18-8 Histology-Driven Therapies for Non-Small Cell Lung Cancer[7,9]

HISTOLOGY	REGIMEN(S)
Non-squamous—EGFR +	Afatinib (Gilotrif) Dacomitinib (Vizimpro) Erlotinib (Tarceva) Gefitinib (Iressa) Osimertinib (Tagrisso)
Non-squamous— EMLA4-ALK Rearrangement	Alectinib (Alecensa) Brigatinib (Alunbrig) Ceritinib (Zykadia) Crizotinib (Xalkori)
Non-squamous—ROS-1 +	Ceritinib (Zykadia) Crizotinib (Xalkori) Entrectinib (Rozlytrek)
Non-small cell—PD-L1 +	Atezolizuumab (Tecentriq) Durvalumab (Imfinzi) Nivolumab (Opdivo) Pembrolizumab (Keytruda)
Non-small cell (squamous or non-squamous)— BRAF V600E Mutation +	Dabrafenib (Tafinlar) + Trametinib Vemurafenib (Zelboraf)
Non-squamous—EGFR – OR unknown	Carboplatin + Paclitaxel + Bevacizumab Carboplatin + Pemetrexed ± Bevacizumab Cisplatin + Pemetrexed ± Bevacizumab Platinum-based doublet
Squamous histology	Gemcitabine + Cisplatin Carboplatin + Pacitaxel + Pembrolizumab

Abbreviations used: EGFR, epidermal growth factor receptor; EMLA4-ALK, echinoderm microtubule associated protein like 4—anaplastic lymphoma kinase.
Adapted from Frieze D, Adams V. Lung Cancer. In: DiPiro J, Talbert R, Yee G, Matzke G, Wells B, Posey L, eds. *Pharmacotherapy: A Pathophysiologic Approach.* 8th ed. McGraw-Hill; 2011:2271–2285; National Comprehensive Cancer Network. NCCN Guidelines (version 3.2020): Non-Small Cell Lung Cancer. Available at: https://www.nccn.org/professionals/physician_gls/pdf/nscl.pdf.

ADVERSE EVENT	ASSOCIATED AGENTS	NOTES
Anemia	Generally, all cytotoxic chemotherapy	Use of erythropoietin stimulating agents Refer to **Chapter 11** for specific details on agents and dosing in malignancy
Infection	Generally, all cytotoxic chemotherapy	Use of colony-stimulating factors ■ Filgrastim and biosimilars ■ Pegfilgrastim and biosimilars ■ Sargramostim—mainly used in hematologic malignancies Anti-infectives may be used as prophylaxis for high-risk indivdiuals
Nausea/vomiting	Generally, all cytotoxic chemotherapy	Agents used dependent on emetic risk of chemo agent (high, moderate, low, minimal risk) Antiemetic regimen typically includes combination of the following, depending on risk level: ■ Aprepitant/fosaprepitant ■ Serotonin (5-HT3) antagonist (-setrons) ■ Corticosteroids ■ Olanzapine Single agents may be used if emetic risk is low; additional options include ■ Metoclopramide ■ Prochlorperazine
Cardiotoxicity	Anthracyclines Anti-HER2 therapies	Dexrazoxane approved for use in secondary prevention of anthracycline associated cardiotoxicity Correlation of anthracycline induced cardiotoxicity with cumulative anthracycline dose Monitor ejection fraction while on these agents Consider dose and/or therapy modification if cardiotoxicity presence or risk outweighs treatment benefit
Diarrhea	May be any agent but irinotecan main agent associated with diarrhea	Acute (within 24 h post-infusion) treatment ■ Atropine SubQ/IV: Maximum cumulative dose of 1.2 mg Delayed (≥24 h post-infusion) treatment (dose-limiting toxicity) ■ Supportive care, loperamide
Neurotoxicity	Bortezomib Ifosfamide Methotrexate Platinums Taxanes Vinca alkaloid	Cisplatin and carboplatin associated with ototoxicity Taxanes associated with peripheral neuropathy Prevention strategies ■ Avoid concomitant administration of exacerbating agents ■ Bortezomib SubQ administration associated with less neurotoxicity ■ Apply maximum dosing strategy outlined in protocol
Pulmonary toxicity	Bleomycin PD-1 inhibitors PD-L1 inhibitors	Prevention strategies ■ Avoid concomitant administration of exacerbating agents/radiation therapy Treatment ■ Discontinue drug

Abbreviations used: HER2, Human epidermal growth factor receptor-2; SubQ, subcutaneous; IV, intravenous.
Adapted from National Comprehensive Cancer Network. NCCN Guidelines (version 3.2020): Breast Cancer. Available at: https://www.nccn.org/professionals/physician_gls/pdf/breast.pdf; Hu LY, Mi WL, Wu GC, Wang YQ, Mao-Ying QL. Prevention and Treatment for Chemotherapy-Induced Peripheral Neuropathy: Therapies Based on CIPN Mechanisms. *Curr Neuropharmacol.* 2019;17(2):184–196; National Comprehensive Cancer Network. NCCN Guidelines (Version 2.2020): Hematopoietic Growth Factors. Available at: https://www.nccn.org/professionals/physician_gls/pdf/breastgrowthfactors.pdf; National Comprehensive Cancer Network. NCCN Guidelines (version 2.2020): Antiemesis. Available at: https://www.nccn.org/professionals/physician_gls/pdf/breastantiemesis.pdf; Meadors M, Floyd J, Perry MC. Pulmonary Toxicity of Chemotherapy. *Semin Oncol.* 2006;33(1):98–105.

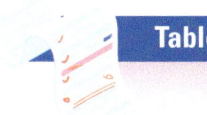

Table 18-10 Immune-Related Adverse Events and Pharmacists' Considerations[14]

IMMUNE-RELATED ADVERSE EVENT	PHARMACIST CONSIDERATIONS
Immune-mediated dermatitis	▪ Counsel on skincare: moisturizers, sunscreen use, avoiding sun ▪ Encourage prompt reporting of symptoms given propensity to become severe during treatment ▪ Review list of medications to rule out concomitant drug interactions or reactions ▪ Initiate topical and/or systemic corticosteroids depending on severity ▪ Clinical pearl: rash may lead to improved responses in metastatic melanoma
Diarrhea and colitis	▪ Counsel on over-the-counter antidiarrheals, proton-pump therapy, pre/probiotics ▪ Initiate systemic corticosteroids depending on severity; consider infliximab/vedolizumab if no response from steroid treatment
Immune-mediated hepatitis	▪ Evaluate use of concomitant medications which may cause increase in liver function tests ▪ Initiate systemic corticosteroids depending on severity ▪ If mycophenolate used for treatment, counsel on enterohepatic recirculation

Immune-mediated pneumonitis	▪ Initiate systemic corticosteroids depending on severity
	  ● Intravenous route preferred for severe or acute immune mediated pneumonitis
	  ● Usual treatment course is 6–8 w; should not exceed 12 w
	▪ Options to consider if refractory to systemic corticosteroids:
	  ● Immunoglobulin (IVIG)
	  ● Interleukin (IL-6) receptor inhibitor
	  ● Infliximab

Immune-mediated endocrinopathies	▪ Recommend starting corticosteroids before thyroid hormone replacement to prevent precipitating adrenal crisis ▪ Follow FT4 for recommendations on thyroid hormone replacement titration ▪ Insulin recommended for type 1 diabetes
Musculoskeletal	▪ Counsel on use of NSAIDs and potential for increased renal dysfunction ▪ Initiate systemic corticosteroids depending on severity
Immune-mediated nephritis and renal dysfunction	▪ Evaluate concomitant renally cleared and nephroxic medications ▪ Initiate systemic corticosteroids depending on severity

General care	▪ Consider supportive prophylaxis medications (if >12 w on steroids)
	  ● Proton-pump inhibitor for GI prophylaxis
	  ● Bactrim for pneumocystis prophylaxis (should be initiated in patients receiving 20 mg systemic corticosteroids daily for >6 w)
	  ● Antifungal prophylaxis
	  ● Calcium + vitamin D

Adapted from Haanen JBAG, Carbonnel F, Robert C, et al. Management of Toxicities From Immunotherapy: ESMO Clinical Practice Guidelines for Diagnosis, Treatment and Follow-Up. *Annals of Oncology*. 2017;28(suppl_4):iv119–iv142.

ADDITIONAL RESOURCES

American Society of Clinical Oncology. Guidelines, tools, and resources. Available at: https://www.asco.org/research-guidelines/quality-guidelines/guidelines.

National Comprehensive Cancer Network. NCCN guidelines (version 6.2020): breast cancer. Available at: https://www.nccn.org/professionals/physician_gls/pdf/breast.pdf.

National Comprehensive Cancer Network. NCCN guidelines (version 2.2020): prostate cancer. Available at: https://www.nccn.org/professionals/physician_gls/pdf/prostate.pdf.

National Comprehensive Cancer Network. NCCN guidelines (version 1.2021): small cell lung cancer. Available at: https://www.nccn.org/professionals/physician_gls/pdf/sclc.pdf.

National Comprehensive Cancer Network. NCCN guidelines (version 8.2020): non-small cell lung cancer. Available at: https://www.nccn.org/professionals/physician_gls/pdf/nscl.pdf.

National Comprehensive Cancer Network. NCCN guidelines (version 2.2020): hematopoietic growth factors. Available at: https://www.nccn.org/professionals/physician_gls/pdf/growthfactors.pdf.

National Comprehensive Cancer Network. NCCN guidelines (version 2.2020): antiemesis. Available at: https://www.nccn.org/professionals/physician_gls/pdf/antiemesis.pdf.

Haanen JBAG, Carbonnel F, Robert C, et al. Management of toxicities from immunotherapy: ESMO Clinical Practice Guidelines for diagnosis, treatment and follow-up. *Annals of Oncology.* 2017;28(suppl 4):iv119–iv142.

REFERENCES

1. Medina P, Shord S. Cancer treatment and chemotherapy. In: DiPiro J, Talbert R, Yee G, Matzke G, Wells B, Posey L, eds. *Pharmacotherapy: A Pathophysiologic Approach.* 8th ed. McGraw-Hill; 2011:2191–2227.

2. Teicher BA. Newer cytotoxic agents: attacking cancer broadly. *Clin Cancer Res.* 2008;14(6):1610–1617.

3. National Comprehensive Cancer Network. NCCN guidelines (version 3.2020): breast cancer. Available at: https://www.nccn.org/professionals/physician_gls/pdf/breast.pdf.Accessed April 28, 2020.

4. Michaud LB, Barnett C, Esteva F. Breast cancer. In: DiPiro J, Talbert R, Yee G, Matzke G, Wells B, Posey L, eds. *Pharmacotherapy: A Pathophysiologic Approach.* 8th ed. McGraw-Hill; 2011:2229–2270.

5. National Comprehensive Cancer Network. NCCN guidelines (version 1.2020): prostate cancer. Available at: https://www.nccn.org/professionals/physician_gls/pdf/prostate.pdf. Accessed April 28, 2020.

6. Norris L, Kolesar J. Prostate cancer. In: DiPiro J, Talbert R, Yee G, Matzke G, Wells B, Posey L, eds. *Pharmacotherapy: A Pathophysiologic Approach.* 8th ed. McGraw-Hill; 2011:2319–2332.

7. Frieze D, Adams V. Lung cancer. In: DiPiro J, Talbert R, Yee G, Matzke G, Wells B, Posey L, eds. *Pharmacotherapy: A Pathophysiologic Approach.* 8th ed. McGraw-Hill; 2011:2271–2285.

8. National Comprehensive Cancer Network. NCCN guidelines (version 3.2020): small cell lung cancer. Available at: https://www.nccn.org/professionals/physician_gls/pdf/sclc.pdf. Accessed April 28, 2020.

9. National Comprehensive Cancer Network. NCCN guidelines (version 3.2020): non-small cell lung cancer. Available at: https://www.nccn.org/professionals/physician_gls/pdf/nscl.pdf. Accessed April 28, 2020.

10. Hu LY, Mi WL, Wu GC, Wang YQ, Mao-Ying QL. Prevention and treatment for chemotherapy-induced peripheral neuropathy: therapies based on CIPN mechanisms. *Curr Neuropharmacol.* 2019;17(2):184–196.

11. National Comprehensive Cancer Network. NCCN guidelines (version 2.2020): hematopoietic growth factors. Available at: https://www.nccn.org/professionals/physician_gls/pdf/growthfactors.pdf. Accessed April 30, 2020.

12. National Comprehensive Cancer Network. NCCN guidelines (version 2.2020): antiemesis. Available at: https://www.nccn.org/professionals/physician_gls/pdf/antiemesis.pdf. Accessed April 30, 2020.

13. Meadors M, Floyd J, Perry MC. Pulmonary toxicity of chemotherapy. *Semin Oncol.* 2006;33(1):98–105.

14. Haanen JBAG, Carbonnel F, Robert C, et al. Management of toxicities from immunotherapy: ESMO clinical practice guidelines for diagnosis, treatment and follow-up. *Annals of Oncology.* 2017;28(suppl_4):iv119–iv142.

CHAPTER 19

Dietary and Herbal Supplements

With medical writing support provided by
Banner Medical LLC Writer: Miriam Opara

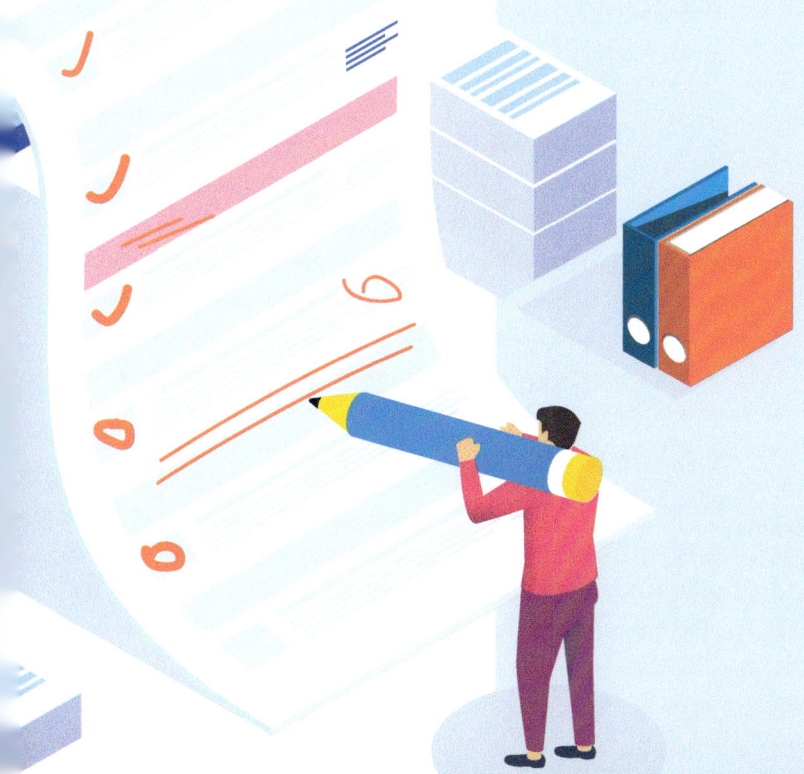

Dietary supplements

Dietary and herbal supplements are regulated by the Dietary Supplement Health and Education Act (DSHEA) of 1994. DSHEA permits structure–function claims on supplements, but no medical claims. There are numerous vitamin supplementations that are recommended for a variety of conditions that can enhance a patient's quality of life.[1]

Vitamin A (retinol) is important for vision. People with high alcohol intake, liver disease, hyperlipidemia, or severe protein malnutrition are more susceptible to adverse effects of excessive vitamin A (nausea, vomiting, headache, vertigo, blurred vision).

Vitamin B6 (pyridoxine) is a coenzyme for the metabolism of amino acids and glycogen.

- **Deficiency:** seborrheic dermatitis, microcytic anemia, convulsions, depression
  - At-risk population: people with chronic alcohol intake or preeclampsia
- **Interactions:** isoniazid, L-dopa

Vitamin B12 (cobalamin) is essential for blood formation and neurological function.

- **Deficiency:**
  - Hematologic effects: anemia (weakness, fatigue, shortness of breath, palpitations)
  - Neurologic effects (tingling, numbness in extremities, visual disturbances)
  - GI effects (loss of appetite, flatulence, constipation)

Biotin is a coenzyme in bicarbonate–dependent carboxylation reactions.

- **Deficiency:** dermatitis, conjunctivitis, alopecia, central nervous system abnormalities
  - At-risk population: people on hemodialysis or peritoneal dialysis

Vitamin C (ascorbic acid) is an antioxidant and a cofactor in enzymatic and hormonal processes, biosynthesis of carnitine, neurotransmitters, collagen, and connective tissue.

- **Deficiency:** scurvy (petechiae, inflamed gums, arthralgia, impaired wound healing, edema, weakness)
  - At-risk population: people who smoke

Vitamin D is involved in bone health and absorption of calcium and phosphorus.

- **Deficiency:** results in inadequate bone mineralization: rickets (children), osteomalacia (adults), increased parathyroid hormone, decreased phosphorus, osteoporosis
  - At-risk population: older adults (produce 4× less vitamin D)
- **Interactions:** glucocorticoids inhibit vitamin D–dependent intestinal absorption causing osteopenia

Vitamin E is an antioxidant and plays a role in metabolic pathways; deficiency is rare.

- **Excessive intake:** hemorrhagic toxicity
  - AREDS is a combination of vitamin C, vitamin E, beta-carotene, copper, and zinc.
  - AREDS is used for eye health and to prevent progression of age-related macular degeneration.

Folate is a coenzyme in the metabolism of nucleic and amino acids.

- **Deficiency:** macrocytic anemia (weakness, fatigue, irritability, headache, palpitation, shortness of breath)
  - At-risk population: pregnant women, people with chronic alcohol intake, people on chronic anticonvulsant therapy or methotrexate therapy

Vitamin K is a coenzyme involved in blood coagulation and bone metabolism. It is poorly transported across the placenta, so a single (0.5 mg–1 mg) shot is recommended for all newborns in the hospital. It is also an antidote for warfarin.

Thiamin (vitamin B1) is a coenzyme in the metabolism of carbohydrates and amino acids.

- **Deficiency:** chronic alcohol consumption (anorexia, weight loss, mental changes, muscle weakness)

Calcium is involved in bone and teeth formation and vascular and neuromuscular function.

- **Deficiency:** osteopenia, osteoporosis, increased risk of fractures
  - At-risk population: older adults
- **Excessive intake:** kidney stones, hypercalcemia with renal insufficiency

Iron is a component of proteins including enzymes, cytochromes, myoglobin, and hemoglobin.

- **Deficiency:** anemia
- **Interactions:** some antacids decrease iron absorption (separate dosing by at least 2 hours), oral contraceptives that contain iron may decrease iron requirement

Magnesium is involved in the development and maintenance of bone and maintaining intracellular levels of potassium and calcium. Phosphorus and calcium intake may decrease magnesium absorption.

- **Deficiency:** hypocalcemia, muscle cramps, seizures
  - At-risk population: people with excessive alcohol intake, people on diuretics, older adults
- **Excessive intake:** diarrhea, metabolic alkalosis, hypokalemia
  - At-risk population: those with impaired renal function

Herbal supplements

Herbal supplements have been used for centuries for various ailments. Herbal supplements may be used alone or in combination with conventional medicine (see Table 19-1).[1-3] Remember, many products lack sufficient evidence and require more research. Patients may still wish to try these agents; therefore, a thorough drug utilization review should occur before recommending them.

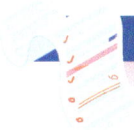

| **Table 19-1** | Common Dietary and Herbal Supplements and Their Purported Use[1-3] |

SUPPLEMENT	INDICATION/USE
NEUROLOGY AND PSYCHIATRY	
5-HTP	Depression
Butterbur	Migraine headache
Caffeine	Headache
Feverfew	Migraine headache
Ginkgo biloba	Anxiety, dementia, schizophrenia
Kava	Anxiety
Melatonin	Insomnia, preoperative anxiety and sedation
St. John's Wort	Depression, somatoform disorders
Valerian	Insomnia
DIGESTIVE SYSTEM	
Ginger	Nausea and vomiting (antiretroviral or pregnancy induced)
Milk thistle	Dyspepsia
Peppermint	Dyspepsia, irritable bowel syndrome
Probiotics	Antibiotic-associated diarrhea, colic, constipation, IBS
Psyllium	Diarrhea, IBS, constipation*

(*continued on next page*)

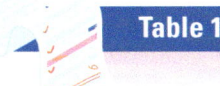

Table 19-1 Common Dietary and Herbal Supplements and Their Purported Use[1-3] (*Continued*)

SUPPLEMENT	INDICATION/USE
IMMUNE MODULATORS	
Echinacea	Common cold
Elderberry	Influenza
Probiotics	Respiratory tract infections, otitis media
WOMEN'S HEALTH	
Black cohosh	Menopausal symptoms
Chaste tree berry	PMS, PMDD
Evening primrose oil	Mastalgia (breast pain)
Fenugreek	Dysmenorrhea, stimulate breast milk production
L-carnitine	Polycystic ovarian syndrome
Phytoestrogens (soy)	Menopausal symptoms
CARDIOVASCULAR SYSTEM	
Coenzyme Q10 (ubiquinone)	Congestive heart failure, prevention of ischemia-reperfusion injury
Fish oil (omega-3 fatty acids)	Hypertriglyceridemia*
Garlic	Atherosclerosis, hyperlipidemia, hypertension
Niacin	Metabolic syndrome, HIV/AIDS–related dyslipidemia
Red yeast rice	Hyperlipidemia, CVD, HIV/AIDS–related dyslipidemia
MUSCULOSKELETAL SYSTEM	
Chondroitin sulfate	Osteoarthritis
Creatinine	Athletic performance
Glucosamine sulfate	Osteoarthritis
S-Adenosyl-L-Methionine	Osteoarthritis
Willow bark	Back pain
ENDOCRINE SYSTEM	
Alpha-Lipoic acid	Increase insulin sensitivity, improve peripheral neuropathy
Cinnamon	Type 2 diabetes
URINARY TRACT AND PROSTATE	
Cranberry	Urinary tract infections
Pygeum	Benign prostatic hyperplasia
WEIGHT LOSS	
Caffeine	Obesity
Conjugated linoleic acid	Obesity

Abbreviations used: CVD, cardiovascular disorder; IBS, irritable bowel syndrome; PMDD, premenstrual dysphoric disorder; PMS, premenstrual syndrome.
*high level of clinical evidence that generally supports recommending for listed indication.

Nonprescription medications can interact with prescription drugs; therefore, the pharmacist must ask about dietary and herbal supplements when evaluating a patient's medication history. Common interactions and complications occur from pharmacokinetic interactions, increased bleeding risk, hepatotoxicity, and cardiotoxicity (see Table 19-2).[1–3]

St. John's Wort is generally used as an antidepressant but has the potential for multiple interactions. St. John's Wort induces CYP3A4, CYP2C19, CYP2C9, CYP1A2, and P-glycoprotein.[1,2] Potential complications with St. John's Wort can occur with oral contraceptives, warfarin, and antidepressants (e.g., SSRIs, SNRIs, MAO inhibitors). St. John's Wort can cause photosensitivity and lower the seizure threshold.[1,2]

Complementary health approaches can be used concomitantly with conventional medicine and offer patients a holistic approach to health. Naturopathy techniques include[4]

- Lifestyle coaching
- Hydrotherapy
- Stress management
- Meditation
- Homeopathy
- Traditional Chinese medicine
  - Acupuncture
  - Cupping
  - Meditation
  - Tai chi
- Chiropractic care
- Ayurveda
- Yoga
- Massage
- Hypnotherapy

Table 19-2	Common Complications with Complementary and Alternative Medicine[1–3]

COMPLICATION	HERB/SUPPLEMENT
Increased risk of bleeding	Garlic
	Ginger
	Ginkgo
	Fish oil
	Willow bark
Hepatotoxicity	Black cohosh
	Echinacea
	Green tea
	Kava
	Saw palmetto
Cardiotoxicity	Bitter orange

ADDITIONAL RESOURCES

Krinsky D, Ferreri S, Hemstreet B, et al. *Handbook of Nonprescription Drugs: An Interactive Approach to Self-Care.* 19th ed. Washington, DC: American Pharmacists Association; 2017.

National Institutes of Health, Office of Dietary Supplements. Dietary supplement fact sheets. Available at: https://ods.od.nih.gov/factsheets/list-all/.

Therapeutic Research Center. Natural medicines. Available at: https://naturalmedicines.therapeuticresearch.com.

REFERENCES

1. National Institutes of Health, Office of Dietary Supplements. Dietary supplement fact sheets. Available at: https://ods.od.nih.gov/factsheets/list-all/. Accessed July 13, 2020.

2. National Institutes of Health, Office of Dietary Supplements. Vitamin and mineral supplement fact sheets. Available at: https://www.ncbi.nlm.nih.gov/pubmed/. Accessed May 27, 2020.

3. Therapeutic Research Center. Natural medicines. Available at: https://naturalmedicines.therapeuticresearch.com. Accessed May 27, 2020.

4. Fleming SA, Gutknecht NC. Naturopathy and the primary care practice. *Prim Care.* 2010;37(1):119–136.

CHAPTER 20

Special Populations

With medical writing support provided by Banner Medical LLC Writers: Jennifer Miller and Miriam Opara

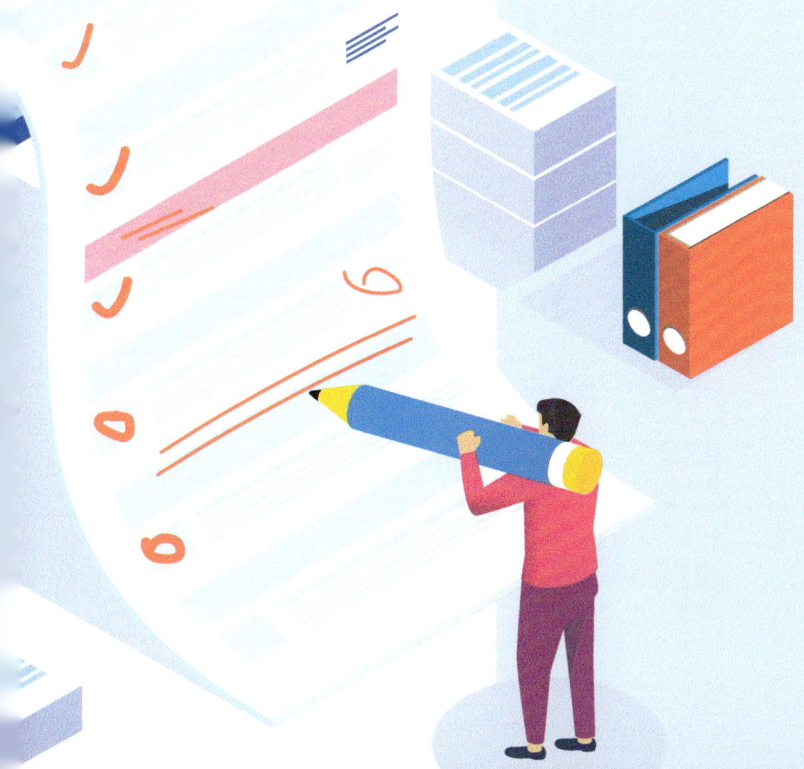

Critical care fluids/electrolytes

Electrolyte disorders are a common complication in critically ill patients and are classified by the affected electrolyte.[1–7]

Sodium is the major extracellular cation. Sodium plays a vital role in maintaining blood volume and blood pressure.

HYPOnatremia (Na <135 mEq/L)
- Hypotonic (most common)
  - Hypovolemia (causes: Na loss + volume depletion; diuretics, diarrhea)
  - Euvolemia (causes: SIADH, thiazide diuretics)
  - Hypervolemia (causes: CHF, renal failure, cirrhosis)

HYPOnatremia treatment
- Rate of correction is dependent on onset, degree, and symptoms
  - Acute onset: increase Na 1–2 mEq/L per hour OR 8–10 mEq/L per 24 hours
  - Chronic: increase Na 0.5–1 mEq/L per hour or <8 mEq/L in 24 hours
- Isotonic saline for hypovolemic hyponatremia
- Hypertonic saline (3% NaCl) for severe hyponatremia
- Vasopressin receptor antagonists
  - Conivaptan approved for euvolemic and/or hypervolemic hyponatremia
  - Tolvaptan approved for euvolemic and/or hypervolemic hyponatremia

HYPERnatremia (Na >145 mEq/L)
- Results from GI losses, hyperglycemia, or diabetes insipidus

HYPERnatremia treatment
- Acute onset: Correct to normal range in ~24 hours
- Chronic onset: Target Na decrease of ~10 mEq/L per day
- Hypotonic fluid (0.45% NaCl, D5W)

Potassium is the major intracellular cation. Potassium plays a role in cell metabolism, myocardial action potential, and synthesis of protein and glycogen.

HYPOkalemia (K <3.5 mEq/L)
- Results from intracellular shifting (e.g., beta-agonists, insulin, alkalosis, hypothermia), potassium losses (e.g., loop or thiazide diuretics, mineralocorticoids, aminoglycosides, amphotericin B), or GI losses

HYPOkalemia treatment
- Potassium replacement at 10–20 mEq/hr
- **Remember,** treat hypomagnesemia

HYPERkalemia (K >5 mEq/L)
- Caused by impaired urinary excretion, extracellular shifting (e.g., beta-blockers, digoxin, succinylcholine, insulin deficiency), or cellular release

HYPERkalemia treatment
- Stabilize cell membrane of cardiac muscle: IV calcium chloride or calcium gluconate
- Intracellular potassium shift
  - Insulin + dextrose, albuterol, sodium bicarbonate
- Eliminate potassium from the body
  - Sodium polystyrene sulfonate
  - Patiromer calcium sorbitex
  - Sodium zirconium cyclosilicate

Phosphorus plays a role in bone formation, cellular membrane composition, metabolism, muscle function, and nerve conduction.

HYPOphosphatemia (PO_4 <2.5 mg/dL)
- Results from decreased intestinal absorption (e.g., diarrhea, vitamin D deficiency), increased utilization, intracellular shift, and increased urinary excretion

HYPERphosphatemia (PO_4 >4.5 mg/dL)
- Results from renal insufficiency, tumor lysis syndrome, rhabdomyolysis, or metabolic acidosis

HYPERphosphatemia treatment
- Phosphate binders
  - Calcium acetate, lanthanum, sevelamer

Magnesium is an important part of cellular membrane action potential, enzymatic cofactor, and biochemical processes.

HYPOmagnesemia (Mg <1.7 mg/dL)
- Results from GI losses or renal losses

HYPOmagnesemia treatment
- IV magnesium for acute replacement
- Oral magnesium for asymptomatic patients

HYPERmagnesemia (Mg >2.3 mg/dL)
- Due to exogenous magnesium administration

HYPERmagnesemia treatment
- Eliminate sources of exogenous magnesium
- IV calcium for cardiovascular and neuro-muscular effects
- Dialysis

Calcium is found in bone and has a function in bone metabolism, smooth muscle contraction, cardiac and neuromuscular functions, and coagulation.

$$Corrected\ Calcium = (normal\ albumin - serum\ albumin) \times 0.8 + serum\ total\ calcium$$

HYPOcalcemia (Ca <8.9 mg/dL)
- Caused by hypoparathyroidism, vitamin D deficiency, hyperphosphatemia, or hypomagnesemia

HYPOcalcemia treatment
- IV calcium gluconate > IV calcium chloride
- Oral for asymptomatic patients
  - Calcium carbonate, calcium citrate

HYPERcalcemia (Ca > 10.1 mg/dL)
- Result of bone resorption or calcium absorption

HYPERcalcemia treatment
- Furosemide, bisphosphonates, calcitonin, dialysis

Drug use during pregnancy and lactation

Teratogenic drugs (see Table 20-1) should be discontinued prior to pregnancy.

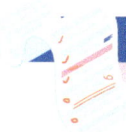

Table 20-1 Teratogenic Medications to Avoid in Pregnancy[8–10]

TERATOGENIC MEDICATIONS	EFFECT
Antineoplastic agents	Causes fetal malformations/anomalies, spontaneous abortions, fetal and/or maternal deaths
Androgens/progestins	Causes virilization
ACEIs	Risk of fetal malformations and impaired fetal renal function
Antithyroid medications	Causes fetal goiter and hypothyroidism
Carbamazepine	Causes neural tube defects and other abnormalities
Isotretinoin	Causes craniofacial heart and central nervous system defects
Phenytoin	Causes cleft lip/palate, microcephaly, hypoplastic phalanges
Tetracyclines	Causes discolored/deformed teeth, bone growth retardation
Thalidomide	Causes phocomelia
Warfarin	Causes fetal abnormalities

Abbreviations used: ACEIs, angiotensin-converting enzyme inhibitors.
Adapted from Shaikh A, Kulkarni M. Drugs in pregnancy and lactation. *Int J of Basic & Clin Pharmacol.* 2013;2:130–135; Cooper WO, Hernandez-Diaz S, Arbogast PG, et al. Major congenital malformations after first-trimester exposure to ACE inhibitors. *N Engl J Med.* 2006;354(23):2443–2451; Arnon J, Meirow D, Lewis-Roness H, Ornoy A. Genetic and teratogenic effects of cancer treatments on gametes and embryos. *Hum Reprod Update.* 2001;7(4):394–403.

Consult individual drug prescribing information or *Drugs in Pregnancy & Lactation* for specific pregnancy/lactation recommendations. Medications to avoid while breastfeeding per the American Academy of Pediatrics include the following:[12]

- Amphetamines
- Aspirin (high dose)
- Buprenorphine
- Bupropion
- Citalopram
- Codeine
- Diazepam
- Diflunisal
- Doxepin
- Fluoxetine
- Fluvoxamine
- Hydrocodone
- Ketorolac
- Lamotrigine
- Lithium
- Oxycodone
- Olanzapine
- Meperidine
- Mirtazapine
- Sertraline
- Venlafaxine

Hypertension is a common complication of pregnancy and choosing safe therapy is essential (see Table 20-2).

Pediatrics

Pediatric age classifications are important when considering drug metabolism and dosing.

- **Pediatric patients:** under 18 years
- **Premature:** born prior to 37 weeks gestation

Table 20-2 Preferred Agents for Treatment of Hypertension in Pregnancy[14]

DRUG CLASS	PREFERRED AGENT/CLASS
Alpha-2 agonist	Methyldopa
Beta-blockers	Labetalol
Calcium channel blockers	Nifedipine
Direct vasodilators	Hydralazine
Diuretics	Thiazides

Adapted from Kattah AG, Garovic VD. The management of hypertension in pregnancy. *Adv Chronic Kidney Dis.* 2013;20(3):229–239.

- **Neonates:** 1 day to 1 month
- **Infants:** 1 month to 1 year
- **Children:** 1 year to 11 years
- **Adolescents:** 12 years to 16 years

Pharmacokinetic parameters differ in pediatric patients (see Table 20-3).

Physiological and disease state differences affect pediatric therapy and drug dosing (see Table 20-4).

Table 20-5 provides a list of common pediatric infectious disease conditions.

The following are drugs/drug classes to avoid in children:

- Tetracyclines: affects bone and teeth development
- Fluoroquinolones: arthropathy, tendinitis, tendon rupture, cartilage erosions in weight bearing joints
- Codeine, promethazine, and tramadol: increases risk for respiratory depression

Vaccine-preventable diseases include

- Measles, mumps, rubella
- Polio
- Pertussis

Transplant

Solid-organ transplant is treatment for those with end-organ failure and improves morbidity and mortality.[20] The main goal of transplant medication is to prevent rejection. Rejection occurs when the body has an immune response to the transplanted organ. **Remember** to assess tissue typing and compatibility for human leukocyte antigen and ABO blood group prior to transplant.

Immunosuppression therapy (see Table 20-6) is given in three phases: induction, maintenance, and treatment.[21] Induction immunosuppression is given before the transplant to prevent acute rejection. Maintenance immunosuppression is provided by the combination of calcineurin inhibitor, antiproliferative agent, and ± steroids.

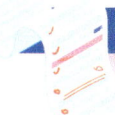

Table 20-3 Pharmacokinetic Parameters in Pediatric Patients[15]

PARAMETER	EFFECTS
Absorption	IM sites: IM dosing of therapeutic agents rarely used in neonates Skin: Increased percutaneous absorption in neonates
Distribution	Decreased plasma protein binding of drugs → **increased volume of distribution** → requires larger dosing of certain medications
Metabolism	Metabolism **slower** in infants versus older children and adults
Elimination	Glomerular filtration, tubular secretion, and tubular reabsorption develop over time from several weeks of age to 1 year after birth

Abbreviations used: IM, intramuscular.
Adapted from Nahata MC, Taketomo C. Pediatrics. In: DiPiro JT, Talbert RL, Yee GC, Matzke GR, Wells BG, Posey LM, eds. *Pharmacotherapy: A Pathophysiologic Approach.* 10th ed. New York, NY: McGraw-Hill; 2017.

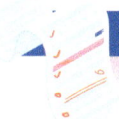

Table 20-4 Various Diseases Affecting Pediatric Therapy[15,16]

DISEASE	EFFECTS
Hepatic disease	▪ Drug clearance is decreased in patients with hepatic disease ▪ Medications can be divided into two categories: 　• Clearance affected by decreased hepatic blood flow: high hepatic extraction ratio (>0.7) → lidocaine, meperidine, morphine, propranolol 　• Clearance affected by hepatocellular function: low hepatic extraction ratio (<0.2) → acetaminophen, chloramphenicol, theophylline
Renal disease	Frequent monitoring of drugs with narrow therapeutic indices should be performed (e.g., aminoglycosides, vancomycin)
Cystic fibrosis	Pediatric patients with cystic fibrosis may require higher doses of certain medications (e.g., penicillin, aminoglycosides, theophylline)
Obesity	Chemotherapy dosing should be based on actual body weight Correction factors used to adjust dosing in obese children

Adapted from Nahata MC, Taketomo C. Pediatrics. In: DiPiro JT, Talbert RL, Yee GC, Matzke GR, Wells BG, Posey LM, eds. *Pharmacotherapy: A Pathophysiologic Approach.* 10th ed. New York, NY: McGraw-Hill; 2017; Schwartz GJ, Work DF. Measurement and estimation of GFR in children and adolescents. *Clin J Am Soc Nephrol.* 2009;4(11):1832–1843.

Speci

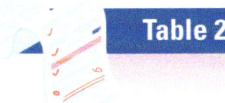

Table 20-5 Management of Common Infectious Disease Conditions in Pediatrics[17–19]

Condition	Management
Bacterial meningitis	Empiric regimens should cover *Group B Streptococcus, Listeria monocytogenes, S. pneumoniae, N. meningitidis,* and *H. influenzae* and are based on age: ■ <1 month: ampicillin + gentamicin ■ >1 month: Vancomycin + ceftriaxone
Acute otitis media	1st line: amoxicillin 90 mg/kg/day for 7–10 days If type 1 penicillin allergy: azithromycin, clarithromycin, clindamycin
Respiratory syncytial virus	Season: November through April Prophylaxis: palivizumab (Synagis) 15 mg/kg IM for qualified patients given monthly for a maximum of 5 doses

Abbreviations used: IM, intramuscular.
Adapted from Lieberthal AS, Carroll AE, Chonmaitree T, et al. The diagnosis and management of acute otitis media. *Pediatrics.* 2013;131(3):e964–e999; Kim K. Acute bacterial meningitis in infants and children. *Lancet Infect Dis.* 2010;10:32–42; Olchanski N, Hansen RN, Pope E, et al. Palivizumab prophylaxis for respiratory syncytial virus: examining the evidence around value. *Open Forum Infect Dis.* 2018;5(3):ofy031–ofy031.

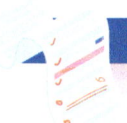

Table 20-6 Immunosuppressant Agents Used in Solid-Organ Transplant[21,22]

INDUCTION THERAPY	
Antithymocyte globulin	(ATGAM; Thymoglobulin)
Basiliximab	CD25 chimeric monoclonal antibody
MAINTENANCE THERAPY	
Calcineurin inhibitor	
Cyclosporine	Goal trough: 100–400 ng/mL
Tacrolimus	Trough goals depend on patient factors, concomitant immunosuppression, and time post-transplant
Antiproliferative agents	
Azathioprine	
Mycophenolate mofetil	
Mycophenolic acid	
Steroids	
Methylprednisolone	
Prednisone	
ADJUVANT AGENTS WITH CALCINEURIN INHIBITORS	
Mammalian target of rapamycin (mTOR kinase inhibitor)	
Everlimus	Goal trough: 3–8 ng/mL
Sirolmus	Trough goals vary depending on organ and immunosuppression regimen
T-CELL CO-STIMULATION BLOCKERS	
Belatacept	Prevents CD28 binding

Adapted from Enderby C, Keller CA. An overview of immunosuppression in solid organ transplantation. *Am J Manag Care.* 2015;21(suppl 1):S12–23; Halloran PF. Immunosuppressive drugs for kidney transplantation. *N Engl J Med.* 2004;351(26):2715–2729.

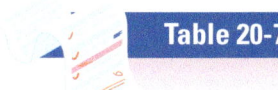

Table 20-7 Adjunct Pharmacologic Agents Used in the Treatment of Obesity[23–25]

DRUG AGENT	NOTES
Bupropion-naltrexone	Bupropion decreases appetite
	Naltrexone decreases food craving
	Can be used long term
Liraglutide	GLP-1 receptor agonist: increases satiety
	Can be used long term
Orlistat	Pancreatic lipase inhibitor: decreases fat absorption
	Can be used long term
Phentermine-topiramate	Phentermine is a sympathomimetic, suppresses appetite
	Topiramate increases satiety and decreases appetite
	Can be used long term
Benzphetamine	Noradrenergic sympathomimetics: release of norepinephrine
Diethylpropion	stimulates the satiety center to decrease appetite
Phendimetrazine	Not recommended for weight loss
Phentermine	If used, use only for short term (<12 weeks)

Abbreviations used: GLP-1, glucagon-like peptide-1.
Adapted from Jensen MD, Ryan DH, Apovian CM, et al. 2013 AHA/ACC/TOS guideline for the management of overweight and obesity in adults. *Circulation.* 2014;129(25)(suppl 2):S102–138; Kim GW, Lin JE, Blomain ES, Waldman SA. Antiobesity pharmacotherapy: new drugs and emerging targets. *Clin Pharmacol Ther.* 2014;95(1):53–66; National Library of Medicine. DailyMed. Available at: https://dailymed.nlm.nih.gov/dailymed/index.cfm. Accessed April 24, 2020.

Weight loss

Overweight and obesity is defined by[23]

- **Underweight:** Body mass index (BMI) <18.5 kg/m^2
- **Normal Weight:** BMI 18.5–24.9 kg/m^2
- **Overweight:** BMI of 25–29.9 kg/m^2
- **Obesity:** BMI ≥30 kg/m^2

Pharmacologic therapy is indicated when

- BMI >30 kg/m^2 OR
- BMI 27–29.9 kg/m^2 + comorbidities who failed to achieve weight loss goal of loss of ≥5% at 3–6 months with lifestyle interventions (see Table 20-7)

ADDITIONAL RESOURCES

Brinkman JE, Dorius B, Sharma S. Physiology, Body Fluids. In: StatPearls Publishing; 2020.

Viera AJ, Wouk N. Potassium Disorders: Hypokalemia and Hyperkalemia. *Am Fam Physician.* 2015;92(6):482–495.

Armstrong C. ACOG Guidelines on Psychiatric Medication Use During Pregnancy and Lactation. *Am Fam Physician.* 2008; 78(6):772–778.

Briggs GG, Freeman RK, Yaffe SJ. *Drugs in Pregnancy and Lactation: A Reference Guide to Fetal and Neonatal Risk.* 10th ed. Wolters Kluwer Health: Lippincott Williams & Wilkins; 2015.

Black CK, Termanini KM, Aguirre O, Hawksworth JS, Sosin M. Solid-organ transplantation in the 21(st) century. *Ann Transl Med.* 2018;6(20):409–409.

Jensen MD, Ryan DH, Apovian CM, et al. 2013 AHA/ACC/TOS Guideline for the Management of Overweight and Obesity in Adults. *Circulation.* 2014;129(25_suppl_2): S102–S138.

REFERENCES

1. DiPiro J, Talbert R, Yee G, Matzke G, Wells B, Posey L. Disorders of calcium and phosphorus homeostasis. In: *Pharmacotherapy: A Pathophysiologic Approach.* 8th ed. New York, NY: McGraw-Hill; 2011:891–907.

2. DiPiro J, Talbert R, Yee G, Matzke G, Wells B, Posey L. Disorders of potassium and magnesium homeostasis. In: *Pharmacotherapy: A Pathophysiologic Approach.* 8th ed. New York, NY: McGraw-Hill; 2011:909–922.

3. Kingley J. Fluid and electrolyte management in pareneteral nutrition. *Support Line.* 2005;27(6):13–22.

4. Lehrich RW, Ortiz-Melo DI, Patel MB, Greenberg A. Role of vaptans in the management of hyponatremia. *Am J Kidney Dis.* 2013;62(2):364–376.

5. Brinkman JE, Dorius B, Sharma S. Physiology, body fluids. In: StatPearls; 2020.

6. Viera AJ, Wouk N. Potassium disorders: hypokalemia and hyperkalemia. *Am Fam Physician*. 2015;92(6):482–495.

7. Watson PE, Watson ID, Batt RD. Total body water volumes for adult males and females estimated from simple anthropometric measurements. *Am J Clin Nutr*. 1980;33(1):27–39.

8. Shaikh A, Kulkarni M. Drugs in pregnancy and lactation. *Int J of Basic & Clin Pharmacol*. 2013;2:130–135.

9. Cooper WO, Hernandez-Diaz S, Arbogast PG, et al. Major congenital malformations after first-trimester exposure to ACE inhibitors. *N Engl J Med*. 2006;354(23):2443–2451.

10. Arnon J, Meirow D, Lewis-Roness H, Ornoy A. Genetic and teratogenic effects of cancer treatments on gametes and embryos. *Hum Reprod Update*. 2001;7(4):394–403.

11. Armstrong C. ACOG guidelines on psychiatric medication use during pregnancy and lactation. *Am Fam Physician*. 2008; 78(6):772–778.

12. Sachs HC, Committee on Drugs. The transfer of drugs and therapeutics into human breast milk: an update on selected topics. *Pediatrics*. 2013;132(3):e796–809.

13. Ward R, Bates B, Benitz W, et al. The transfer of drugs and other chemicals into human milk. *Pediatrics*. 2001;108(3): 776–789.

14. Kattah AG, Garovic VD. The management of hypertension in pregnancy. *Adv Chronic Kidney Dis*. 2013;20(3):229–239.

15. Nahata MC, Taketomo C. Pediatrics. In: DiPiro JT, Talbert RL, Yee GC, Matzke GR, Wells BG, Posey LM, eds. *Pharmacotherapy: A Pathophysiologic Approach*. 10th ed. New York, NY: McGraw-Hill; 2017.

16. Schwartz GJ, Work DF. Measurement and estimation of GFR in children and adolescents. *Clin J Am Soc Nephrol*. 2009;4(11):1832–1843.

17. Lieberthal AS, Carroll AE, Chonmaitree T, et al. The diagnosis and management of acute otitis media. *Pediatrics*. 2013;131(3): e964–e999.

18. Kim K. Acute bacterial meningitis in infants and children. *Lancet Infect Dis*. 2010;10:32–42.

19. Olchanski N, Hansen RN, Pope E, et al. Palivizumab prophylaxis for respiratory syncytial virus: examining the evidence around value. *Open Forum Infect Dis*. 2018;5(3):ofy031–ofy031.

20. Black CK, Termanini KM, Aguirre O, Hawksworth JS, Sosin M. Solid organ transplantation in the 21st century. *Ann Transl Med*. 2018;6(20):409–409.

21. Enderby C, Keller CA. An overview of immunosuppression in solid organ transplantation. *Am J Manag Care*. 2015;21(suppl 1): S12–23.

22. Halloran PF. Immunosuppressive drugs for kidney transplantation. *N Engl J Med*. 2004;351(26):2715–2729.

23. Jensen MD, Ryan DH, Apovian CM, et al. 2013 AHA/ACC/TOS guideline for the management of overweight and obesity in adults. *Circulation*. 2014;129(25)(suppl 2):S102–138.

24. Kim GW, Lin JE, Blomain ES, Waldman SA. Antiobesity pharmacotherapy: new drugs and emerging targets. *Clin Pharmacol Ther*. 2014;95(1):53–66.

25. National Library of Medicine. DailyMed. Available at: https://dailymed.nlm.nih.gov/dailymed/index.cfm. Accessed April 24, 2020.